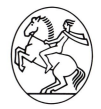

M. Sindou, R. Abbott, and Y. Keravel (eds.)

Neurosurgery for Spasticity

A Multidisciplinary Approach

Springer-Verlag Wien New York

Marc P. Sindou, M.D.

Department of Neurosurgery, Hôpital Neurologique Pierre Wertheimer, Lyon, France

I. Richmond Abbott, M.D.

Department of Neurosurgery, New York University Medical Center, New York, U.S.A.

Yves Keravel, M.D.

Department of Neurosurgery, Hôpital Henri Mondor, Creteil, France

© 1991 by Springer-Verlag Wien

Phototypesetting by Thomson Press (India) Ltd, New Delhi
Printed in Germany by Konrad Triltsch GmbH, Würzburg

Printed on acid-free paper

With 110 Figures

ISBN 3-211-82225-9 Springer-Verlag Wien-New York
ISBN 0-387-82225-9 Springer-Verlag New York-Wien

Dedication

This book is dedicated to those **patients** whom we were unable to help because of a lack of sufficient knowledge and experience.

We would also like to dedicate this work to the **pioneers** in the neurosurgical treatment of spasticity, whose efforts have strongly influenced us in treating spasticity.

– Otfrid Foerster (1873–1941), a German neurologist from Breslau who was trained by Wernicke, Pierre-Marie and Babinski and then was influenced by the works of Jackson and Sherrington. With this strong background he was able to apply physiologic principles to neurologic diseases, devising soundly based procedures such as dorsal rhizotomies for the treatment of spasticity.

– Claude Gros (1915) a Frenchman from Montpellier who is to be credited with leading a group which resurrected sensory rhizotomies for treating spasticity. He and his group devised modifications which avoided the unacceptable side-effects of complete limb sensory rhizotomies. One of his major contributions was the differentiation of "useful" from "harmful" spasticity and the use of intraoperative nerve root stimulation to achieve this differentiation. His group also noted that rhizotomies not only had an effect at the spinal segment which they innervated but also at segments at a distance: e.g., a decrease in arm tone after rhizotomies in the cauda equina.

– Victor Fasano (1920) an Italian living in Torino who with his pupils developed the functional dorsal rhizotomy to treat Little's disease or spastic cerebral palsy. They advanced the notion of cutting those sensory rootlets responsible for motor activity outside of its spinal segment's myotome, so called "diffusion" of motor activity.

Acknowledgments

The editors want to especially acknowledge the ANPP Foundation (Paris) and Mrs. Helene Ollat (M.D.), its scientific director, for their generous support which allowed the contributors to meet together in Saint-Paul-de-Vence, France, to prepare this book.

Foreword

M.R. Dimitrijevic

Division of Restorative Neurology and Human Neurobiology, Baylor College of Medicine, Houston, Texas, U.S.A.

I feel very privileged to be given the opportunity of this foreword by the editors to share some opening remarks with the readers of this book.

Spasticity is a common finding in chronic neurological disorders after traumatic or hemorrhagic insults, vascular insufficiency, tumorous damages, degenerative or demyelinating diseases, as well as hereditary conditions. Children and adults, in poor and wealthy societies, in developed and underdeveloped countries, are suffering from muscular stiffness, feeling of muscle soreness and tightness, and experience difficulty in overcoming their motor disabilities.

Past studies on the underlying mechanisms of spasticity in humans after spinal cord injury and brain hemisphere lesions have taught us that the basic neurobiological properties of the nervous system respond to lesion by reorganizing synapses, creating new connectivities and a variety of residual functions of the partially affected structures. We can find a great variety in the different underlying mechanisms of spasticity even when there are clinical findings of identical clinical features.

Spasticity is not only a manifestation of increased muscle tone and hyperexcitability of the tonic and phasic stretch reflex, but also motor activity under the impaired control of the brain. The goal of contemporary medicine, therefore, is not only to improve the control of spasticity in order to diminish spasms, but also to restore movement for the improvement of volitional activity, posture and gait.

In all these past years, while taking care of many patients with severe spasticity in our Houston Program of Restorative Neurology, we have learned that there is no one method which is effective in all patients. There are many different methods which can be effective in many different patients and, even so, not forever. From time to time a method, modality or intervention, needs to be added to another that once had a therapeutic effect but is no longer effective.

Different modalities of treatment are available: physical, pharmacological, and surgical. Among the many interventions, we are going to choose according to medical resources and expertise. We will take into account the patient's clinical condition, his style of life, and above all his goals.

This book represents a very comprehensive review by highly renowned experts in the field of contemporary neurosurgery for the control of spasticity. We shall read the description of a wide range of interventions, starting with those that use surgery to place stimulating electrodes or catheters for the local delivery of drugs, to end with a series of surgical interventions having the goal to modify the anatomy of the stretch reflex organization. Someone could question the need for so many interventions. The answer is that they all are necessary and that we expect to develop even more in the future. The book will conclude by discussing which are the most appropriate procedures for adults and for children.

Before the central part of the book, which is especially devoted to the practical management of spasticity, there are several introductory chapters, acknowledging that there are different kinds of spasticity and different neurological syndromes, without neglecting to explore the contemporary views on the neuroanatomical, neurophysiological and neurochemical bases of spasticity.

All along the book, the authors emphasize on the great need for a collaborative, multidisciplinary effort, particularly if we think that in the future there will be around the world specialized services for the evaluation, assessment and treatment of spasticity by neurosurgeons, orthopedic surgeons, clinical neuropharmacologists, clinical neurophysiologists, restorative neurologists, specialists in rehabilitation and physiatrists.

Contents

Introduction

M. Sindou (Lyon), **R. Abbott** (New York), and **Y. Keravel** (Paris–Creteil)

The sequelae of neurological diseases are an increasingly important component of the clinical neuroscientist's practice. And spasticity is one of the commonest of these effects. While spasticity can be useful in compensating for lost motor strength, it frequently becomes harmful and leads to further functional losses. When not controllable by physical therapy, it requires consideration of more aggressive treatment. Over the past two decades, many advances have been made in the treatment of this complaint through functional neurosurgery. Therefore the editors of this book have asked a number of renowned experts in the field to present the current state of knowledge relating to the assessment and treatment of spasticity.

Neuroanatomical, physiological and chemical mechanisms of tone are first outlined in order to establish a basis for subsequent therapeutic discussions. Then the main clinical and neurophysiological methods of assessing and quantifying spasticity in children and adults are discussed. Basic principles of pharmacologic treatment are summarized to give the reader a general overview of the nonsurgical techniques available.

Methods involving neurostimulation of the spinal cord, cerebellum, and brain are critically reviewed, with particular attention to their remaining indications.

There is an extensive discussion of the bases and techniques of pharmacologic treatments using intrathecal baclofen administered by an implanted pump. Preliminary results of this treatment are reported.

The classical neuroablative procedures and their recent modifications using microsurgical techniques and intraoperative neural stimulation are described as they apply to the peripheral nerves, spinal roots, dorsal root entry zone, spinal cord, cerebellum, and cerebrum.

Short practical chapters are devoted to the spastic bladder and its treatment, and to orthopedic procedures for correcting the consequences for spasticity.

Finally, guidelines are given for treatment for adults and children functionally debilitated by their spasticity. Along all these chapters the importance of using a multidisciplinary team to work with the spastic patient is stressed.

This book is designed to be of use not only to neurosurgeons, but to all specialists involved in the management of spasticity: neurologists, pediatricians, physiatrists, clinical neurophysiologists, orthopedic surgeons, urologists, and physiotherapists. It is the hope of the editors that **Neurosurgery for Spasticity** will provide a useful – if not complete – summary of current knowledge concerning spasticity and its treatment, and will enable any clinician treating this condition to understand and employ all currently available techniques.

Fundamental bases of spasticity

Neuroanatomical bases of spasticity

D. Jeanmonod

Labor für funktionelle Neurochirurgie, Neurochirurgische Klinik, Zürich, Switzerland

Introduction

A *detailed clinical analysis of spastic conditions* shows that spasticity is not one homogeneous phenomenon. There are multiple clinical presentations of it, in particular: 1) in its selective distribution over different muscle groups in a given limb, 2) in its selective response to various natural stimuli, 3) in its time course characteristics, with the absence, but more often with the presence, of a spasticity-free interval of a few months after the lesion, and 4) in the location of the causative lesion(s). These lesions have been seen in regions as widely spread and diverse as the central and premotor cortices or their cortico-spinal fibres, the brain stem motor centres or their descending pathways, and the spinal cord.

The same diversity can be observed in a study of the *experimental models* of spasticity. Mention can be made (Wiesendanger 1985) of: 1) the decerebrate rigidity, coming up immediately after an intercollicular section and probably best related to the "release" phenomenon of Sherrington, 2) the spinal cord transection model, 3) the bilateral cortical lesions of areas 4 and 6, and 4) the spinal interneuronal rigidity, due to the ischaemic loss of spinal cord interneurons and a consecutive motoneuronal hyperactivity. 2, 3, and 4 characteristically are delayed in their appearance.

The clinical neurophysiological studies related to spasticity have been mainly concentrated on the segmental and intersegmental reflex activities (Dimitrijevic et al. 1967a, b, 1968, 1970, Fasano et al. 1979, Barolat-Romana et al. 1980, Delwaide 1985, Pierrot Deseilligny et al. 1985) and have analyzed a host of different mechanisms there, as well as variations in these activities in spastic states. Some authors have,

in addition, implicated the loss of balance between excitatory and inhibitory descending influences on the spinal cord (Dimitrijevic 1988), or have proposed the study of the long latency, supposedly transcortical, reflexes in spasticity (Delwaide 1985) and mainly rigidity (Dimitrijevic 1988). These human studies find support in many experimental works on the physiology of segmental and intersegmental reflex activities and the influences on them of descending projections (Laporte 1963, Lundberg 1979, 1982, Baldissers et al. 1981).

There has been an immense diversity of *surgical approaches* to spasticity proposed on the basis of these very different working hypotheses.

In face of such a variety, the ultimate goal of the neuroanatomist, although far from being reached, will be to provide a specific *neuroanatomy* for each of the different spastic syndromes, i.e. what pathways or centres are destroyed by the causal lesion, and what are the remaining untouched structures involved in the appearance of this given form of spasticity. This presentation will be based exclusively on studies, a selection of which is given in the reference list, using modern tract tracing techniques (silver impregnation of degenerated terminals, transport of horseradish peroxydase, fluorescent dies or radioactive amino-acids). The great majority of the data discussed here have been collected from experiments on primates, with a smaller number from the cat. Six Figs. will be offered, each including a selection of acceptably well established connections between the different components of the systems studied. An arrow in these Figs. between centres A and B means that A projects axons, without interposing synaptic relay, directly to B. A two-headed arrow indicates a reciprocal projection, from A to B and B to A.

Suprasegmental motor levels

It is possible and useful, on the basis of their connections, to subdivide the suprasegmental motor areas into two main subunits, the striatal and the cerebellar systems. Although the first one has been assigned roles in the determination of direction and amplitude of movements resulting from complex motor programming, and the second in the coding for learned motor skills and synergia, both of them have also been implicated in more basic, postural and tonic, manifestations. An extensive amount of data have been collected on the connections of these two systems (Nauta et al. 1966, 1978, Macchi et al. 1977, Carpenter 1981, Carpenter et al. 1981, 1982, Kuypers 1981, Wiesendanger 1983, Schell et al. 1984, Nieuwenhuys et al. 1988).

The striatal system

Central in this system are the projections (thicker arrows in Fig. 1) going from the whole neocortex to the striatum, the pallidum, some thalamic nuclei, and then back (Fig. 2) to the premotor and prefrontal cortices. The thalamic nuclei concerned are the nucleus ventralis anterior (VA), the nuclei ventralis lateralis pars anterior (VLa), and medialis (VLm) and also the centrum medianum (CM). *This loop system thus conveys information from all the neocortex back only to the frontal cortex.* Some data (see below) recently indicates that this might be performed more through parallel loop systems than in a purely converging manner.

From this central loop many other shorter loops branch, as shown in Fig. 1: CM projects back to the striatum and nucleus subthalamicus. The substantia nigra is reciprocally connected to the striatum, but also receives pallidal input and sends fibres to the thalamus. The nucleus subthalamicus has reciprocal connections with the pallidum and projects to the nigra. The nucleus tegmenti pedunculopontinus, a part of the mesencephalic reticular formation, has been shown recently to have afferents, and probably even reciprocal

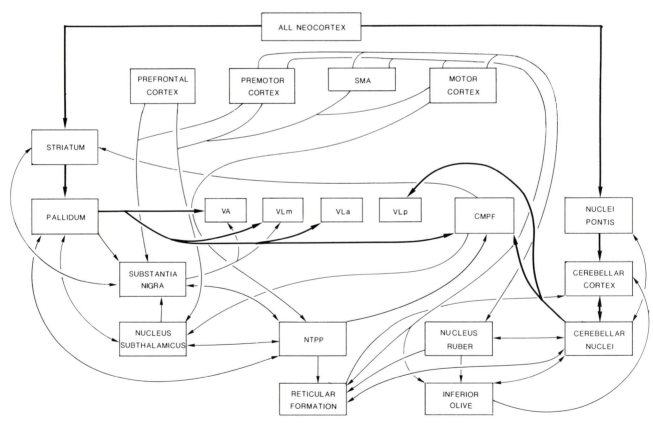

Fig. 1. *Suprasegmental motor levels: the striatal and the cerebellar systems.* Cortical areas are in the superior part of the figure, the thalamus is central, the striatal system is on the left handside and the cerebellar system on the right handside. *CMPF* centrum medianum and nucleus parafascicularis; *NTPP* nucleus tegmenti pedunclopontinus; *SMA* supplementary motor area; *VA* nucleus ventralis anterior of the thalamus; *VLa* nucleus ventralis lateralis pars anterior of the thalamus; *VLm* nucleus ventralis lateralis pars medialis of the thalamus; *VLp* nucleus ventralis lateralis pars posterior of the thalamus

efferent connections with the substantia nigra, the subthalamic nucleus and the pallidum; it also sends fibres to CM. Descending cortical projections from frontal areas have been shown to go to the nigra, the nucleus subthalamicus and the nucleus tegmenti pedunculopontinus. The outputs of the striatal system are either through the corticospinal system, or through the reticular formation. The relative importance of these 2 outputs has been much discussed but is still uncertain.

The cerebellar system

A similar general organization can be described for the cerebellar as for the striatal system. Central in the cerebellar system are the projections (thicker arrows in Fig. 1) from the whole neocortex to the pontine nuclei, the cerebellar cortex, the cerebellar nuclei, the nucleus ventralis lateralis pars posterior of the thalamus (VLp), and then back (Fig. 2) to the motor cortex. There are, moreover, projections from the cerebellar nuclei to the intralaminar thalamic nuclei. *This loop system thus conveys information from all neocortex back only to the motor cortex.* It remains to be elucidated if this information processing is performed in a converging or in a parallel manner.

From this central loop many other shorter loops branch, as displayed in Fig. 1, interconnecting, often reciprocally, the cerebellar cortex and nuclei with the red nucleus, the inferior olive and the pontobulbar reticular formation. Descending cortical projections from frontal areas go to the red nucleus, the inferior olive and the reticular formation. In hominidae and especially in man, the corticorubral and particularly the rubrospinal tracts are very small, and the red nucleus has to be conceived of in these species as a member of the cerebellar system, much more than a station in a descending corticorubrospinal pathway. The inportant outputs the cerebellar system are, however, numerous, through its many connections with the reticular formation, the descending projections from the cerebellar nuclei, and the corticospinal tract from area 4.

Thalamocortical organization

This part has been individualized (Fig. 2) from the two preceding ones only for the sake of clarity of presentation. It comprises, in fact, portions of both the striatal and cerebellar systems. An addition has been made of some data on thalamocortical sensorimotor relationships.

There has been, and there still is much *debate about the exact cortical distribution of the output of the thalamic nuclei VA and VL.* Most difficulties have arisen because of uncertainties in the delineation of subdivisions of nuclei VA and of nucleus VLm. Figure 2 shows pallidal and nigral projections to these nuclei, with an isolated input from the pallidum to VLa. The cerebellar nuclei send fibres only to the posterior part of this nucleus, VLp. This one projects them onto the motor cortex (Jones 1983, 1985), whereas VLa, VLm and Va go to premotor and mainly supplementary motor areas, and VLm and nucleus dorsomedialis (DM) to more anterior, prefrontal, zones. Fibres have however also been claimed to go from parts of VA to the prefrontal cortex and from parts of VLp, DM, CM and VLm to the supplementary motor area. (Schell et al. 1984, Wiesendanger et al. 1985, Alexander et al. 1986). Based on anatomical and physiological data, there has emerged the concept of a parallel processing of information inside the striatal system (De Long et al. 1981, 1984, Alexander et al. 1986): a given cortical area would send information to particular portions of the striatum, pallidum, substantia nigra and thalamus. The thalamus would then close the loop by projecting back to this cortical area. Many such parallel loops would exist, separated from each other inside all their subcortical synaptic stations. Alexander et al. (1986) mention a motor loop, an oculomotor loop, and associational and limbic loops.

The right handside of Fig. 2 displays some data about *somatosensory afferents to the thalamus* (Grant et al. 1973, Boivie et al. 1981, Jones 1983, 1985). Spinothalamic multimodal information is conveyed monosynaptically to VLp, and a central region in the nucleus ventralis posterior (VP) called the "VP core". Proprioceptive input from the dorsal column nuclei, the nucleus Z and the nucleus cuneatus externus is projected to the "VP shell", which surrounds its core. The dorsal column nuclei send also, presumably, tactile fibres to the VP core. The VP shell is reciprocally connected to the proprioceptive cortical areas 3a and 2, whereas the VP core relates to the tactile areas 3b and 1. Somatosensory information has thus many pathways at its disposal to influence more or less directly the motor cortical areas. These pathways are possible candidates in the search for an anatomical substrate to the physiological long latency reflexes. The proprioceptive information has thus the

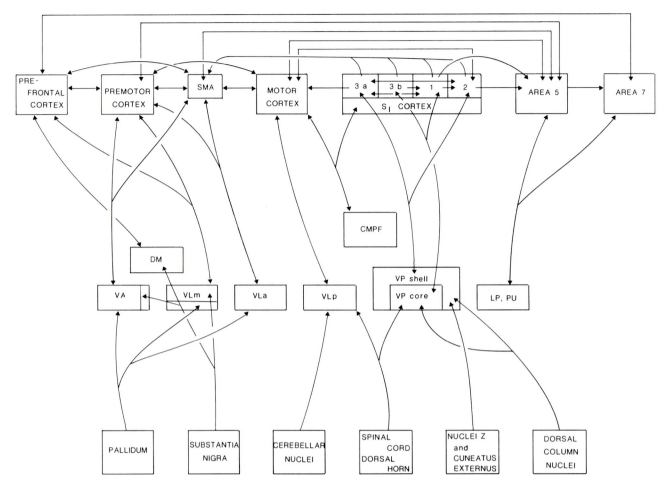

Fig. 2. *Suprasegmental motor levels: the thalamocortical connections.* Cortical areas are at the top of the figure, thalamic nuclei are intermediate, and the afferents to the thalamus are at the bottom. Cortical areas are numbered according to Brodmann. *CMPF* centrum medianum and nucleus parafascicularis; *DM* nucleus dorsomedialis of the thalamus; *LP* nucleus lateralis posterior of the thalamus; *PU* pulvinar; *SMA* supplementary motor area; *VA* nucleus ventralis anterior of the thalamus; *VLa* nucleus ventralis lateralis pars anterior of the thalamus; *VLm* nucleus ventralis lateralis pars medialis of the thalamus; *VLp* nucleus ventralis lateralis pars posterior of the thalamus; *VP* nucleus ventralis posterior of the thalamus

possibility of a quick access to the motor cortex either through the VLp, or through the VP shell and areas 3a or 2.

Figure 2 includes finally some *corticocortical frontoparietal connections which are most often reciprocal* (Bowker et al. 1981). They are to be considered as important substrates for the tight relationships which exist between the "motor" and the "sensory" domains. Attention may also be drawn to the projections of the centrum medianum and nucleus parafascicularis which go to both the pre- and post-central cortices.

A word might be added concerning the homologies between the monkey (Jones 1985) and the human (Hassler 1982) thalamic nuclei:
1) Hassler's nucleus ventralis caudalis corresponds to the animal

VP, although finer subdivisions inside these two nuclei are much more difficult to correlate.
2) Hassler's nucleus ventralis intermedius should correspond to a portion of the animal VLp (possibly the nucleus ventralis posterior lateralis pars oralis VPLO of Olschewski), the rest of VLp being then the homologue of the human nucleus ventralis oralis pars posterior.
3) Hassler's nucleus ventralis oralis pars anterior and nucleus lateropolaris would correspond respectively to the animal VLa and VA.

Descending projections

Extensive and numerous studies of the anatomy of the descending cortical and subcortical projections are available (Kuypers 1981, 1982, Walberg 1982). The following description (Fig. 3) has been essentially based on the works of Kuypers (1981, 1982).

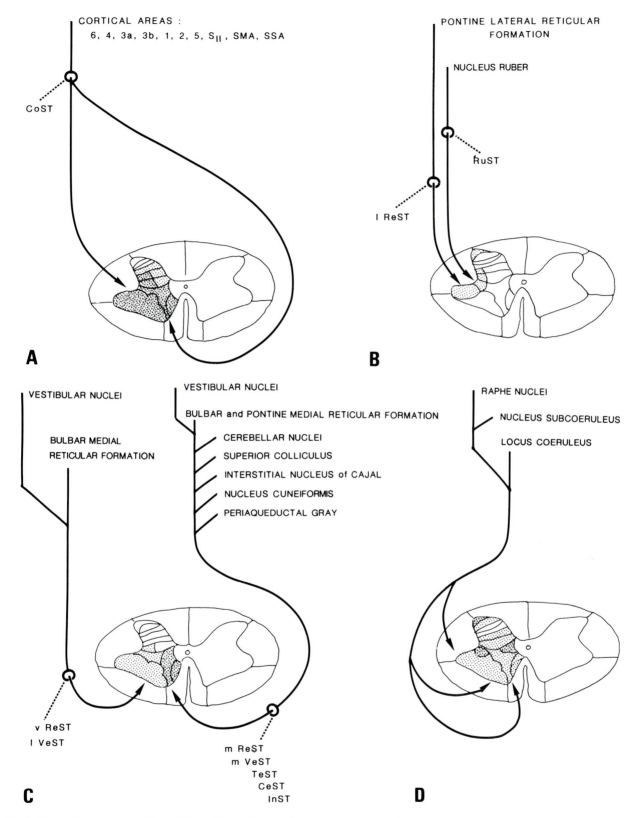

CORTICAL AREAS :
6, 4, 3a, 3b, 1, 2, 5, S$_{II}$, SMA, SSA

CoST

A

PONTINE LATERAL RETICULAR FORMATION

NUCLEUS RUBER

RuST

l ReST

B

VESTIBULAR NUCLEI

BULBAR MEDIAL RETICULAR FORMATION

VESTIBULAR NUCLEI

BULBAR and PONTINE MEDIAL RETICULAR FORMATION

CEREBELLAR NUCLEI

SUPERIOR COLLICULUS

INTERSTITIAL NUCLEUS of CAJAL

NUCLEUS CUNEIFORMIS

PERIAQUEDUCTAL GRAY

v ReST
l VeST

m ReST
m VeST
TeST
CeST
InST

C

RAPHE NUCLEI

NUCLEUS SUBCOERULEUS

LOCUS COERULEUS

D

Fig. 3. *Descending projections.* From left to right and top to bottom are represented the corticospinal system (**A**), the lateral brainstem system (**B**), the medial brainstem system (**C**), and the monoaminergic system (**D**). This figure does not give information about the crossed and/or uncrossed nature of the 4 systems (see text). Cortical areas are according to Brodmann. The heavily shaded areas correspond to the main terminations of the 4 systems, the lightly shaded areas to the zones of lighter projection. The position of the arrowhead indicates the funiculus, or funiculi, where the axons of each system are located. The spinal grey substance has been subdivided into ten laminae according to Rexed (for their labelling, see Fig. 4). *SMA* supplementary motor area; *SSA* supplementary sensory area; *CeST* cerebellospinal tract; *CoST* corticospinal tract; *InST* interstitiospinal tract; *l, v* and *m ReST* lateral, ventral and medial reticulospinal tracts; *RuST* rubrospinal tract; *TeST* tectospinal tract; *l* and *m VeST* lateral and medial vestibulospinal tracts

The corticospinal system

Large areas of the frontoparietal cortex give rise to corticospinal fibres, i.e. areas 6, 4, 3a, 3b, 1, 2, 5, SII, and the supplementary motor and sensory areas (Fig. 3A). The majority of these fibres project contralaterally onto the spinal cord, a minority remain ipsilateral. The two fibre groups travel respectively in the dorsolateral and ventral funiculus, to descend onto a large extent of the spinal cord grey substance, from lamina IV to lamina IX. This system has been unequivocally shown to code for *individual fine movements of the fingers.*

The lateral brain stem system

The red nucleus and the lateral pontine reticular formation are the main origins of this system (Fig. 3B), which projects contralaterally through the dorsolateral funiculus onto lamina I and the lateral part only of laminae V, VI, VII and IX. This system subserves the possibility of performing *independent flexion or extension movements of the elbow and hand.*

The medial brain stem system

Widespread mes-, met-, and myelencephalic origins to this system have been demonstrated (Fig. 3C), mainly the reticular formation, the vestibular and cerebellar nuclei and the tectum. The fibres travel in both the ventrolateral and ventral funiculi, bilaterally or ipsilaterally, with the exception of the tectal fibres, which project contralaterally. The innervated spinal cord area corresponds to the lateral part of lamina VI and laminae VII, VIII and IX, with a preference for the medial part of lamina VII and lamina VIII. The functions of this system can be summarized as follows: *maintenance of the erect position and righting, body and head orientation, body-limb interaction, synergistic global movements of a limb.*

The monoaminergic system

The raphe nuclei, the locus coeruleus and the nucleus subcoeruleus are the origin of a newly discovered descending projection. It travels in the dorsolateral, ventrolateral and ventral funiculi and descends ipsilaterally on neurons in the whole spinal grey matter, except laminae III and IV, with a preference for lamina I and a lateral and a medial zone in the zona intermedia and ventral horn (Fig. 3D).

Although some data have appeared, showing that this monoaminergic system *can mediate inhibition or excitation of spinal cord neuronal pools* (Lundberg 1982, Chen et al. 1987), a precise conceptualization of its function has, to our knowledge, not yet emerged. Some authors would indicate a role in the setting of various states of "*motor preparedness*" *of spinal cord neurons.*

Peripheral afferents to the spinal cord

It has been shown in man (Sindou 1972, Sindou et al. 1974), that the peripheral afferents present with a special organization as they near the dorsal root entry zone (DREZ): the fine, group III and IV fibres first collect themselves in the most superficial parts of the rootlet. The medially placed fine fibres then travel laterally across the DREZ to join the lateral ones, in the ventrolateral border of the DREZ. The large-diameter afferents remain central in the DREZ, moving either medially to enter the dorsal funiculus, going ventrally and medially to enter the dorsal horn, or travelling ventrally to join the ventral horn.

The destination of each group (I to IV) of peripheral afferent fibers has been studied in detail (Brown 1981, Cervero 1986), and is summarized in Fig. 4A. The fine, group III and IV, fibres project to laminae I, II, III and V and X, the larger group II and I fibres are destined mainly to laminae III, IV, V, VI, VII and IX. Among these are the Ia proprioceptive fibres projecting directly onto the motoneurons in layer IX and constituting the anatomical basis of the monosynaptic reflex arc. It is noteworthy that all laminae receive direct peripheral afferent information, except lamina VIII. There is a good correlation between the anatomical data of the destination of the different groups of fibres, their functional role, and the main function ascribed physiologically to some laminae (Willis 1985): for example laminae I and II receive fine, nociceptive, fibres and are known to play a significant role in *nociception.* Lamina IV receives group II fibres and is *tact-related.* The multireceptive lamina V receives *all fibre groups.* Finally, the mainly *proprioceptive* lamina VI receives only large, group I and II, fibre afferents.

Spinal cord ascending projections

The spinal cord ascending projections are presented in Fig. 4B. Laminae III and IV are the main origins

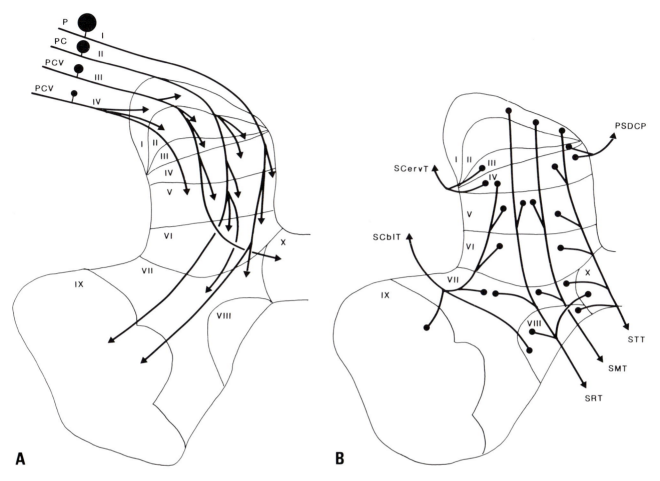

Fig. 4. *Peripheral afferents to the spinal cord (A) and spinal cord ascending projections (B).* The presynaptic large-diameter fibres ascending in the dorsal funiculus are not depicted. The laminae of Rexed are indicated, from I to X. Peripheral afferent fibre types are shown on the left handside, from I to IV. **(A)** Shows the laminar distribution of peripheral afferent terminals. **(B)** Shows the laminar origin of the ascending tracts, without providing information on their crossed or uncrossed nature. P is for proprioceptive, C for cutaneous and V for visceral afferents. *PSDCP* postsynaptic dorsal column pathway; *SCbIT* spinocerebellar tracts; *SCervT* spinocervical tract; *SMT* spinomesencephalic tract; *SRT* spinoreticular tract; *STT* spinothalamic tract

of *the spinocervical tract and the postsynaptic dorsal column pathway*, which travel cranially and ipsilaterally in respectively the dorsolateral and dorsal funiculi. The main function of these tracts, either tactile or nociceptive, is still disputed (Willis 1985). *The spinocerebellar tracts* find origin in a vast number of cord laminae (IV–IX) (Grant 1982), the main one being probably lamina VI and the associated nucleus of Clarke. These tracts ascend ipsi- and contralaterally to the cerebellum in both the dorsolateral and ventrolateral funiculi. *The spinothalamic, spinomesencephalic and spinoreticular tracts* all travel in the ventrolateral and ventral funiculi. The spinothalamic tract arises from many cord laminae (I, IV–VIII), ascends mainly contralaterally (74–95%) and reaches both the specific nucleus ventralis posterior and the

medial thalamus. It has been shown to contain cells conveying cutaneous innocuous and noxious, proprioceptive and visceral stimuli (Willis 1985, 1986). The spinomesencephalic tract arises from laminae I, V and VII, ascends, mainly contralaterally, to the superior colliculus, the nucleus intercollicularis, the nucleus cuneiformis and the periaqueductal gray matter. Its exact function is still discussed, but it may well contribute to nociceptive information processing (Willis 1985, 1986). The spinoreticular tract arises mainly from deep laminae (VII, VIII and X) and ascends both ipsi- and contralaterally to the pontobulbar reticular formation. It probably plays a significant role in rostral and caudal feedback processing of nociception, as well as in some motor adjustments (Willis 1985, 1986).

Spinal cord interneurons

The *zona intermedia* of the spinal cord grey substance can be defined anatomically (Kuypers 1981) as the lateral half of laminae V and VI and the whole of laminae VII and VIII. It is in this domain that physiologists have extensively studied the function of many types of propriospinal interneurons which have been shown to control intersegmental reflex activities. An authoritative review of the available anatomical data on these propriospinal neurons is available (Kuypers 1981).

As shown in Fig. 5, the propriospinal neuronal pool has to be subdivided into 3 subgroups, the short, intermediate and long propriospinal neurons. The *short propriospinal neuron* cell bodies are located in

the lateral part of laminae V, VI and VII. Their axons travel in the dorsolateral and ventrolateral funiculi and reach up to 6–8 cord segments, to finish in the lateral parts of laminae V, VI, VII and IX, where the distal, mainly flexor motoneurons are situated. The *intermediate propriospinal neurons* are located mainly in the central part of lamina VII. Their axons travel in the ventrolateral funiculus and extend to a subtotal number of cord segments, for example from cervical to lumbar, or thoracic to sacral ones. The destination of these axons is to central parts of lamina VII and adjacent motoneurons in lamina IX. The *long propriospinal neurons* are located in the medialmost part of lamina VII and in lamina VIII. Their axons travel in the ventral funiculus to reach the whole extent of the spinal cord segments. They end, at all these

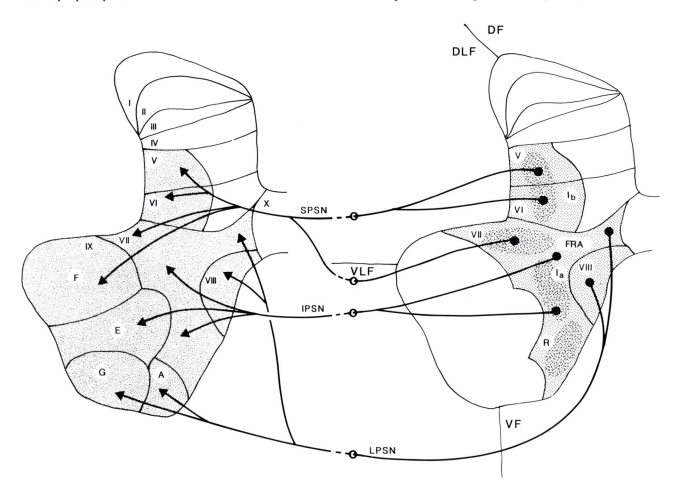

Fig. 5. *Spinal cord interneurons.* Origin (right shaded area) and destination (left shaded area) of the spinal cord interneurons, subdivided in short (SPSN), intermediate (IPSN) and long (LPSN) propriospinal neurons. The initial trajectory of the various axons indicate the funiculus (funiculi) they travel in. The interrupted line and circle represent the passage to other cord segmental levels. The laminae of Rexed are indicated from I to X. Under IX, F is for motoneurons to flexors, E to extensors, G to girdle muscles and A to axial ones. DF dorsal funiculus; *DLF* dorsolateral funiculus; *VLF* ventrolateral funiculus; *VF* ventral funiculus. The 4 heavily shaded oval domains on the right indicate the physiologically determined location of some interneuronal pools: *Ib* Ib interneurons; *FRA* flexor reflex afferent interneurons; *Ia* Ia reciprocal inhibition interneurons; *R* recurrent inhibition interneurons, or Renshaw cells

levels, in the same laminae as the ones they originate from, and in the ventral portions of lamina IX, where axial and proximal motoneurons have been identified.

Extensive physiological studies (Lundberg 1979, 1982, Baldissera et al. 1981) have prompted the creation of the term "premotor zone", an area where interneurons collect converging information from multiple descending and peripheral origins and process them to the motoneuronal pool.

The right handside of Fig. 5 contains darkly shaded oval areas inside the zona intermedia, which represent the locations of the most important physiologically identified interneuronal pools. It can thus be seen that the Ib interneurons are located in the lateral part of laminae V and VI, the flexor reflex afferent interneurons in the dorsolateral part of lamina VII, the Ia reciprocal inhibition interneurons in the central part of lamina VII, and the Renshaw recurrent inhibition interneurons in the ventralmost part of the same lamina.

Plasticity

Many studies are available now to illustrate the powerful plasticity which is present during development, in young postnatal animals. Plasticity in the adult nervous system clearly also exists, but has been shown to be much less dramatic. It is mainly characterized by short distance (i.e. restricted to the dendritic field of one cell) sprouting of one afferent type onto postsynaptic sites vacated because of a lesion of other afferents to the same cell (see Tsukahara 1981 for references). Such studies were rendered possible thanks to the differential recognition of two synapse types at least on one given type of cell, as was done in the septal area, nucleus interpeduncularis, nucleus ruber and hippocampal formation. The time course characteristics of this phenomenon was shown to be between 2 weeks and many months (Tsukahara 1981).

In the spinal cord, the existence of plasticity has for a long time been and is still hotly disputed. Goldberger and collaborators (Goldberger et al. 1982) have extensively studied plasticity in the hemisected cord, deafferented cord and spared root models using silver impregnation techniques in cats, and confirmed the positive initial data presented by McCouch et al. (1958). They have thus described a plasticity characterized by an increase of the number of terminals which do not trespass the borders of the normal termination zone of the given projection. This plasticity obeys strict hierarchical laws, the sprouting

from a spared root blocking for example the one from descending fibres. They have moreover correlated these anatomical data with functional recoveries. Micevych et al. (1986) have studied the spared root and hemisected cord model in the cat, but using horseradish peroxydase tracing. They see no evidence of sprouting in these conditions and interpret the data of Goldberger et al. as technologically false positive results. Devor et al. (1986) have brought convincing, although initially disputed physiological arguments for a reorganization through sprouting of the somatotopic map of the dorsal horn after peripheral nerve sections, with a time course of 2–4 weeks in the cat and 4 days in the rat. Kucera et al. (1985) have studied with autoradiography the ipsilateral corticomotoneuronal projections after subtotal lesions of the bulbar pyramid in 2 monkeys. The lesion caused loss of manual dexterity which recovered partially in 4–6 weeks. They find tentative evidence in one monkey that new connections from the ipsilateral motor cortex to some distal motoneurons might well have developed.

Two arguments can be brought forward to indicate a significant influence of spinal cord plasticity on the development of spasticity. First, the time course characteristics of all plastic events (from a few weeks to many months) would seem well fitted to the often present spasticity free interval of a few months after the causative lesion. This indeed would very much call for a mechanism "en route", up to the moment that its consequences become clinically significant, more than for a "release" (disinhibition) phenomenon which ought to be immediate, or for a denervation hypersensitivity, which should be immediate, and then stabilize or wear off. Moreover, spasticity, after having increased progressively, tends to stabilize then in a new steady state, which could be a manifestation of the reoccupation by sprouts of all formerly vacated postsynaptic sites.

Second, the lateral part of laminae V and VI and the whole lamina VII seem ideally organized to harbour short distance sprouting phenomena. As shown in Figs. 5 and 6, these laminae receive altogether peripheral afferents and descending projections, and contain neurons taking part in ascending projections to suprasegmental levels as well as propriospinal neurons. Short distance sprouting for vacated postsynaptic sites could well take place inside these laminae and remain undemonstrated or doubtfully proved. A definitive answer could only be expected

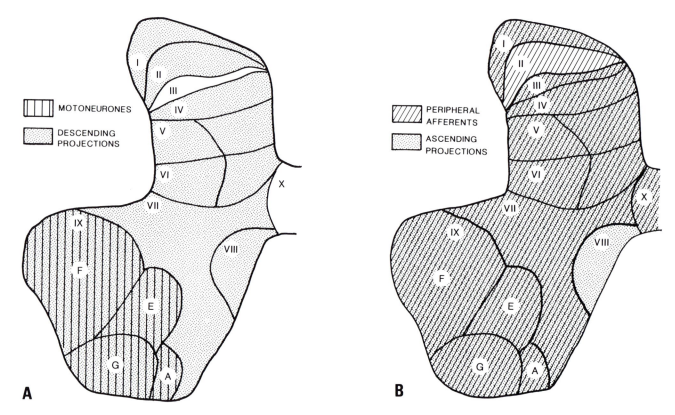

Fig. 6. *Spinal cord grey matter.* Laminar distribution of 4 populations: the motoneuronal pool and descending projections (**A**), and the peripheral afferents and ascending projections (**B**). The laminae are labelled according to Rexed. For the meaning of F, E, G and A, see Fig. 5

when two given synaptic types – for example from a peripheral afferent and a descending axon – are identified on a given cell dendritic field and their distribution is studied before and after a lesion.

Conclusion

We think that neuroanatomical data, as summarized here, will play a crucial role in our endeavours for a better understanding of the different types of clinical spasticities. These data will constitute a base on which the following fundamental questions, among others, will possibly be answered: What are the respective roles of the striatal and cerebellar systems in tone regulation mechanisms and in pathological hypertonias?

What are the exact influences of the long latency, probably transcortical sensorimotor, reflexes in the genesis of spasticity?

How do different lesions in the four descending projection systems correlate with different forms of spasticities?

At an even finer level, the exact physiopathological and morphological mechanisms that give rise to

spasticity remain also to be elucidated. Three such mechanisms must be mentioned: 1) the "release" or *disinhibition phenomenon* of Sherrington, due to an immediate physiological and morphological imbalance after a loss of inhibition and a maintenance of excitation, 2) *plastic changes*, as the short distance sprouting discussed above, with its delayed time course, and 3) *neuronal hyperactivities*, which would follow, again with a delay, the partial or total deafferentation of motoneurons and/or interneurons. It is to be hoped that more studies in the future will uncover which of these mechanisms, alone or in combination, is/are significant in the genesis of the different types of spasticity.

Acknowledgements

We wholeheartedly acknowledge the technical help of Mr. Daldos in the production of all the figures of this chapter, and the secretarial help of Mrs. V. Cucci.

References

Alexander GE, De Long MR, Strick PL (1986) Parallel organization of functionally segregated circuits linking basal ganglia and cortex. Annu Rev Neurosci 9: 357–381

Baldissera F, Hultborn H, Illert M (1981) Integration in spinal neuronal systems. In: Brooks VB (ed) Handbook of physiology, section 1 (Nervous system), vol 2. Williams and Wilkins, Baltimore, pp 509–595

Barolat-Romana G, Davis R (1980) Neurophysiological mechanisms in abnormal reflex activities in cerebal palsy and spinal spasticity. J Neurol Neurosurg Psychiatry 43: 333–342

Boivie J, Boman K (1981) Termination of a separate (proprioceptive?) cuneothalamic tract from external cuneate nucleus in monkey. Brain Res 224: 235–246

Bowker RM, Coulter JD (1981) Intracortical connectivities of somatic sensory and motor areas. Multiple cortical pathways in monkeys. In: Woolsey CN (ed) Cortical sensory organization, vol 1. Multiple somatic areas. Humana Press, Clifton, New Jersey, pp 205–239

Brown AG (1981) Organization in the spinal cord. Springer, Berlin Heidelberg New York Tokyo

Carpenter MB (1981) Anatomy of the corpus striatum and brain stem integrating systems. In: Brooks VB (ed) Handbook of physiology, section 1 (Nervous system), vol 2. Williams and Wilkins, Baltimore, pp 947–987

Carpenter MB, Batton RR III (1982) Connections of the fastigial nucleus in the cat and monkey. Exp Brain Res [Suppl] 6: 250–287

Carpenter MB, Carleton SC, Keller JT, Conte P (1981) Connections of the subthalamic nucleus in the monkey. Brain Res 224: 1–29

Cervero F (1986) Dorsal horn neurons and their sensory inputs. In: Yaksh TL (ed) Spinal afferent processing. Plenum Press, New York London, pp 197–216

Chen DF, Bianchetti M, Wiesendanger M (1987) The adrenergic agonist tizanidine has differential effects on flexor reflexes of intact and spinalized rat. Neuroscience 23: 641–647

De Long MR, Georgopoulos AP (1981) Motor functions of the basal ganglia. In: Brooks VB (ed) Handbook of physiology, section 1 (Nervous system), vol 2. Williams and Wilkins, Baltimore, pp 1017–1055

De Long MR, Alexander GE, Georgopoulos AP, Crutcher MD, Mitchell SJ, Richardson RT (1984) Role of basal ganglia in limb movements. Hum Neurobiol 2: 235–244

Delwaide PJ (1985) Electrophysiological testing of spastic patients: its potential usefulness and limitations. In: Delwaide PJ, Young RR (eds) Clinical neurophysiology in spasticity. Elsevier, Amsterdam New York, pp 185–203

Devor M, Wall PD (1986) Spinal plasticity after nerve injury: mediolateral localization of rewired cells. Exp Brain Res [Suppl] 13: 142–149

Dimitrijevic MR (1988) Spasticity and rigidity. In: Jankovic J, Tolosa E (eds) Parkinson's disease and movement disorders. Urban and Schwarzenberg, Baltimore Munich, pp 385–394

Dimitrijevic MR, Nathan PW (1967a) Studies of spasticity in man. 1. Some features of spasticity. Brain 90: 1–30

Dimitrijevic MR, Nathan PW (1967b) Studies of spasticity in man. 2. Analysis of stretch reflexes in spasticity. Brain 90: 333–358

Dimitrijevic MR, Nathan PW (1968) Studies of spasticity in man. 3. Analysis of reflex activity evoked by noxious cutaneous stimulation. Brain 91: 349–368

Dimitrijevic MR, Nathan PW (1970) Studies of spasticity in man. 4. Changes in flexion reflex with repetitive cutaneous stimulation in spinal man. Brain 93: 743–768

Goldberger ME, Murray M (1982) Lack of sprouting and its presence after lesions of the cat spinal cord. Brain Res 241: 227–239

Grant G (1982) Spinocerebellar connections in the cat with particular emphasis on their cellular origin. Exp Brain Res [Suppl] 6: 466–473

Grant G, Boivie J, Silfvenius H (1973) Course and termination of fibres from the nucleus Z of the medulla oblongata. An experimental light microscopical study in the cat. Brain Res 55: 55–70

Hassler R (1982) Architectonic organization of the thalamic nuclei. In: Schaltenbrand G, Walker AE (eds) Stereotaxy of the human brain. Thieme, Stuttgart New York, pp 140–180

Jones EG (1983) The nature of the afferent pathways conveying short-latency inputs to primate motor cortex. In: Desmedt JE (ed) Motor control mechanisms in health and disease. Raven Press, New York, pp 263–285

Jones EG (1985) The thalamus. Plenum Press, New York London

Kucera P, Wiesendanger M (1985) Do ipsilateral cortico-spinal fibers participate in the functional recovery following unilateral pyramidal lesions in monkeys? Brain Res 348: 297–303

Kuypers HGJM (1981) Anatomy of the descending pathways. In: Brooks VB (ed) Handbook of physiology, section 1 (Nervous system), vol 2. Williams and Wilkins, Baltimore, pp 597–666

Kuypers HGJM (1982) A new look at the organization of the motor system. In: Kuypers HGJM, Martin GF (eds) Anatomy of descending pathways to the spinal cord. Elsevier, Amsterdam New York, pp 381–403

Laporte Y (1963) Activité réflexe de la moelle épinière. In: Kayser C (ed) Physiologie, vol 2. Flammarion, Paris, pp 376a–ay

Lundberg A (1979) Multisensory control of spinal reflex pathways. Prog Brain Res 50: 11–28

Lundberg A (1982) Inhibitory control from the brain stem of transmission from primary afferents to motoneurons, primary afferent terminals and ascending pathways. In: Sjölund B, Björklund A (eds) Brain stem control of spinal mechanisms. Elsevier, Amsterdam, pp 179–224

Macchi G, Bentivoglio M, D'Atena C, Rossini P, Tempesta E (1977) The cortical projections of the thalamic intralaminar nuclei restudied by means of the HRP retrograde axonal transport. Neurosci Lett 4: 121–126

McCouch GP, Austin GM, Liu CN, Liu CY (1958) Sprouting as a cause of spasticity. J Neurophysiol 21: 205–216

Micevych PE, Rodin BE, Kruger L (1986) The controversial nature of the evidence for nueroplasticity of afferent axons in the spinal cord. In: Yaksh TL (ed) Spinal afferent processing. Plenum Press, New York London, pp 417–443

Nauta WJH, Mehler WR (1966) Projections of the lentiform nucleus in the monkey. Brain Res 1: 3–42

Nauta HJW, Cole M (1978) Efferent projections of the subthalamic nucleus: an autoradiographic study in monkey and cat. J Comp Neurol 180: 1–16

Nieuwenhuys R, Voogd J, van Huijzen C (1988) The human central nervous system. Springer, Berlin Heildelberg New York Tokyo

Pierrot-Deseilligny E, Mazières L (1985) Spinal mechanisms underlying spasticity. In: Delwaide PJ, Young RR (eds) Clinical neurophysiology in spasticity. Elsevier, Amsterdam New York, pp 63–76

Schell GR, Strick PL (1984) The origin of thalamic inputs to the arcuate premotor and supplementary motor areas. J Neurosci 4: 539–560

Sindou M (1972) Etude de la jonction radiculo – médullaire postérieure. La radicellotomie postérieure sélective dans la chirurgie de la douleur. Medical Thesis

Sindou M, Quoex C, Baleydier C (1974) Fiber organization at the posterior spinal cordroolet junction in man. J Comp Neurol 153: 15–26

Tsukahara N (1981) Synaptic plasticity in the mammalian central nervous system. Annu Rev Neurosci 4: 351–379

Walberg F (1982) Paths descending from the brain stem – an

overview. In: Sjölund B, Björklund A (eds) Brain stem control of spinal mechanisms. Elsevier, Amsterdam, pp 1–27

Wiesendanger M (1983) Cortico-cerebellar loops. Exp Brain Res [Suppl] 7: 41–51

Wiesendanger M (1985) Is there an animal model of spasticity? In: Delwaide PJ, Young RR (eds) Clinical neurophysiology in spasticity. Elsevier, Amsterdam, pp 1–12

Wiesendanger R, Wiesendanger M (1985) The thalamic connections with medial area 6 (supplementary motor cortex) in the monkey (macaca fascicularis). Exp Brain Res 59: 91–104

Willis WD Jr (1985) The pain system. Karger, Basel

Willis WD Jr (1986) Ascending somatosensory systems. In: Yaksh TL (ed) Spinal afferent processing. Plenum Press, New York London, pp 243–274

Correspondence: Dr. D. Jeanmonod, Labor für funktionelle Neurochirurgie, Neurochirurgische Klinik, Universitätsspital Zürich, Rämistrasse 100, CH-8091 Zürich, Switzerland

Neurophysiological bases of spasticity

M. Wiesendanger

Institut de Physiologie, Université de Fribourg, Switzerland

Introduction

Spasticity is an ill-defined term. Lance (1980) proposed an operational and relatively straightforward definition: "*Spasticity is a motor disorder characterized by a velocity-dependent increase in tonic stretch reflexes (muscle tone) with exaggerated tendon jerks, resulting from hyperexcitability of the stretch reflex, as one component of the upper motor neuron syndrome.*" This definition not only emphasizes the reflex nature of tone and spasticity, but also suggests that hypertonia is just one component of a more complex motor disorder that may be subsumed under the term "spastic syndrome". In this contribution, I will argue that the reflex-notion of tone does not provide sufficient pathophysiological background for understanding the motor disorder of spasticity. Tone and posture is a prerequisite function for purposeful movements, often set in anticipation of goal-directed movements; what matters for the patient is how altered muscle tone is also expressed in voluntary movements. This chapter will first deal with these two aspects of tone, i.e. its *reactive* (*reflexive*) and its *prospective* (*anticipatory*) nature. Then the reflex nature of tone, emphasizing the multi-modal afferent contribution and the variability of the resulting motoneuronal output as they depend on the *gain and the threshold of spinal neurones* regulated from segmental as well as supraspinal sources, will be discussed. This brings us to the classic concept, first proposed by Sherrington (1947), that exaggerated reflexes are caused by a release from supraspinal inhibition thus resulting in an *imbalance* in favor of an exaggerated excitatory state at spinal level. This notion was derived from the observation that hypertonia is an immediate consequence of decerebration. However, in most human cases of spasticity, increased tone and hyperreflexia develop gradually over weeks or months, after a period of depressed spinal activity. The possible underlying mechanisms, which are obviously important for the *adaptive changes* that occur during the long-term development of hypertonia, will finally be discussed.

The reactive and prospective nature of tone and posture

Since Sherrington's demonstration that the stiffness of a decerebrate animal is maintained by segmental afferents, tone (and therefore spasticity) has been viewed as a reflex phenomenon (Fulton 1951). This concept that has dominated clinical neurology. To quote Granit (1979), "tone became defined as postural reflexes adjusting body to ground and parts of the body to one another". Accordingly, posture is an adequately distributed tonic innervation that is reflexly evoked and maintained by afferent inputs including neck and labyrinthine afferents. Classically, these postural reflexes are studied by means of the perturbation paradigm, mainly conducted in man standing on a platform that can be tilted predictably or unpredictably for the subject. Such posturographic studies (that include multiple electromyographic and mechanographic recordings) revealed three major issues (Nashner and McCollum 1985): 1. In the unpredictive, reactive mode, perturbations often result in widespread synergies that are triggered by a combination of sensory afferents and that are more complex than the classical spinal reflexes such as the monosynaptic stretch reflex. 2. When a standing subject is performing an active limb movement, the displacement of the moving limb is accompanied by a stabilizing synergy that is as wide-spread as the one produced by passive perturbations and that often even *precedes* the intended movement (Massion 1984). 3. In a situation when subjects expect a perturbation, they tend to 'set' the excitability of the muscles likely to be perturbed thus augmenting the reflex gain in anticipation (Evarts 1984). It is thus clear that the reactive mode of postural operation is not sufficient to explain the exquisitely fine-tuned postural control in man. Whenever possible, *we prepare tone and posture in anticipation.*

Since the discovery of tonogenic centers in the brainstem (Rhines and Magoun 1946) and their influence on gamma-motoneurons (Granit 1955), the notion of a subtle central 'bias' of tone has emerged: *tone seen as a state.* It is in Granit's words "a kind of slight excitation, i.e. subliminal or liminal activation of motoneurons". The further anatomical discovery of slow-conducting, relatively diffuse projections to the spinal cord, that use aminergic transmitters, triggered a great amount of electrophysiological investigations about the possible role of these "non-classical" descending pathways in motor control (Holstege and Kuypers 1987). Granit (1979) proposed that "monoaminergic mobilization" is causing "a new state of motor preparedness in the spinal cord". Recent experiments have demonstrated that both serotonergic (Hounsgaard et al. 1986) and noradrenergic (Chen et al. 1987) fiber systems projecting to the spinal cord indeed exert a tonic control of motoneurons. These tone-setting mechanisms would be adequate to maintain tone over a longer time range.

It is thus clear that tone is tightly associated with voluntary movements as a physical necessity for stabilizing posture whenever we move. Prospective, or anticipatory, control of posture is an essential task of the central nervous system that is as important as the reactive, reflex-type of control coming into play when the perturbations are unexpected. Given this enlarged view of tone and posture, it follows that spasticity has also to be studied and evaluated in the context of purposeful acts: an antispastic therapy will be useful for the patient if it improves the capacity to perform purposeful movements.

There are reasons, however, to test reflexes in spastic subjects. First, they allow one to obtain a quantitative measure of hyperreflexia. Monosynaptic reflexes as well as polysynaptic cutaneous reflexes are extensively used for this purpose. Secondly, reflex testing (especially by means of H-reflexes) have revealed a number of abnormal changes that can be related to spinal circuits and which have become increasingly accessible to investigations in human subjects. Interestingly, most

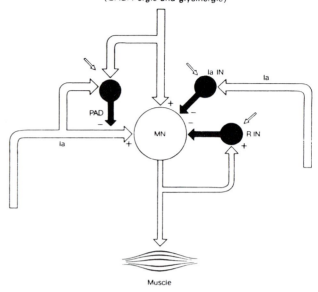

Fig. 1. Inhibitory circuits in the spinal cord: possible sites for pharmacological treatment of spasticity by agonists of inhibitory transmitters. *PAD* Interneuron producing presynaptic inhibition; *IaIN* postsynaptic inhibition by Ia interneuron on motoneuron (MN); *RIN* inhibitory Renshaw interneuron (from Wiesendanger 1989)

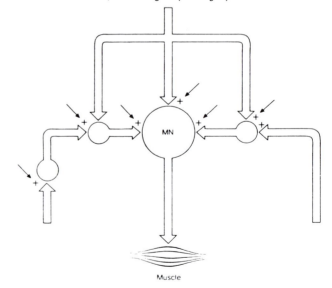

Fig. 2. Excitatory interneurons interposed in the reflex and descending actions to motoneurons (MN). Synaptic transmission is by means of excitatory amino acid transmitters. In spasticity, this transmission can be depressed by antagonists of excitatory transmitters (from Wiesendanger 1989)

studies have been on inhibitory circuits including presynaptic inhibition, inhibition from Ib- and from group II-afferents, recurrent inhibition, reciprocal inhibition. Some of these circuits were found to be depressed, to a variable degree and variable from patient to patient (for reviews cf. Pierrot–Deseilligny 1985, Delwaide 1985, Wiesendanger 1985). These deficiencies seem not to be specific for spasticity; they are nevertheless important since they provide clues for the problem of how normal tone may be restored in spastic patients. Thus, hyperreflexia may be depressed by agonists of the inhibitory transmitters (glycine and GABA) or by antagonists of excitatory amino acid transmitters. Antispatic drugs presently used appear to have one or the other action, or both (cf. Davidoff 1989, for review). A representation of the circuits and the involved transmitters is provided in Figs. 1 and 2.

The appealing idea that an increased drive to the gamma-motoneurons may be causally related to hyper-active stretch reflexes in spastic patients (Granit 1955) could not be substantiated by means of recording the activity of spindle afferents with microelectrodes positioned into peripheral nerves of spastic patients (Hagbarth et al. 1973). Since only a small number of patients have been tested, the possibility remains, however, that an increased excitability of the gamma-loop contributes to hyperactive stretch reflexes in some patients. Even if the excitability of the gama-loop is not increased, blocking of the loop (e.g. by means of differential nerve block) may help to decrease the stretch reflex.

Supraspinal control of reflex pathways: the concepts of release and imbalance

It is now a well established fact that descending fiber systems and segmental afferents have an extensive convergence onto the same interneurones of the spinal cord. Accordingly, it was demonstrated that the segmental reflexes are strongly modifiable by central commands. The anatomy of this circuitry has been discussed by Jeanmonod in this volume. The pathology leading to spasticity is variable from case to case with some descending fiber systems being more affected than others. It is therefore not surprising that transmission in spinal circuits are affected differently from case to case. In view of the clinical term "pyramidal syndrome" which is used sometimes synonymously with the term "spastic syndrome", it is worth mention-

ing that pure lesions of the pyramidal tract (which are exceedingly rare in human pathology) do not result in spasticity in subhuman primates (Wiesendanger 1981, 1984).

The notion of a supraspinal "checking" of spinal reflexes led to the concept that interruption of these controls is followed by a "release" of reflexes and an imbalance in favour of an enhanced spinal excitability (Fulton 1951). This concept holds for the special case of decerebrate rigidity since midbrain lesions usually lead to an immediate hypertonia. In most acute capsular or spinal lesions, the well-known result is, however, a severe depression of all propriospinal functions. It is doubtful, therefore, that in these cases, spasticity, which develops gradually over weeks or months after a period of spinal depression, can be explained simply in terms of "release" (i.e. disinhibition) of spinal circuits. Instead, the slow time course strongly points to compensatory long-term changes at the spinal level as an adaptive process in response to the degeneration of descending fibers.

The hypothesis of a long-term spinal reorganization in chronic spasticity

It is well known from experimental studies that lesions interrupting the afferent inflow to neural centres lead to profound reorganization of the partly denervated structure (Wiesendanger 1989). Two mechanisms have been discovered that are characterized by long-term changes in the synaptic transmissions: 1. *Collateral sprouting* from intact stem fibers with occupation of vacated synaptic sites in the course of degeneration. 2. *Receptor supersensitivity* of neurons as a response to a loss of synaptic inputs (Figs. 3 and 4). Both mechanisms develop with a time course that would be compatible with the development of spasticity following an acute lesion. Although these causes for spasticity have been discussed for a long time (McCouch et al. 1958, Benecke et al. 1984), no concrete direct evidence is thus far available from human spastic cases. It is interesting in this context that massive destruction of spinal interneurons in man – e.g. by infiltrating glioma (Rushworth et al. 1961) as well as in cats (Wiesendanger 1967), has been shown to cause a slowly developing, severe hypertonia. The hyperactive motoneurons would have lost many afferent synaptic contacts in these cases.

Obviously, studies of long-term changes in the spinal cord following lesions of descending fiber systems

A   **B**

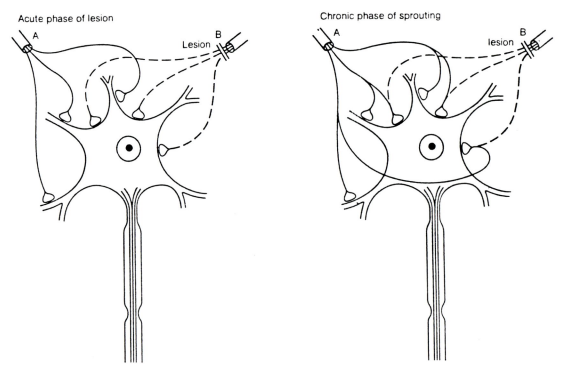

Fig. 3. The phenomenon of collateral sprouting. (**A**) Presynaptic fiber terminals degenerate as a consequence of lesion B, and synaptic sites are vacated. (**B**) The intact fiber terminals from source A form new preterminal collaterals which occupy the vacated synaptic sites

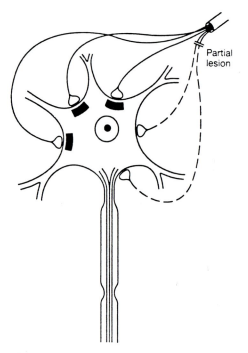

Fig. 4. The phenomenon of denervation supersensitivity: partial degeneration of presynaptic terminals leads to an increased post-synaptic receptor sensitivity of intact synapses to the released transmitter

have to be pursued in order to test the hypothesis of receptor supersensitivity and collateral sprouting as causative factors of spasticity.

Conclusion

From the clinical-therapeutic point of view, applied neurophysiological studies in spastic subjects will have to concentrate on the interplay of tone and posture with voluntary movements. The therapeutic aim is to restore a muscle tone of an adequate amount for the performance of volitional movements, not too much and not too little. Ideally, tone should only be reduced to the extent that it is not acting as a brake on intended movements, otherwise the patient, rendered too flaccid, looses postural support (the "spastic crutch"). There-fore, it appears imperative that spasticity be assessed in the context of purposeful motor acts, such as walking, bicycling, grasping etc. (Conrad et al. 1985). With few exception (for example severe spontaneous spasms), an antispastic therapy should primarily be aimed at improving voluntary movements rather than reflexes. Therefore, the emphasis of such analyses will have to focus on abnormal temporal patterns of muscle activity such as overshooting activity, irradiation of activity cocontractions (rather than reciprocal patterns), associative movements, triggered spasms, dystonia, and disturbances in postural support. Complete restoration of normal patterns of activity will of course rarely occur and the degree to which it does depend on the amount of spared supraspinal control. Nevertheless, some preliminary results obtained with small doses of Baclofen continuously administered intrathecally are rather encouraging in that voluntary movements were "unmasked" under the therapy, improving also the capacity for recruiting muscles more selectively than before the therapy (Penn 1989).

An enlarged view of "spasticity" in the context of voluntary movements calls for a new definition of this term. The following might be more relevant with respect to therapeutic strategies: *Spasticity is a movement disorder that develops gradually in response to a partial or complete loss of supraspinal control of spinal cord function. It is characterized by altered, activity patterns of motor units occurring in response to sensory and central command signals which lead to co-contractions, mass movements and abnormal postural contol.*

References

Benecke R, Conrad B, Meinck H-M (1984) Neue Erkenntisse zur Pathophysiologie der Spastizität. In: Conrad B, Benecke R, Bauer HJ (Hrsg) Die klinische Wertung der Spastizität. Schattauer, Stuttgart New York, S 17–30

Chen D-F, Bianchetti M, Wiesendanger M (1987) Involvement of noradrenergic systems in the modulation of cutaneous reflexes. In: Benecke C, Conrad B, Marsden CD (eds) Motor disturbances I. Academic Press, pp 179–186

Conrad B, Benecke R, Meinck H-M (1985) Gait disturbances in paraspastic patients. In: Delwaide P, Young RR (eds) Clinical neurophysiology of spasticity. Elsevier, Amsterdam, pp 155–174

Davidoff RA (1989) Actions of antispastic drugs. In: Emre M, Benecke R (eds) Spasticity: the current status of research and treatment. Parthenon, Carnforth, pp 115–124

Delwaide PJ (1985) Electrophysiological testing of spastic patients: its potential usefulness and limitations. In: Delwaide PJ, Young RR (eds) Clinical neurophysiology in spasticity. Elsevier, Amsterdam, pp 185–203

Evarts E (1984) Hierarchies and emergent features in motor control.

In: Edelman GM, Gall WE, Cowan WM (eds) Dynamic aspects of neocortical function. Wiley, New York, pp 557–579

Fulton JF (1951) Physiology of the nervous system, 3rd edn. Oxford University Press, New York, pp 157–193

Granit R (1955) Receptors and sensory perception. Yale University Press, New Haven London

Granit R (1979) Somme comments on 'tone'. In: Granit R, Pompeiano O (eds) Reflex control of movements. Elsevier, Amsterdam (Prog Brain Res 50: 17–29)

Hagbarth KE, Wallin G, Löfstedt L (1973) Muscle spindle responses to stretch in normal and spastic subjects. Scand J Rehabil Med 5: 156–159

Holstege JC, Kuypers HGJM (1987) Brainstem projections to spinal motoneurons: an update commentary. Neuroscience 23: 809–821

Hounsgaard J, Hultborn H, Kiehn O (1986) Transmitter-controlled properties of alpha-motoneurones causing long-lasting motor discharge to brief excitatory inputs. Prog Brain Res 64: 39–49

Lance JW (1980) Symposium synopsis. In: Feldman RG, Young RR, Koella WP (eds) Spasticity: disordered motor control. Year Book Medical Publ, Chicago London, pp 485–500

Massion J (1984) Postural changes accompanying voluntary movements. Normal and pathological aspects. Hum Neurobiol 2: 261–267

McCouch GP, Austin GM, Liu CN, Liu CY (1958) Sprouting as a cause of spasticity. J Neurophysiol 21: 205–216

Nashner LM, McCollum G (1985) The organization of human postural movements: a formal basis and experimental synthesis. Behav Brain Sci 8: 135–172

Penn RD (1989) Intrathecal medications for spasticity. In: Emre M, Benecke R (eds) Spasticity: the current status of research and treatment. Parthenon, Carnforth, pp 125–129

Pierrot-Deseilligny E, Mazières L (1985) Spinal mechanisms underlying spasticity. In: Delwaide PJ, Young RR (eds) Clinical neurophysiology in spasticity. Elsevier, Amsterdam, pp 63–76

Rhines R, Magoun HW (1946) Brain stem facilitation and cortical motor response. J Neurophysiol 9: 219–229

Rushworth G, Lishman WA, Hughes JT, Oppenheimer DR (1961) Intense rigidity of the arms due to isolation of motoneurones by a spinal tumor. J Neurol Neurosurg Psychiatry 24: 132–142

Sherrington C (1947) The integrative action of the nervous system, 2nd edn. Yale University Press, New Haven

Wiesendanger M (1967) Morphological, electrophysiological and pathological aspects of interneurones. Electroencephalogr Clin Neurophysiol [Suppl] 25: 45–58

Wiesendanger M (1981) The pyramidal tract. Its structure and function. In: Towe A, Luschei E (eds) Handbook of behavioral neurobiology, vol 5. Plenum, New York, pp 401–491

Wiesendanger M (1984) Pyramidal tract function and the clinical 'pyramidal syndrome'. Hum Neurobiol 2: 227–234

Wiesendanger M (1985) Is there an animal model of spasticity? In: Delwaide PJ, Young RR (eds) Clinical neurophysiology of spasticity. Elsevier, Amsterdam, pp 1–12

Wiesendanger M (1989) Neurobiology of spasticity. In: Emre R, Benecke R (eds) Spasticity – the current states of research and treatment. Parthenon, Carnforth, pp 45–61

Correspondence: Prof. M. Wiesendanger, Université de Fribourg, rue du Musée 5, CH-1700 Fribourg, Switzerland

Neurochemical bases of spasticity

H. Ollat

Association pour la Neuro-Psycho-Pharmacologie, Paris, France

Introduction

The neurobiochemical substratum of spasticity is highly complex and remains poorly understood. However, it is possible to throw some light on it using data from functional neuroanatomy and pharmacological studies of antispastic drugs. In this chapter we will look at the neurobiochemistry of control exerted at the segmental (spinal) level, then at those exerted at the supraspinal levels.

The neurochemistry of segmental control of motor neurone activity

Motor neurons (MN) are under the local influence of Ia fibers innervating the muscle spindles, interneurons and Renshaw cells (Henneman and Mendel 1981, Massion 1984).

1. Ia afferent fibers from muscle spindles respond to muscular stretching and excite monosynaptically MN innervating the same muscle from which these Ia fibers arise as well as MN going to synergist muscles (stretch reflex or myotatic reflex).

The neurotransmitters are unknown but excitatory aminoacids (glutamate, aspartate) *may be involved.*

2. Spinal interneurons may facilitate or inhibit MN activity (Jankowska and Lundberg 1981).

2.1 Several types of excitatory interneurons have been identified:

- interneurons located in the intermediary zone, which mediate signals delivered by descending pathways (including the cortico-spinal pathway);
- interneurons activated by nociceptive afferent fibers, which excite flexor MN (flexion reflex, Fig. 1a);
- interneurons activated by Ib afferent fibers from Golgi tendon organs, which excite antagonists MN of the stretched muscle (inverse myotatic reflex, Fig. 1b);
- short propriospinal neurons activated by descending pathways and sending ascending collaterals to the nucleus reticularis lateralis which in turn project to the cerebellum.

In each case, the neurotransmitters are unknown.

2.2 Inhibitory interneurons are essentially glycinergic. Some are GABAergic or encephalinergic. Several types are wellknown:

- the interneurons of reciprocal inhibition (Ia inhibitory interneurons) are localized in lamina VII of the spinal gray matter. They receive multiple convergent excitatory signals (Ia fibers activated by stretch of antagonists muscles; peripheral afferents from all sources and of all modalities; descending pathways) and inhibitory signals (Renshaw cells, collateral branches of spinal MN) (Fig. 1c).
- the interneurons of the inverse myotatic reflex are located in lamina V–VI. They are activated by Ib afferent fibers (which innervate Golgi tendon organs and signal the strength of muscular contraction), by peripheral afferents and by the cortico- and rubro-spinal pathways. They are inhibited by the dorsal reticulo-spinal pathways and by the noradrenergic descending pathways (Fig. 1b).
- the interneurons activated by nociceptive afferent fibers decrease the activity of extensor MN (flexion reflex, Fig. 1a). The neurotransmitters used by nociceptive fibers are still being debated; however there is strong evidence – immunohistochemical and electrophysiological – pointing to the major role of glutamate, substance P, ATP, and Calcitonine-Gene-Related-Peptide (Besson and Chaouch 1987).
- GABAergic interneurons have a presynaptic inhibi-

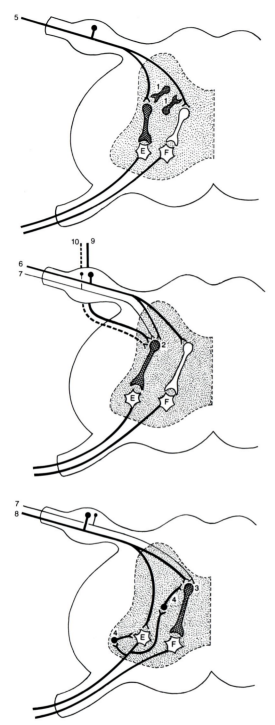

Fig. 1. a Flexor reflex. **b** Inverse myotatic reflex. **c** Reciprocal inhibition. White interneurons are excitatory. Black interneurons are inhibitory. *E* Extensor motor neuron; *F* Flexor motor neuron; *1* inhibitory interneuron acting on presynaptic terminal of primary afferent fibers; *2* Ib inhibitory interneuron; *3* Ia inhibitory interneuron; *4* Renshaw cell; *5* nociceptive afferent fiber; *6* Ib afferent fiber innervating Golgi tendon organ in extensor muscles; *7* peripheral afferent fibers (skin, muscles, joints); *8* Ia afferent fiber innervating muscles spindles in extensor muscles; *9* dorsal reticulo-spinal tract and noradrenergic pathways; *10* cortico- and rubro-spinal tracts

tory action on primary afferent fibers with which they make axono-axonal synapses (Besson and Chaouch 1987, Hamill et al. 1983, Hamon 1987) (Fig. 1a). The receptors involved are probably essentially of GABA-A type; their activation triggers the opening of a chloride channel directly coupled to the receptor; the resulting Cl^- transmembrane current is in accordance to its electrochemical gradient; in the case of afferent terminals, an outward current, with a depolarization of the membrane occurs (as shown by the occurrence of slow potentials derived from juxtaspinal dorsal roots). The final result is a decrease in the release of neurotransmitters by the afferent terminal, thus a decrease of the message delivered to the spinal cord (Hamon 1987). For other afferent fibers, GABAergic presynaptic inhibition is probably mediated by GABA-B receptors. Their activation induces a decrease in an inward calcium current and a decrease in neurotransmitter release by the terminal afferent.

The direct action of GABAergic interneurons on motor neurons has a different mechanism. In this case activation of GABA-A receptors and opening of chloride channels induce an inward Cl^- current with hyperpolarization of the membrane and an inhibitory post-synaptic potential or reduced MN excitability. Activation of GABA-B receptors also induces hyperpolarization of the membrane by activation of a K^+ channel (Andrade et al. 1986).

Table 1 sums up the differential characteristics between GABA-A and GABA-B receptors.
– encephalinergic (and dynorphinergic) neurons, located in the superficial laminae of the dorsal horn, exert inhibitory effects on nociceptive transmission at spinel level and are mediated by three types of opiate receptors (mu, delta and kappa).

Whether this inhibition is pre- or post- synaptic is still under discussion (Besson and Chaouch 1987). It must be added that interneurons of presynaptic inhibition may be activated by peripheral afferents and by bulbo-spinal monoaminergic pathways (the receptors involved are probably of alpha-2 type for noradrenergic pathways and of $5HT_1$ type for serotonergic pathways – Davies and Quinlan 1985, Howe et al. 1983, Roberts 1984).

3. Renshaw cells (Fig. 1a) are glycinergic interneurons and, in some cases, GABAergic. They are specifically activated by recurrent collateral branches of the spinal motor neurons. These synapses are cholinergic with

Table 1. GABA-A and GABA-B receptors. Differential characteristics

	GABA-A	GABA-B
Physiological agonist	GABA	GABA
Ligands		
muscimol	selective agonist	weak agonist
isoguvacine	agonist	0
(-)baclofen	0	selective agonist
bicuculline	selective antagonist	0
phaclofen	0	selective antagonist
delta-amino-valeric acid	agonist	antagonist
Modulation of binding		
$Ca^{2+} - Mg^{2+}$	independent	dependent
GTP	0	↘
{ Benzodiazepines	↗	0
{ Barbiturates		
{ Convulsivants	↘	0
Effector	Cl^- conductance ↗	K^+ conductance ↗ conductance Ca^{2+} ↘ adenylate-cyclase ↘

two responses: the first is mediated by nicotinic receptors, and the second by muscarinic receptors. Renshaw cells have an inhibitory effect (membrane hyperpolarization) on their target cells: i.e., alpha and gamma motor neurons, Ia inhibitory interneurons, other Renshaw cells, cells from which the ventral spino-cerebellar tract arises. Their activity is modulated by peripheral afferents and descending pathways (Massion 1984).

The neurochemistry of supra-segmental controls acting on motor neuron activity

1. Descending pathways arising from supra-spinal structures. The origins routes, synaptic physiology and target cells of these pathways are well known (Table 2 from Armand 1982, Kuypers 1982) as are their resultant effects on MN activity; as a rule they excite their target cells (motoneurons, inhibitory and excitatory interneurons) but their resultant effects are different. For example:

– the lateral reticulo-spinal tract facilitates the activity of flexor MN and inhibits the activity of extensor MN; the median reticulo-spinal tract has an opposite effect;

– the rubro-spinal tract has a predominantly excitatory effect on flexor MN and an equal inhibitory and excitatory effect on extensor MN;

– the lateral vestibulo-spinal tract facilitates the activity of antigravity MN.

In contrast *the neurotransmitters* involved in descending pathways are poorly known.

Only a few reticulo-spinal tracts have been neurochemically characterized; there are *noradrenergic fibers*, arising from the Locus Coeruleus, sending their signals to the MN via alpha-1 adrenergic receptors (Chen et al. 1987, Ono et al. 1986) and *serotonergic fibers*, arising from raphe nuclei. *These monoaminergic pathways facilitate the MN activity*. It is interesting to recall that they decrease the nociceptive transmission in the dorsal horn. The limbic system (emotions, affectivity...), which projects both to the Locus Coeruleus and raphe, is thus able to control simultaneously but in an opposite manner motor activity and pain perception.

Moreover, various peptides (substance P, cholecystokinin, TRH, encephalins...) are often co-localized with serotonin. This coexistence probably endows raphe-spinal neurons with very specific effects. These same peptides are present in terminal arborisations of the descending pathways, but the origin and function of the fibers where they have been found have not yet been identified.

2. The circuitry of the motor thalamus. The activity of the descending pathways is in its turn modulated by two circuits which are articulated through the

Table 2. Descending pathways which control activity of motor neurons

Type	Descending pathway	
	Origin	Name
Ventro-medial pathways		
* Target spinal cells	nucleus giganto-cellularis	latero reticulo-spinal tract
– interneurons of ventro-medial		
intermediary zone (lamina VIII)	pontic medial reticular formation	medial reticulo-spinal tract
– motor neurons for axial muscles and		
proximal muscles of limbs	superior colliculus (deep layers)	tecto-spinal tract
* Modality of ending		
– bilateral	lateral vestibular (Deiters) and	lateral vestibulo-spinal tract
– multisegmental	medial vestibular nuclei	
	primary motor cortex	direct cortico-spinal tract (ventral)
	non primary motor cortex	
	somesthesic cortex	
Dorso-lateral pathways		
* Target spinal cells		
– interneurons of dorso-lateral		
intermediary zone (laminae V–VII)	magnocellular red nucleus	
– motor neurons for distal muscles of	(controlateral)	rubro-spinal tract
muscles		
* Modality of ending		
– unilateral	primary motor cortex	
– paucisegmental	non primary motor cortex	crossed cortico-spinal tract (lateral)

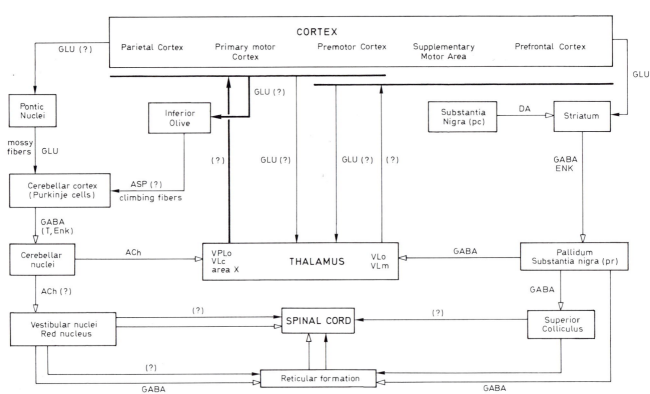

Fig. 2. Circuits of motor thalamus. *Black* excitatory afference; *White* inhibitory afference; *ACh* acetyl-choline; *ASP* aspartate; *DA* dopamine; *Enk* enkephalins; *GABA* gamma-amino-butyric acid; *GLU* glutamate; *T* taurine; *?* not precisely known; *VLc* ventral lateral nucleus of thalamus, caudal part; *VLm* ventral lateral nucleus of thalamus, median part; *VLo* ventral lateral nucleus of thalamus, oral part; *VPLo* ventral posterolateral nucleus of thalamus, oral part; *area X* nucleus ventralis intermedius medialis of thalamus

thalamus: the cerebello-thalamo-cortical and the pallido-thalamo-cortical circuits, which are schematically depicted in Fig. 2.

These two circuits are parallel, with different thalamic and cortical relays, but have clear analogies in all respects: e.g. organization, neurochemistry function (Wise and Strick 1984).

Precise analysis of the functional neurochemistry of motor thalamic circuits is not the topic of this chapter exclusively devoted to spasticity; but it is necessary to recall their existence and their complexity to avoid viewing spasticity as a simple dysregulation of local spinal circuits.

Conclusion

The neurochemical mechanisms of spasticity are very complex, due to 1) the diversity of the neuronal circuits involved and of their neurotransmitters 2) the feedbacks which take place and 3) the interactions between the different circuits. It is possible, however, to state some of the principles for the pharmacological treatment of spasticity.

1. Reduction of stretch and flexor reflexes, by presynaptic inhibition of their afferent fibers.

2. Depression of excitability of motor neurons

– either by reduction of excitatory effects and/or potentiation of inhibitory effects of the descending pathways not greatly involved in motor activity;
– or by potentiation of the inhibitory effects of interneurons.

The "ideal" treatment of spasticity will have to: first, redress the balance inside spinal circuits without unbalancing supra-spinal circuits; second decrease the reflex activity of motor neurons while simultaneously facilitating their voluntary activity. We have to admit that our current knowledge in neurochemistry is unable to resolve these problems.

References

Andrade R, Malenka RC, Nicoll RA (1986) A G protein couples serotonin and GABA-B receptors to the same channels in hippocampus. Science 234: 1261–1265

Armand J (1982) The origins, course and terminations of corticospinal fibers in various mammals. In: Kuypers HGJM, Martin GF (eds) Descending pathways to the spinal cord. Prog Brain Res 57: 329–360

Besson JM, Chaouch A (1987) Peripheral and spintal mechanisms of nociception. Physiol Rev 67: 67–186

Chen DF, Bianchetti M, Wiesendanger M (1987) The adrenergic agonist tizanidine has differential effects on flexor reflexes of intact and spinalized rat. Neuroscience 23: 641–647

Davies J, Quinlan JE (1985) Selective inhibition of responses of feline dorsal horn neurones to nixious cutaneous stimuli by tizanidine (DS 103–282) and noradrenaline: involvement of alpha 2-adrenoceptors. Neuroscience 16: 673–682

Hamill OP, Bormann J, Sakmann B (1983) Activation of multiple-conductance stade chloride channels in spinal neurones by glycine and GABA. Nature 305: 805–808

Hamon H (1987) Les récepteurs GABA dans le système nerveux central. Aspects biochimiques et pharmacologiques. L'Encéphale 13: 159–163

Henneman E, Mendell LM (1981) Functional organization of the motoneuron pool and its inputs. In: Brooks VB (ed) Handbook of physiology: the nervous system, vol 2. Motor control. American Physiological Society, Washington DC

Howe JR, Wang JY, Yaksh TL (1983) Selective antagonism of the antinociceptive effect of intrathecally applied alpha-adrenergic agonists by intrathecal prazosin and intrathecal yohimbine. J Pharmacol Exp Ther 224: 552–558

Jankowska E, Lundberg A (1981) Interneurons in the spinal cord. TINS 4: 230–233

Kuypers HGJM (1982) A new look at the organization of the motor system. In: Kuypers HGJM, Martin GF (eds) Anatomy of descending pathways to the spinal cord. Prog Brain Res 57: 381–403

Massion J (1984) Fonctions motrices. Encycl Med Chir Neurologie (17002 D10) 11: 28 pages

Ono H, Matsumoto K, Kato K, Miyamoto M, Mori T, Nakamura T, Oka J, Fukuda H (1986) Effects of tizanidine, a centrally acting muscle relaxant, on motor systems. Gen Pharmacol 17: 137–142

Roberts MHT (1984) 5 HT and antinociception. Neuropharmacology 23 (12B): 1529–1536

Wise SP, Strick PL (1984) Anatomical and physiological organization of the non primary motor cortex. TINS 7: 442–446

Correspondence: Prof. H. Ollat, Directeur Scientifique, Association pour la Neuro-Psycho-Pharmacologie, 16, boulevard de Charonne, F-75020 Paris, France

Assessment of spasticity

Clinical features of spasticity

Ph. Frerebeau with the collaboration of **F. Segnarbieux, F. Ohanna**, and **J.F. Ronzier**

Department of Neurosurgery, C.H.R. Saint Eloi-Gui de Chauliac, University of Montpellier, France

Introduction

Spasticity is one of the major component of the upper motor neuron syndrome. It may arise in patients suffering from a multitude of lesions which include the sensori-motor cortical area and its descending tracts, centers in the brain stem and their descending pathways, and the spinal cord itself (Wiesendanger 1985). Hyperexcitability of the stretch-reflex continues to be considered as the basic phenomenon causing the increase in muscle tone, in addition to the pathological proprioceptive reflexes.

1) Wherever the site of its causal lesion, *disturbance of the descending motor control system* influences the reactivity of peripheral afferents. An extensive modification of the segmental afferent information system and of the integrative system of the spinal cord interneuronal pool explains the excitability of flexor reflexes and their powerful influence on the motor performance of spastic patients (Dimitrijevic and Nathan 1967).

2) The *level of release of supra-spinal descending control* determines the specific clinical pattern of spasticity. According to Lawrence and Kuypers (1986), two main systems must be considered in this control: the ventro-median system including the medial pontine-, reticulo-, vestibulo- and tecto-spinal pathways, mainly involve in posture regulation; the lateral system including cortico- and rubro-spinal pathway, implicated in finer skilled movements (Struppler 1985).

From these data and results of experimental work it seems possible to differenciate two main types of spasticity:

– *Cerebral spasticity*, as seen in two different animal models:

Large and even bilateral lesions of area 4 and 6 in the monkey, interrupting the drive of the premotor cortex on the mesencephalon, produce a pattern of decortication. In this variety, the predominant disinhibition of the rubro-spinal system increase the influence of tonic neck and vestibular reflexes.

Decerebrate rigidity produced by intercollicular section rostral to the vestibular nuclei, displays a predominantly increased extensor tone with phasic and tonic components of the exagerated stretch reflex (Sherrington 1940).

– *Spinal spasticity*, as seen in the experimental spinal animal. Similar to human trauma, cord transection is followed by a period of spinal shock. Later, with a delay implicating a phase of neural reorganization, there occurs a phase of increased intrinsic spinal activity with both exaggeration of proprioceptive and afferent flexor reflexes, confirmed by mono- and polysynaptic reflex clinical studies (Hultborn and Malmstem 1983).

Comparing experimental and clinical data, one can deduce that magnitude and associated responses of spasticity depend mainly on the site of the causal lesion.

3) Extensive and combined lesions cause *associated neurological impairment*: these deficits mainly motor weakness, combined with spasticity in the agonist/antagonist coupled muscle groups are the main cause of functional disability (Hoffer 1976).

4) The *chronology of the lesion* is important in two ways: age of patients at the onset of spasticity, as with the special pattern of the spastic child related to

cerebral palsy; time course of the acquisition of the lesion, especially in adults.

Spastic hemiplegia

A hemispheric lesion in an adult, following a stroke or trauma, can result in spasticity developing over a varying interval (Rondot 1968). "Pyramidal hypertonicity", investigated by Foix and Chavany as early as 1924, appears initially in the arms and the lower face. Classically, spasticity develops firstly in the fingers and wrist flexors, and later in the proximal arm resulting in the well known posture: an elevated and internally rotated shoulder, adducted arm, half-flexed elbow, clenched fingers and thumb adducted into the palm. For the lower limb, spasticity develops in plantar and toes flexors, knee extensors, and hip adductors and internal rotators. Enhanced spasticity on standing may partly compensate for the weakness but interferes with walking.

Evolution of the handicap depends on the central lesion: in cases of progressive recovery, the first voluntary movements are facilitated by spasticity (Twitchell 1951), and must be carefully identified during the assessment. In cases of permanent deficit, spasticity remains associated with negative signs such as weakness, disturbed higher cortical functions, and other abnormalities of motor control like syncinetic movements, grasping reflex, rigidity, athetosis.

Functional evaluation requires a multidisciplinary approach, the most important point being to identify the dominant harmful pattern. For the upper limb, the scapulo-humeral sub-luxation and the distal trophic lesions are initially improved by spasticity. Later on spasticity impaires the position and prehensive function of the hand. Zancolli (1978) has devised a classification scheme which can be useful for describing extensor function of the fingers and wrist in the spastic. Equino-varus and proximal stiff leg lead often to a major gait impairment. Using a computerized analysis in a kinesiology laboratory, Winters (1987) has grouped patients according to contraction patterns in their legs: in the first group, a dominant extensor weakness results in a drop foot during swing phase inspite of adequate ankle dorsi-flexion. In the main group 2, a permanent spastic plantar flexion persists throughout the gait cycle, with a forced hyperextension of the knee in the terminal stage. The other groups are related to a stiff-legged gait with limited flexion of the knee (group 3), and hip (group 4). A triple flexed leg is an unusual but harmful pattern.

Spinal spasticity

"Spinal spasticity" is widely used by clinicians to describe involuntary or partially controlled movements which can be seen frequently after partial or complete, sudden or gradual lesions of the spinal cord. According to Maury (1981), the following can be noted: 1) Spasm reflexes induced by different stimuli like a pinch, touch, joint mobilisation, bladder filling. 2) Spontaneous spasms without evident extero- or interoceptive stimuli. 3) Stretch reflexes, characterized by a velocity-dependent increase in passive resistance to stretch with exaggerated tendon jerk. 4) Inadequate motor control, specifically seen in incomplete paraplegia, like delay in muscle contraction and relaxation. If the abnormal stretch reflex is due to a disorder of the monosynaptic organization, the other disturbances are probably related to an abnormal polysynaptic reflex organization.

In fact, the distinction of these causative factors remains less evident in clinical observation. For example it is frequently difficult to appreciate the stretch reflex, considering cutaneous contact as a factor of spasm recruitment. The various tone disturbances are also influenced by common factors like emotional status, ambient temperature, and bladder filling. Therefore, spinal spasticity supports multifactorial causes which should be taken into account when therapeutic management is considered.

The pathophysiology of spinal spasticity can be related: 1) to an *intrinsic hyperexcitability of the stretch reflex* mainly resulting from a decrease in presynaptic inhibition (Azouvi et al. 1989, Cadilhac et al. 1977, Delwaide et al. 1989, Gros 1979, Lawrence and Kuypers 1986, Struppler 1985, Young et al. 1987), 2) to an *imbalance between mono- and polysynaptic reflexes*, resulting frequently from an increase of spinal cutaneous reflexes which produces flexor or extensor spasms, 3) to *spinal re-structuring* when segmental motoneuron afferents are increased by axonal sprouting or by histochemical modifications (Azouvi et al. 1989), 4) to *morphological modifications* of the muscle motor unit itself, considering a conversion from type 1 (slow) to type 2 (fast fatigable) fibers (Ohanna 1987); the mechanism underlying these modifications remains obscure.

In clinical practice, one will see:

1) *An initial phase of spinal shock,* commonly observed after an acute lesion. A persistant activity in anal and urethral sphincter, and a flexor response of the big toe (Guillen sign) is usually observed (Maury 1981). Regarding the return of the H-reflex activity, the mean time of the spinal shock does not exceed ten hours (Cadilhac et al. 1977). The reflex activity does not arise simultaneously at each level, but is carried out from distal to proximal site and appears earlier for somatic centers than for vegetative ones (Maury 1981). Spasticity occurs later in complete cervical lesions than in dorsal ones, and earlier and more intensely in incomplete lesions.

2) *Monosynaptic disorganization.* The stretch reflex is dominant on the adductor and anti-gravity muscle groups, rarely giving a major disability. The main problem occurs later on, due to a disorganization of the reciprocal inhibition causing interference with antagonist muscles during movement (Maury 1981, Young et al. 1987). Severe spasticity may often be complicated by contractures; this usually causes sustained muscle activity over a shortened range due to muscle stiffness and atrophy, resulting from loss in their visco-elastic properties.

3) *Polysynaptic disorganization.* The polysynaptic reflexes are organized over multiple spinal segments. Loss of the modulating mechanisms by the interneuron spinal pool and descending motor pathways produces flexor, extensor or alternative modes of spasms. Induced spontaneously or by various stimuli, they are the main cause of handicap, but, in practice, they can be considered as useful or harmful spasms (Gros 1979). Extensor spasms are frequently the more useful, facilitating standing with or without orthesis. In some tetraplegic patients, a stimulus on the anterior aspect of the thigh could induce extension of the wrist allowing prehension by a tenodesis effect. In addition, spasms are useful in preventing venous thrombosis, facilitating expectoration, and reducing osteoporosis. Harmful spasms occur frequently, such as sudden extensor spasms which may jeopardize positions in the wheelchair. Even after a long stabilization, abrupt modification of the reflex activity may occur after current complications (bed sores, bladder infection). Painful flexor spasms can extend to the trunk, inducing spinal deformities, respiratory embarrassement or voiding difficulties. Such painful spasms can remain fixed even if the main pathological cause is cured, indicating the plasticity of the spinal cord mechanisms (Hoffer 1976).

4) *Bladder dysfunction and spasticity.* In paraplegic patients, the detrusor and sphincter activities may undergo a different evolution. Usually the neural reorganization, arising from sacral short loop reflexes, is sufficient to produce normal reflex micturition (Costa et al. 1976). Nevertheless, the urethral sphincter presents the same reflex organization as the lower limbs, with mono- and polysynaptic activity (Ohanna 1987). In our experience we observed an evolution from synergic to dysinergic bladder in 40% of patients. The study of the sacral reflex related to the lower limbs reflex activity and to the effect of intrathecal injection of morphine and baclofen, demonstrated the role of polysynaptic reflexes as the main cause of dysinergic bladder. Increase in polysynaptic activity led to a simultaneous contraction of detrusor and urethral sphincter, with difficulties in micturition, high pressure voiding, and rapid deterioration of the lower urinary tract.

The spastic child

Cerebral palsy includes a number of disabilities resulting from developmental or perinatal injury of the immature brain. The definition implies a non progressive but multi-level disturbance of nervous system functions, with motor control and posture abnormalities associated with other cerebral dysfunctions. Spasticity is a major sign dominating the main categories of cerebral palsy: Hemiplegia, Di- and Quadriplegia, and Mixed Quadriplegia with its associated disorders leading to a total body involvement.

Two main problems characterize the evolution of the spastic varieties of cerebral palsy:

1) *The functional disorders due to joint muscle imbalance.* In 96 patients of a personal series (Ronzier 1977), spasticity was predominant in hip adductors (89%), knee flexors (57%) and ankle flexors (85%). Weakness was dominant in the antagonist muscle groups: Gluteus (45%), Quadriceps femoris (30%) and Triceps surae (25%).

2) *Evolution of the growing spastic muscle.* During bone growth, adaptation of muscle longitudinal growth by addition of sarcomere units, is able to maintain an optimal length tension relationship (Tardieu 1964). In spastic patients, the lack of lengthening by active mobilization and stretching by weakened antagonist muscle groups, leads progressively to fibrous shortening. The hypothesis of a

defective adaptation mechanism has been studied by Tardieu (1964) using the measurement of angular displacement as a function of the passive torque applied to the ankle.

The specific motor pattern of a spastic cerebral palsied child is the result of muscle imbalance: Children stand up with slightly bent knees and legs held closely together; in severe cases, the legs are crossed, giving a scissor type gait. With ankle equinus, internally rotated feet and partial contact of the sole and toes on the ground, the gait becomes digitigrade. With improving ambulation, the conflict between the gravity and postural support turns the equinovarus deformity into a varus foot. A progressive hip subluxation and dislocation can also occur in those with spastic hip musculature. The study of late results after rehabilitation in our series (Ronzier 1977) shows the high frequency of muscle shortening and joint deformities: 40% hip flexion deformity; 44% adduction deformity and pelvic obliquity; 12% hip dislocation; 36% knee deformity, 31% equinus and 38% equinovalgus deformity; with a total of 104 orthopaedic procedures required to repair these deformities.

References

Azouvi Ph, Roby-Brami A, Tougeron A, Dizien O, Bussel B (1989) La spasticité: physiologie et therapeutiques non chirurgicales. In: Bardot A, Pelissier J (eds) Neuro-orthopédie des membres inférieurs chez l'adulte. Masson, Paris, pp 1–8

Cadilhac J, Georgesco M, Benezech J, Duday H, Dapres G (1977) Potentiel évoqué somesthésique et reflexe d'Hoffman dans les lésions médullaires aiguës. Intérêt physiopathologique et pronostic. Electroencéphalogr Clin Neurophysiol 43: 160–167

Costa P, Ohanna F, Martinazzo J, Grasset D (1986) La dyssynergie vésico-sphinctérienne du paraplégique central. Reflexion physiopathologique. J Urol 92(3): 147–152

Delwaide PJ, Olivier E, Fornarelli M (1989) Les myorelaxants. In: Dehan H, Dordan G (eds) Le médicament en neurologie. Doin, Paris, pp 405–418

Dimitrijevic MR, Nathan PW (1967) Studies in spasticity in man: some features of spasticity. Brain 90: 1–30

Gros C (1979) Spasticity clinical classification and surgical treatment. Adv Tech Stand Neurosurg 6: 55–97

Hoffer MM (1976) Basic considerations and classifications of cerebral palsy. In: Instructional course lectures, vol 6. The American Academy of orthopedic surgeons. Mosby, St. Louis, pp 96–106

Hultborn M, Malmstem J (1983) Changes in segmental reflexes following chronic spinal hemisection in the cat. Increased monosynaptic and polysynaptic ventral root discharges. Acta Physiol Scand 199: 405–422

Kasdon David L, M.D. F.A.C.S. (1986) Controversies in the surgical management of spasticity. Clin Neurosurg 33: 523–529

Lacert Ph, Picart A (1985) La spasticité: étude clinique. Annales de Réadaptation et de Médecine Physique 28: 195–202

Lawrence DG, Kuypers HG (1986) The functional organisations of the motor system in the monkey. I. The effect of bilateral pyramidal lesions. II. The effect of the descending brain stem pathway. Brain 91: 1–36

Maury M (1981) La paraplégie chez l'adulte et chez l'enfant. Flammarion: 1–733

Ohanna F (1987) Plasticité de l'unité motrice chez le paraplégique: approche histo-enzymologique, neurophysiologiqu et biomécanique: Mémoire d'études et de recherche en biologie humaine. Faculté Médecine Montpellier (juin 1987), pp 1–105

Rondot P (1968) Etudes cliniques et physiopathologiques des contractures. Rev Neurol 118: 321–342

Ronzier JF (1977) La spasticité des membres inférieurs chez l'enfant I.M.C., conséquences fonctionnelles et problèmes thérapeutiques. Thèse Montpellier, France

Shaffer JW (1983) Hand and upper extremities. In: Thompson GH, Rubin IL, Bileyker RM (eds) Comprehensive management of cerebral palsy, pp 227–230

Sherrington C (1940) On the distribution of the sensory nerve roots. In: Denny Brown (ed) Selected writings of Sir Charles Sherrington, chapter 2. Hoeber, New York, pp 1–532

Struppler A (1985) Some aspects of spasticity as revealed by clinical neuro-physiology. In Delwaide PJ, Young RR (eds) Restorative neurology: clinical neurophysiology in spasticity, Elsevier, Amsterdam New York Oxford, pp 95–106

Tardieu GV (1964) Les feuillets de l'infirmite motrice cérébrale. Ass Nat Infirmes Moteurs Cerebraux, Paris

Twitchell TH (1951) The restoration of motor function following hemiplegia in man. Brain 74: 443–481

Vidal M (1982) L'infirme moteur cerebral spastique. Masson, Paris

Wiesendanger M (1985) Is there an animal model of spasticity? In: Delwaide PJ, Young RR (eds) Clinical neurophysiology in spasticity, vol 1. Elsevier, Amsterdam New York Oxford, pp 1–12

Winters TF, Gage JR, Hicks R (1987) Gait patterns in spastic hemiplegia in children and young adults. J Bone Surg 69A: 437–441

Wolpaw JR (1987) Operant conditioning of primate spinal reflexes: the H-reflex. J Neurophysiol 57(2)

Young RR, Allen W, Wiegner (1987) Spasticity. Clin Orthop 219: 50–62

Zancolli EA (1979) Structural and dynamic basis of hand surgery. Lippincot, Philadelphia

Correspondence:Prof. Ph. Frerebeau, Department of Neurosurgery, C.H.R. Saint Eloi-Gui de Chauliac, University of Montpellier, F-34059 Montpellier Cedex, France

Clinical assessment of spasticity

M.R. Dimitrijevic

Division of Restorative Neurology and Human Neurobiology, Baylor College of Medicine, Houston, Texas

Introduction

Spasticity and rigidity are common neurological findings in movement disorders, and share the characteristic clinical feature of increased muscle tone. In clinical neurology, *spasticity* is described as increased resistance to passive movement due to a lower threshold of tonic and phasic stretch reflexes (Holmes 1946). *Rigidity* is a more uniform and continuous resistance of muscle to passive stretching. Unlike spasticity, rigidity is a condition in which muscle tone is increased in both agonist and antagonist muscle groups, and muscle stiffness is manifest throughout the entire range of movements. Two types of rigidity can be distinguished: the plastic type, in which resistance to passive movement is smooth, such as that experienced in bending a piece of lead; and "cogwheel rigidity", when tremor is superimposed on muscle stiffness.

Because spasticity and rigidity do share some clinical features, it is important to describe other clinical characteristics of upper motor neuron dysfunctions. Patients with spasticity also display changes in posture, muscle weakness, and impairment of automatic and volitional motor activities. In patients with rigidity, the delay in movement initiation should be noted, as should slowness in execution, difficulty with complex movements, postural deformities and loss of postural stability.

Tendon jerks are exaggerated in patients with spasticity and of lower amplitude in rigidity. However, when spasticity reveals features of sustained contraction during passive stretch, passive tendon jerks will be suppressed. *The so-called "clasp-knife phenomenon" in* spasticity is apparent with the sudden release of resistance of the maximally elongated muscle. *This clear distinction between spasticity and rigidity may become less obvious when the patient suffers from both disorders,* as can happen in closed head injuries, stroke and other conditions. Therefore, in clinical practice, it is common to find less striking features of spasticity and rigidity.

Neurologists are well prepared to trace even the most minimal clinical signs of spasticity and motor disorders characterized by a velocity-dependent increase in tonic stretch reflexes ("muscle tone") accompanied by exaggerated tendon jerks (Young 1980). However, when the purpose is not only to recognize spasticity but also to assess and describe the extent of its presence, *it is then important to record all exaggerated tonic stretch reflex findings* and describe the conditions in which spasticity was recorded.

The extent and degree of spasticity can be determined by the site, strength and rate of the applied stretch reflex stimulus. Spasticity depends upon the initial muscle tone, length of responding muscle groups, the subject's position, posture, state of relaxation and other ongoing activity within the

Table 1. Assessment of spasticity

1. Position while lying and posture while standing	
2. Rate of passive tonic stretch	1, 2, 3, 4
Irradiation to non-stretched muscles	1, 2, 3
Vibratory tonic reflex	1, 2, 3, 4
3. Phasic stretch reflex	1, 2, 3
Effect of repetition	1, 2, 3
Effect of reinforcement	+ or −
Effect of volitional activity	+ or −
4. Withdrawal reflex	1, 2, 3
Effect of repetition	1, 2, 3
Effect of suppression	+ or −
5. Volitional activity	1, 2, 3, 4

central nervous system. Actually, the evaluation of spasticity is a very simple clinical task. However, in order to achieve a reliable qualitative assessment which can then be compared to the assessment obtained in reevaluation, *it is necessary to follow a standardized protocol.* This is especially true when the purpose of such an assessment is to evaluate the result of treatment, or the control of spasticity, as is the case in this book on "neurosurgery for spasticity".

Examination of muscle tone

An essential prerequisite for the examination of muscle tone is that the patient should be placed in a *supine, comfortable, lying position.* We have found that by keeping the subject in such a position, for five to ten minutes before examination, it is easier to determine the extent of alteration, spontaneous spasms, and involuntary movement.

After examination in the lying position of tonic stretch reflexes by manual passive stretches, elicitation of tendon jerks, and clonus, the subject is placed in a *supported or unsupported sitting position,* depending upon his condition. Then the examination of tonic and phasic stretch reflexes of the available muscle groups is carried out.

The examination of muscle tone and its possible modification through changes in body posture is completed by assessing the *subject's ability to stand and walk.* Polaroid cameras make it easy and very practical to take pictures of patients at regular intervals and during various recording conditions. These pictures can be compared at a later date. In clinical terms, muscle tone is described as the degree

of resistance to passive movement and, as such, passive muscle stretch is actually an artifact but sensitive method for examination (Holmes 1946). A more natural condition, on the other hand, is the continuous muscle contraction used for the maintenance of upright posture. We highly recommend, therefore, that when assessing muscle tone, one should add to the passive manual stretch a systematic evaluation of how the subject's position and posture can modify muscle tone, deformities, etc.

Manual passive stretch

A manual passive stretch maneuver consists of lengthening and shortening the muscles corresponding to a particular joint while passively moving the joint.

Muscle resistance to stretch is evaluated at different rates. When spasticity is mild, only the muscles which are stretched at a high rate will resist. In moderate spasticity, resistance to passive movement is noticed when stretch is applied at a slower rate. The resistance can be so pronounced as to stop movement and when the force of the stretch is increased, resistance suddenly generates the so-called clasp-knife phenomen. In severe spasticity, resistance to stretch can be so strong that it is difficult or impossible to mobilize entire muscle groups (Pedersen 1969).

When assessing muscle tone by manual muscle stretch, in addition to describing when resistance is felt and how strong it is, it is also useful to describe how many different rates of passive stretch can be accomplished. In cases of mild spasticity, it is usually

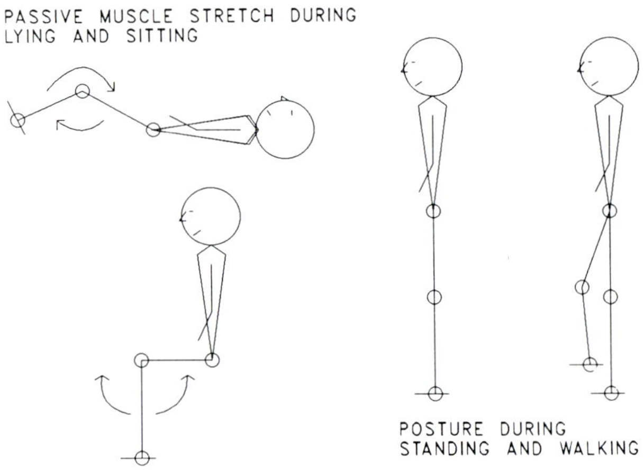

PASSIVE MUSCLE STRETCH DURING
LYING AND SITTING

POSTURE DURING
STANDING AND WALKING

Fig. 1

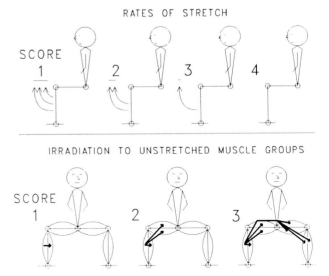

RATES OF STRETCH

SCORE 1 2 3 4

IRRADIATION TO UNSTRETCHED MUSCLE GROUPS

SCORE 1 2 3

Fig. 2

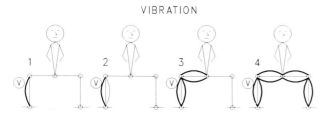

VIBRATION

Fig. 3

possible to elicit three different rates, slow, moderate, and fast and such a response can be scored by 1; when two different rates of stretch (i.e., slow and moderate) are present the score is 2; and when only one rate of stretch (i.e., slow) is possible, such a maneuver is scored 3. In score 4, muscle resistance is so severe that no passive movement can be elicited.

In addition to assessing how many rates of stretch can be achieved, the simultaneous recording of *additional muscle groups that respond* either ipsi or contralaterally can provide further information for the assessment of spasticity. Moreover, as we have already mentioned, before and after the assessment in the lying position, observations on the effects of changing the position of the body on the muscle stretch response can be noted in the scoring system.

Another alternative to assess tonic stretch reflex is the *study of the effect of vibration on the tendon or muscle belly*. The vibrator which can produce frequencies between 80–100 Hz and a displacement of 1–3 mm, when placed over the tendon or belly of skeletal muscles will elicit the so-called vibratory tonic

stretch reflex (Dimitrijevic et al. 1977). This approach is of particular value when the subject has severe contractures which restrict the manual muscle stretch. It has been shown in subjects with different degrees of spasticity due to spinal cord injury, that the severity of spasticity assessed by manual muscle stretch corresponds to the size of induced vibratory tonic reflex. Similar to the manual muscle stretch, the size of the response can be scored by number 1 when the response is restricted to the vibrated muscle, by number 2 when it irradiates to all ipsilateral muscle groups and by 3 when it irradiates to both sides.

Tendon jerks

Hyperactive tendon jerks manifest exaggerated phasic stretch reflexes. This can be easily elicited by percussion of the tendon with a reflex hammer, especially for the achilles, patellar, biceps and triceps tendons. However, when spasticity is present, percussion with the reflex hammer of various muscles of the upper and lower limbs, as well the neck and trunk, can elicit reflex responses, even in muscles without well defined tendons. To those most frequently and conventionally used, one should add the short flexors of the toes, the abductors and adductors of the thigh, and the abdominal, paraspinal, styloradial, deltoid, pectoral, rhomboid and trapezius muscles.

It is essential to describe the *threshold of the phasic stretch reflex*. Repetitively elicited stretch reflexes (20–30 times) allow us to find out if responses are restricted to the stretched muscles at the threshold

THRESHOLD FOR SINGLE MUSCLE RESPONSE –   1

SUPRATHRESHOLD FOR UNILATERAL MULTIMUSCLE RESPONSE –   2

SUPRATHRESHOLD FOR BILATERAL MULTIMUSCLE RESPONSE –   3

Effect of reinforcement influence (present/absent)

Effect of minimal volitional activity

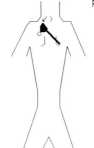

REPETITIVE REGULAR STIMULATION

Steadily decreasing   (1)

Constant response   (2)

Steadily decreasing   (3)

Fig. 4

level, and when a stronger stimulus in the reflex stretch response starts to irradiate to other muscle groups.

Finally, the comparison between the lying and sitting positions of the body when major tendon jerks are elicited must be examined. *Reinforcement maneuvers* (i.e., forceful closing of the eyes, clenching of the jaw, making a fist) must be assessed as well, even when the phasic stretch reflex is exaggerated.

The *effect of minimal volitional activity on* the amplitude and pattern of phasic stretch reflex responses is also a source of useful information.

Other components of the upper motor neuron syndrome

Spasticity and hyperexcitability of the stretch reflex are only minimal components of the dysfunctions of the upper motor neuron (Young 1980). A complete evaluation of spasticity must include the assessment of cutaneomuscular withdrawal reflexes as well as the status of volitional and automatic motor activity.

The most clinically used *withdrawal reflex* is movement induced by nociceptive cutaneous stimulation. Brisk or long lasting withdrawal movement, flexed or extended toes, toe and ankle movement, or movement in all three joints of the ankle, knee and hip, can help in describing the amplitude of the plantar reflex movement. The effect of regular and constant nociceptive stimulation can reveal different behaviour in repetitively elicited reflex responses, i.e., progressively declining amplitude, constant amplitude or even progressively increasing amplitude (Dimitrijevic 1973). The irradiation of the response to the contralateral leg is also a part of the evaluation of spasticity

VOLITIONAL ACTIVITY

Single and multijoint	Multijoint only	Trace movement	No movement
1	2	3	4

Fig. 6

using withdrawal reflex. Usually, the nociceptive stimulus is essential to elicit the withdrawal reflex, but in certain cases of spasticity it is sufficient to apply a non painful touch. Therefore, in the assessment of the withdrawal reflex, it is important to have information about the kind of stimulus that was used as well as the site of stimulation. Finally, while eliciting the withdrawal reflex, we ask the subject to volitionally suppress and then facilitate the reflex response. The effective performance of one or both motor acts provides further information about the severity of upper motor neuron dysfunctions. In this same way one can examine any other withdrawal, skin-muscular reflex response in any part of the body.

The presence or absence of *volitional motor activity* in the subject with spasticity is an important clue to determine the degree of upper motor neuron dysfunction. While there can be severe paralysis with minimal spasticity, the opposite is true that there can be severe spasticity with relatively well preserved volitional motor activity. Therefore, it is important to describe the degree of volitional activity preserved during both single joint and multi-joint movements. When there is no movement in the single joint, the pattern of multi-joint movements is preserved. Further

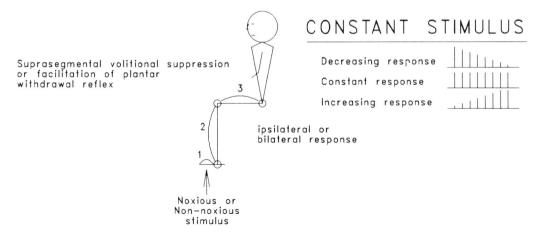

Suprasegmental volitional suppression or facilitation of plantar withdrawal reflex

ipsilateral or bilateral response

Noxious or Non-noxious stimulus

CONSTANT STIMULUS

Decreasing response

Constant response

Increasing response

Fig. 5

deterioration of volitional motor activity will lead to the presence of only traces of movement and finally to complete paralysis with absence of any volitionally induced movement.

Conclusion

From the clinical standpoint, spasticity can be assessed satisfactorily and accurately in order to compare the findings in the same subject during the evolution of the neurological disease or the effect of the treatment of spasticity. It is important to carry out the examination of tonic and phasic stretch reflexes systematically and to document their amplitude and patterns with a scoring system which can be easily compared. In addition, it is very useful to have information on the

other motor neuron dysfunctions (as in the case of withdrawal reflexes) and the status of volitional motor activity.

References

Dimitrijevic MR (1973) New developments in electromyography and clinical neurophysiology, vol 3. Withdrawal reflexes. Karger, Basel, pp 744–750

Dimitrijevic MR, Spencer WA, Trontelj JV, Dimitrijevic MM (1977) Reflex effects of vibration in patients with spinal cord lesions. Neurology 27(11): 1078–1086

Holmes G (1946) Introduction to clinical neurology, 3rd edn. Churchill Livingstone, Edinburgh London

Pedersen E (1969) Spasticity: mechanisms, measurement, management. Publication No. 752. Charles C Thomas, Springfield,Illinois

Young RR (1980) Spasticity: disordered motor control. Epilogue: a view toward the future – restorative neurology. Year Book Medical Publishers, Chicago London, pp 495–500

Correspondence: Prof. M.R. Dimitrijevic, M.D., D.Sc., Division of Restorative Neurology and Human Neurobiology, Baylor College of Medicine, One Baylor Plaza, Houston, Texas 77030, U.S.A.

Clinical neurophysiological assessment of spasticity

J. Zidar[1] and M.R. Dimitrijević[2]

[1]Institute of Clinical Neurophysiology, University Medical Center, Ljubljana, Yugoslavia, and [2]Division of Restorative Neurology and Human Neurobiology, Baylor College of Medicine, Houston, Texas, U.S.A.

Introduction

It is possible to approach the neurophysiological assessment of spasticity in two ways. The most straightforward and simple one is to document clinical phenomena, for example exaggerated tonic and phasic stretch reflexes. The other approach is based on description of the underlying spinal and supraspinal mechanisms of spasticity. Both of them are successful in quantifying spastic phenomena and are therefore useful for assessment of the efficacy of different forms of treatment.

Spasticity is detected by passively moving the limb segment about the joint and noting the resistance offered by the muscles. This hyperexcitability of the stretch reflex is velocity-dependent and is accompanied by the increased deep tendon reflexes. Spasticity is only one component of the upper motoneuron syndrome, the others are hyperactive flexion reflexes and decreased dexterity or loss of strength (Lance 1980). The increased muscle tone results from an increase in the excitability of alpha motoneurons. Motoneurons have a lowered threshold for excitation and excessive and prolonged responses not only to proprioceptive input (neurophysiological characteristic of spasticity) but to all stimuli. Thus activity in skin or visceral afferents can cause excessive activation of many muscles.

At the spinal level there are several possible mechanisms which can cause increased excitability of the alpha motoneurons. Exaggerated stretch reflexes may for example result from muscle spindle hyperactivity, from decreased presynaptic inhibition of Ia terminals, from decreased reciprocal inhibition, or from decreased inhibition from Ib afferents. Other spinal mechanisms may also contribute.

Many *descending pathways* either facilitate or inhibit already mentioned segmental reflex mechanisms. Magoun and Rhines (1947) proposed that spasticity is of supraspinal origin and the result of an impaired balance between facilitatory and inhibitory descending influences through the spinal cord. This is certainly true in the decerebrate cat, which is the most frequently used animal model of spasticity. Lesions of the corticospinal neurons do not cause spasticity or increase tendon reflexes in the affected limbs (Patton and Amassian 1960, Phillips 1973, Asanuma 1981, Wiesendanger 1981). It is therefore likely that spasticity arises not from damage to the corticospinal tract but from damage to corticobulbar or descending brain stem pathways.

Clinical neurophysiological methods are available which can measure many different mechanisms of spasticity. Firstly, clinical phenomena, which are a reflection of heightened alpha motoneuron excitability, can be quantified. Secondly, several methods for evaluation of segmental mechanisms of spasticity are available. And thirdly, supraspinal influences on spinal cord reflex mechanisms can be studied.

Clinical neurophysiological methods for documentation and quantification of clinical phenomena

If continuous, as in case of muscle vibration or during passive limb movements, muscle stretch evokes a tonic stretch reflex (Hagbarth and Eklund 1966, Lance et al. 1973), while brief taps to muscle tendons abruptly stretch the intramuscular spindle receptors and evoke so called phasic stretch reflexes. These reflexes are increased in spastic conditions. When the tendon jerks are exaggerated, it is frequently possible to elicit clonus, which is actually a phasic stretch reflex repeated six to seven times a second. Spastic patients also have other components of upper motoneuron dysfunction. Responses to cutaneous stimulation are abnormally prolonged and may activate most of the muscles of the same as well as of the opposite limb. Most commonly studied is the response to stimulation of the sole of the foot (Dimitrijević and Nathan 1969).

Procedures of clinical value for measurement of electrical and mechanical features of tendon jerks will be described in this section. Assessment of muscle hypertonia by the pendulum test, by passive stretch with isokinetic dynamometer, and by vibratory-induced tonic reflexes will also be mentioned. Measurements of electrophysiological parameters of withdrawal reflexes will be outlined, though, strictly speaking, such reflexes are not included in the definition of spasticity. Finally measurements of motoneuronal overactivity will be discussed.

Tendon jerk

In spastic patients tendon jerks are elicited at weaker stimulus intensities than in subjects with normal muscle tone. Electromyographically, the jerks show larger amplitudes than in the normal and are followed by after-discharge of the motor units. The synchronous discharge of the motor units immediately following the tap on the tendon is often slightly longer-lasting than in the normal. To be useful in clinical practice the procedure should be standardized (Toft et al. 1989).

Sizes of tendon jerks can be measured from electromyographic responses or from recordings of mechanical events. EMG recordings are simpler.

For this purpose surface electrodes are applied over muscle bellies in a standardized way. An electrodynamic hammer is used for eliciting reflex responses and for triggering an oscilloscope where EMG responses are displayed. It is important to note that tendon jerks can easily be elicited from many different muscles (Moody and Dimitrijević 1964, Dimitrijević et al. 1980).

The parameters usually measured are *threshold force for eliciting a reflex* and *maximal amplitude of the tendon jerk* (*T-wave*). Another useful parameter is the *ratio between the maximum amplitude of the T-wave and of the muscle response to supramaximal motor nerve stimulation* (*M-wave*). This ratio measures the proportion of population of motor units which respond to stretch. The ratio is close to 1 in severely spastic patients and is much smaller in normals (Fig. 1). As already mentioned, well synchronized T-wave in spastic patients may be followed by prolonged motor unit firing, either in a tonic way or in bursts (Dimitrijević and Nathan 1967). The amout of after-discharges can be quantified. Its significance will be commented upon later.

H-reflex

The H-reflex is the electrically elicited equivalent of the tendon jerk, both being mediated through activation of motoneurons by the primary spindle afferents. In normal adults, the H-reflex study is restricted mostly to the soleus and flexor carpi radialis muscles. In upper motor neuron lesions the H-reflex may be elicited in muscles where normally it is rarely seen (e.g. intrinsic hand muscles, tibialis anterior, peroneal muscles).

The *Hmax/Mmax ratio* that is the ratio of maximal

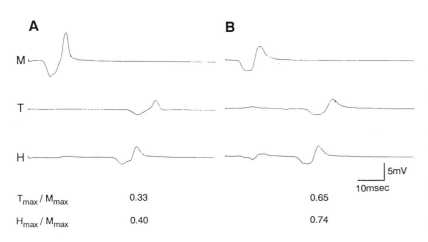

Fig. 1. Ratios between the T and M-wave and between the H and M-wave maximal amplitudes. Responses of gastrocnemius muscles from a normal volunteer (**A**) and from a hemiplegic patient (**B**) are shown. M-waves were elicited by supramaximal electrical stimulation of the tibialis posterior nerve in the popliteal fossa, H-waves by much weaker stimulation at the same site, and T-waves by taps to the Achilles tendons. Relative sizes of the T and H-waves in comparison to the M-wave (the T to M-wave and H to M-wave ratios), which are measures of motoneuronal excitability, are significantly bigger in spastic muscles

H-reflex and M-wave amplitudes, is a good indicator of spasticity, especially in the soleus muscle. Electrical stimulation of the tibial nerve gives first a short latency (6 m sec) response, which is muscle response to motor nerve stimulation M, and a second one, of longer latency (30 m sec), which is the Ia monosynaptic reflex H (Hoffman). When intensity of stimulation is increased, first the H and later the M waves reach a maximum. The ratio Hmax/Mmax is normally 0.5. In spastic cases, this ratio rises up to 0.8 due to hyper-excitability of alpha motoneurons (Fig. 1).

Motoneurons which discharge in the H-reflex undergo excitability changes, which last for up to 5 seconds. The nature and the degree of these changes may be assessed by measuring the *H-wave excitability curve* (or *H-wave recovery curve*). This is constructed by introducing a conditioning stimulus at various intervals preceding a test stimulus (Taborikova and Sax 1968). In normal adults, two electrical shocks applied on the tibial nerve need to be separated by at least 100 to 150 m sec, to give identical H responses. In spastic patients this delay is shorter and the second H-reflex reaches higher amplitude than the first one. This means that the late period of facilitation begins earlier and is enhanced in spastic patients.

Since the electrical stimulus was easier to control than the mechanical, the H-reflex was more extensively used in studies of spasticity. There are only a few accessible sites, however, where the H-reflex can be elicited, and this is a disadvantage in comparison to the tendon jerk.

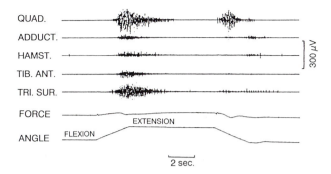

Fig. 3. Isokinetic dynamometry. Response of a spastic spinal cord injured patient to passive extension and flexion of the knee at 30 degrees per second. A modified Cybex II isokinetic dynamometer was used. Knee extension did not immediately result in reflex activation of muscles. In contrast, knee flexion directly caused a burst of EMG activity in the stretched muscle and was accompanied by resisting torque

Passive stretch

A very simple measurement of the resistance to passive stretch is the *pendulum test* (Boczko and Mumenthaler 1954, Bajd and Vodovnik 1984). The proximally supported leg is dropped from horizontal position to move freely at the knee-joint (Fig. 2). Several oscillations are observed before the leg stays still. The amplitude, rate and number of oscillations can be quantified. All of them are diminished in spastic patients.

Recently, *force measurements under controlled isokinetic movements* were introduced to measure the resistance to passive stretch (Knutsson and Mårtensson 1980). This method can be used in many upper and lower extremity muscles (Fig. 3).

Tonic vibration reflex

Vibration of a muscle or tendon through the skin elicits slow muscle contraction (tonic vibration reflex) by stimulating muscle spindles. In this it resembles continuous direct muscle stretch. Due to the simplicity in practical application it serves as an important tool for the assessment of muscle tone. *It can be reduced or even absent in spastic patients* (Lance et al. 1973, Ashby and Verrier 1975, Dimitrijević et al. 1977) (Fig. 4). Measurements of the amplitude of the response and its duration, the type of onset and the irradiation of activity of motor units to non-vibrated muscles can all be important for quantification of spasticity.

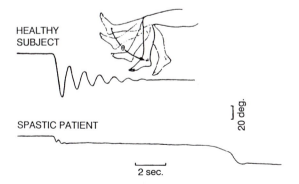

Fig. 2. Pendulum test. Knee angle measurements from healthy volunteer and from a 24 year old male with chronic spinal cord injury at the T10 level. Normal trace consists of several oscillations which are not accompanied by muscle activity. Spastic pattern shown is of a tonic type with characteristic slow flexion of the knee due to the tonic stretch reflex in the quadriceps muscle

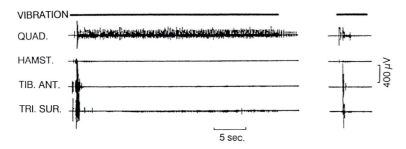

Fig. 4. Tonic vibration reflex. Vibration was applied to the quadriceps muscle in a spinal cord injured patient. In healthy subjects vibration elicits response isolated to the vibrated muscle. Responses build up slowly are persistent and have low amplitudes. The figure, however, shows the response that began with a large initial burst of activity and was followed by low amplitude tonic response for the rest of the time. When vibratory stimulus was short-lasting the muscle responded only phasically. Notice the spread of EMG activity to non-vibrated muscles

Plantar withdrawal reflex

Stroking the ball and the hollow of the sole of the foot elicits flexion of the first toe in normals and dorsiflexion of the first toe and possible abduction of the others in patients with upper motor neuron lesions. This so-called Babinski response is very important sign in clinical neurology. It is usually accompanied by flexion of the whole limb and can occasionally be elicited also with light touch instead of noxious stimulation (Dimitrijević and Nathan 1969). Therefore, *the threshold for the response is decreased and its size is increased in the upper motor neuron syndrome.* EMG recordings of the plantar response can also be of some help for confirmation that the clinically observed

response is not merely a voluntary withdrawal (VanGijn 1975, 1976). Dorsiflexion of the first toe is abnormal if caused by activity in extensor hallucis longus and if simultaneously other flexor muscles are activated. For quantification of the plantar withdrawal response surface EMG recordings are used and stimulation is performed by electrical stimulation of the plantar surface of the foot (Fig. 5).

Motoneuronal overactivity

It has already been noted that the basic physiologic abnormality underlying spasticity is increased excitability of motoneurons. Regardless of its origin any input to motoneurons will produce excessive and

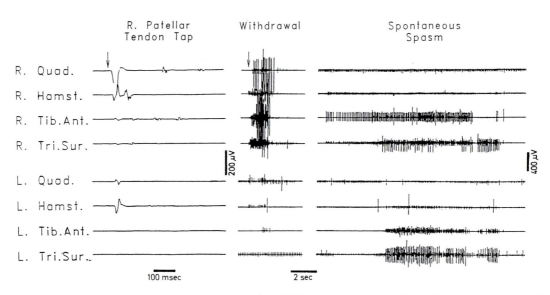

Fig. 5. Motoneuronal overactivity. Simultaneous surface EMG recordings from 8 different lower limb muscles in 3 patients with chronic spinal cord lesions. Electromyographic afterdischarges and spread of activity to different ipsilateral and contralateral muscles are shown after the right patellar tendon tap and after mechanical stimulation of the right foot plantar surface. An example of spontaneous spasm is also shown

prolonged activity which can be observed in the contractions of many limb muscles. To quote Nathan (1980), "The motoneuron is an adding machine. It sums the excitatory and inhibitory inputs that it receives; it receives these from muscles, tendons, skin, viscera, and also distant inputs from the brain. In accordance with what it receives in this way, inhibitory and excitatory, it fires off impulses. How often it fires depends on everything that happens in the nervous system." After-discharge and activation of many distant muscles after a segmental input can be explained by longitudinal and horizontal spread of excitation through the propriospinal interneuronal system. This sytem has thus an ability to enormously increase the number of reflexly activated neuronal population. *Motoneuronal overactivity and spread of the activity to many distant motoneuronal pools is one of the most characteristic features of spasticity.*

In quantifying spasticity it is often more correct to measure the amplitude and frequency of occurrence of the so-called *spontaneous or reflexly induced spasms*, as the spasms would interfere with measurements of the tendon jerks, the H-reflexes, etc.

All these aspects of motoneuronal overactivity can be documented and quantified by *multiple channel surface electromyographic recordings* of motor unit activity. Such measurements can be done simultaneously with the assessment of tendon jerks, H-reflexes, tonic stretch reflexes, and flexor withdrawal reflexes where after-discharges and the irradiation of activity to several different segmental levels is frequently

observed (Fig. 5). The excitability of motoneurons of different muscles as influenced by stimulation of various skin areas or by vibration of muscles of the trunk or lower extremities can also be studied using repetitively induced myotatic reflexes.

Also important for quantitative description of spasticity is the fluctuation in its features over minutes, hours, days or months. Fluctuation depends on many different factors, as for example on the patient's position, fullness of bladder, the immediately preceding exercise, patient stress and his general health and state of alertness. Also important are the level and the extent of the lesion and the cause of the upper motoneuron dysfunction. Therefore *the assessment of spasticity must describe the characteristic fluctuations when tested in a standardized protocol.*

Clinical neurophysiological methods for assessment of spinal mechanisms underlying spasticity

Spinal mechanisms of spasticity as studied in humans were the subject of a review by Pierrot-Deseilligny and Mazieres (1985). The authors divide them in those with evidence against them (fusimotor hyperactivity, decreased group II inhibition, decreased recurrent inhibition), in those with evidence in their favour (decreased presynaptic inhibition of Ia terminals, decreased inhibition of antagonistic muscles), and in other possible mechanisms, which have never been explored (alpha motoneuron hyperexcitability and decrease of Ib inhibition) (Fig. 6).

In animal experiments it was found that fusimotor hyperactivity, while increasing sensitivity of muscle spindle primary endings, contributes to rigidity

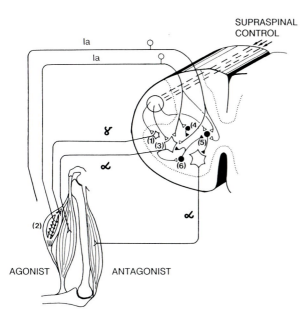

Fig. 6. Schematic diagram representing the following possible spinal mechanisms of spasticity: A) Fusimotor hyperactivity. Hyperexcitability of the stretch reflex could result from hyperactive gamma motor neurons possibly due to supraspinal facilitation (1). This increases muscle spindle sensitivity (2) producing an increase in Ia fibre discharge to muscle stretch which in turn increases output of alpha motor neurons (3). B) Decrease in presynaptic inhibition of Ia terminals. Ia discharge produced by muscle stretch is normally partially blocked by presynaptic inhibition which is produced by axo-axonal synapses and mediated by interneurons (4). Reduction of this inhibition would result in hyperactive stretch reflexes. C) Decreased reciprocal Ia inhibition. Normally voluntary contraction of the synergist muscle occurs simultaneously with active inhibition of antagonist muscle. This inhibition successfully prevents the occurrence of a stretch reflex in the antagonist muscle, which could otherwise be triggered by Ia discharge during stretch. The main mechanism of active inhibition is reciprocal Ia inhibition [Ia fibres from synergist inhibit antagonist motoneurons through Ia inhibitory interneurons (5)]. Voluntary contraction · facilitates transmission in the Ia inhibitory pathway by direct facilitation of these Ia interneurons. Ia inhibitory interneurons are inhibited by synergist-coupled Renshaw cells (6). Failure of Ia reciprocal inhibition causes malfunctioning of spastic patients

(Eldred et al. 1953). There is so far no evidence that the same mechanism operates also in human spasticity (Hagbarth et al. 1973). Microneurography is the only available method for testing gamma hyperactivity in humans but is probably of no practical value for clinical neurophysiological evaluation of patients.

Much simpler is the method for testing presynaptic inhibition of Ia terminals as demonstrated by a decrease in H-reflex in soleus muscle when vibrating the Achilles tendon. (Delwaide 1971). This effect was found to be diminished in most spastic patients (Delwaide 1973) indicating a decrease in presynaptic inhibition.

Clinical methods for studying Ib inihibition and recurrent inhibition also exist (Pierrot-Deseilligny and Bussel 1975, Pierrot-Deseilligny et al. 1981). In most

spastics there is no change in recurrent inhibition (Katz and Pierrot-Deseilligny 1982).

Finally, reciprocal inhibition can be studied by use of test stimuli to agonist nerves to elicit H-reflex responses with appropriately timed conditioning stimuli to the antagonistic muscle group nerve (Tanaka 1974). Studies in patients revealed that a malfunction in reciprocal Ia inhibition, caused by supraspinal mechanism, does exist in man (Katz and Pierrot-Deseilligny 1982, Tanaka 1983).

Clinical neurophysiological assessment of the residual suprasegmental control

Increased alpha motoneuron hyperexcitability which is very likely a direct consequence of abnormal functioning of spinal circuits may result either from residual descending control of segmental

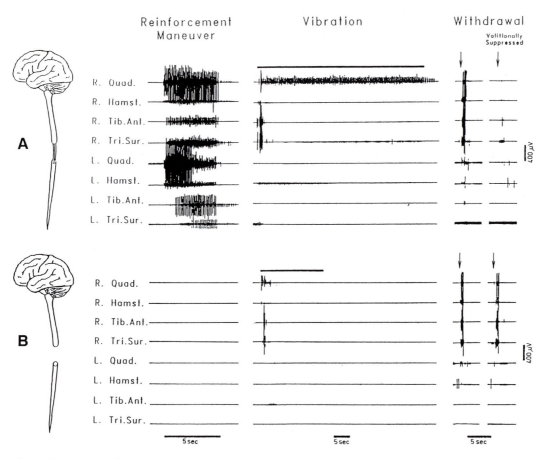

Fig. 7. Clinical neurophysiological assessment of the residual suprasegmental control. Polyelectromyographic recordings from the lower limb muscles in patients who were clinically recognized as having complete spinal cord injury. Responses to reinforcement maneuver (neck flexion), vibration, and to mechanical plantar stimulation are shown. On the basis of results of these tests patients can be further subdivided according to the level of the preserved descending influence. Two major groups are recognized, neurophysiologically incomplete (**A**) and neurophysiologically complete (**B**) spinal cord injuries. Note characteristic inability of reinforcement maneuver in patient with neurophysiologically complete spinal cord lesion (**B**) to activate motor units below the level of the lesion. This patient also showed barely any response to vibration and was not able to volitionally suppress the withdrawal response to mechanical plantar stimulation. The reverse pattern, however, occurred in a patient with neurophysiologically incomplete spinal cord lesion (**A**)

spinal pathways and/or from local (biochemical, histological, synaptic) changes at the spinal level (Pierrot-Deseilligny and Mazieres 1985). Only the first of the proposed mechanisms will be considered here, since for the assessment of the second there are no clinical neurophysiological methods of practical value available.

That spasticity is the clinical expression of preserved brain influences can be inferred from the fact, that in most severe chronic spinal cord injuries tendon jerks are only moderately enhanced while tonic stretch components are absent (Dimitrijević 1985). In another group of patients in whom clinical examination also reveals complete spinal cord lesion and who may show a marked degree of tonic and phasic hypertonia, it is always possible to demonstrate partially preserved descending brain influences. The method which is useful for demonstration and quantification of the residual suprasegmental motor control is that of *polyelectromyographic recordings* from different limb muscles.

Reinforcement maneuvers (e.g. forceful closing of the eyes, clenching of the jaw, making a fist) which depend on the supraspinal control can induce excessive motor unit activity in several muscle groups of otherwise completely paralyzed patients (Dimitrijević et al. 1981) (Fig. 7). In neurophysiologically incomplete spinal cord lesions, reinforcement maneuvers will also have a conditioning effect on responses to test stimuli, such as tendon jerks or H-reflexes.

Another means to demonstrate the preserved supraspinal influences in spinal cord injured patients is the evaluation of the *tonic muscle stretch reflex* (Dimitrijević et al. 1977). This reflex *is under the influence of the bulbo-spinal system* and could only be elicited, if this system is at least partially functioning. The presence of the tonic stretch reflex in clinically complete spinal cord injured patients is thus a sign of a incomplete lesion (Fig. 7).

Suprasegmental suppression of the segmental activity also occur in paralyzed spinal cord injured patients. It can be documented by recording the *withdrawal reflex induced by noxious plantar stimulation while the patient attempts to volitionally supress it* (Cioni et al. 1986) (Fig. 7).

The importance of the observation that supraspinal influence can be preserved even when there is no clinical evidence for it, is in its possible use for modification of the spasticity. These residual physiological mechanisms can possibly be activated to suppress the circuits involved in the generation of spasticity.

Concluding remarks

Clinical neurophysiological techniques to assess spasticity are rarely applied in routine work. The reason could be that they are numerous, rather complex, and have not been properly standardized.

We would like to propose a method based on polyelectromyography, which we think is practical and gives reliable quantitative information to the clinician (Dimitrijevic et al. 1980). Muscle activity is studied in relaxation and during the following test maneuvers: reinforcement maneuvers, cutaneous stimulation, attempts at volitional activation, passive stretch, tendon taps, clonus activation, vibration of tendons, plantar stimulation, and cortical stimulation for more direct evaluation of the functional integrity of the corticospinal tract. To do this, a poly-electromyograph is used with surface electrodes placed over the motor points of selected muscles (in our laboratory we routinely record from 16 muscle groups). The actual recording time for the entire protocol is not longer than 60 minutes and the procedure is well standardized.

Although this method is particularly pertinent for categorization of patients according to their neuro-control status, we found it very useful also for assessment of different modes of treatment of spasticity.

References

Asanuma H (1981) The pyramidal tract. In: Brooks WB (ed) Handbook of physiology. The nervous system, vol 2. Motor control. American Physiological Society, Bethesda, pp 203–233

Ashby P, Verrier M (1975) Neurophysiological changes following spinal cord lesions in man. Can J Neurol Sci 2: 91–100

Bajd T, Vodovnik L (1984) Pendulum testing of spasticity. J Biomed Eng 6: 9–16

Boczko M, Mumenthaler M (1954) Modified pendulousness test to assess tonus of thigh muscles in spasticity. Neurology 8: 846–851

Cioni B, Dimitrijević MR, McKay WB, Sherwood AM (1986) Voluntary supraspinal suppression of spinal reflex activity in paralysed muscles of spinal cord injury patients. Exp Neurol 93: 574–583

Delwaide PJ (1971) Etude Experimentale de l'Hyperreflexie Tendineuse en Clinique Neurologique. Arschia, Bruxelles, pp 1–324

Delwaide PJ (1973) Human monosynaptic reflexes and presynaptic inhibition. An interpretation of spastic hyperreflexia. In: Desmedt JE (ed) New developments in electromyography and clinical neurophysiology, vol 3. Karger, Basel, pp 508–522

Dimitrijević MR (1985) Spasticity. In: Swash M, Kennard C (eds) Scientific basis of clinical neurology. Churchill Livingstone, New York, pp 108–115

Dimitrijević MR, Nathan P (1967) Studies of spasticity in man. 2. Analysis of stretch reflexes in spasticity. Brain 91: 333–358

Dimitrijević MR, Nathan P (1969) Studies of spasticity in man. 3.

Analysis of reflex activity evoked by noxious cutaneous stimulation. Brain 94: 17–90

Dimitrijević MR, Spencer WA, Trontelj JV, Dimitrijević MM (1977) Reflex effects of vibration in patients with spinal cord lesions. Neurology 27: 1078–1086

Dimitrijević MR, Gregorič MR, Sherwood AM, Spencer WA (1980) Reflex responses of paraspinal muscles to tapping. J Neurol Neurosurg Psychiatry 43: 1112–1118

Dimitrijević MR, Dimitrijević MM, McKay WB, Sherwood AM (1981) Supraspinal influence on motor unit activity in paralysed muscles: effects of reinforcement maneuvers. Arch Phys Med 62: 540

Eldred E, Granit R, Merton PA (1953) Supraspinal control of the muscle spindles and its significance. J Physiol (London) 122: 498–523

Hagbarth KE, Eklund G (1966) Motor effects of vibratory stimuli in man. In: Granit Nobel Symposium I. Muscle afferents and motor control. Almquist and Wiksell, Stockholm, pp 177–182

Hagbarth KE, Wallin G, Löfstedt L (1973) Muscle spindle responses to stretch in normal and spastic subjects. Scand J Rehab Med 5: 156–159

Katz R, Pierrot-Deseilligny E (1982) Recurrent inhibition of alpha-motoneurons in patients with upper motor neuron lesions. Brain 105: 103–124

Knutsson E, Mårtensson A (1980) Dynamic motor capacity in spastic paresis and its relation to prime-mover dysfunction, spastic reflexes and antagonistic co-activation. Scand J Rehab Med 12: 93–106

Lance JW (1980) Symposium synopsis. In: Feldman RG, Young RR, Koella WP (eds) Spasticity: disordered motor control. Year Book Medical Publishers, Chicago, pp 485–494

Lance JW, Burke D, Andrews CJ (1973) The reflex effects of muscle vibration. In: Desmedt JE (ed) New developments in electromyography and clinical neurophysiology, vol 3. Karger, Basel, pp 444–462

Magoun HW, Rhines R (1947) Spasticity: the stretch-reflex and extrapyramidal systems. Charles C Thomas Publ, Springfield Illinois

Moody JR, Dimitrijević MR (1964) An electromyogrphic study of tendon reflexes in progressive muscular dystrophy in man. Brain 87: 511–520

Nathan PW (1980) Factors affecting spasticity. Int Rehabil Med 2: 27–30

Patton HD, Amassian VE (1960) The pyramidal tract; its excitation and functions. In: Field J (ed) Handbook of physiology and neurophysiology. American Physiological Society, Washington DC, pp 837–861

Phillips CG (1973) Pyramidal apparatus for control of the baboon hand. In: Desmedt JE (ed) New developments in electromyography and clinical neurophysiology, vol 3. Karger, Basel, pp 136–144

Pierrot-Deseilligny E, Bussel B (1975) Evidence for recurrent inhibition by motoneurones in human subjects. Brain Res 88: 105–108

Pierrot-Deseilligny E, Mazieres L (1985) Spinal mechanisms underlying spasticity. In: Delwaide PJ, Young RR (eds) Clinical neurophysiology in spasticity. Elsevier Science Publishers BV, Amsterdam New York Oxford, pp 63–76

Pierrot-Deseilligny E, Morin C, Bergego C, Tankov N (1981) Pattern of group Ib projections from ankle flexor and extensor muscles in man. Exp Brain Res 42: 337–356

Taborikova H, Sax DS (1968) Motoneurone pool and the spinal H-reflex. J Neurol Neurosurg Psychiatry 31: 354–361

Tanaka R (1974) Reciprocal Ia inhibition during voluntary movement in man. Exp Brain Res 21: 529–540

Tanaka R (1983) Reciprocal Ia inhibitory pathway in normal man and in patients with motor disorders. In: Desmedt JE (ed) Motor control mechanisms in health and disease. Raven Press, New York, pp 433–441

Toft E, Sinkjaer G, Espersen GT (1989) Quantitation of the stretch reflex. Technical procedures and clinical applications. Acta Neurol Scand 79: 384–390

VanGijn J (1975) Babinski response: stimulus and effector. J Neurol Neurosurg Psychiatry 38: 180–186

VanGijn J (1976) Equivocal plantar responses: a clinical and electromyographic study. J Neurol Neurosurg Psychiatry 39: 275–282

Wiesendanger M (1981) The pyramidal tract, its structure and function. In: Towe AL, Luschei ES (eds) Handbook of behavioral neurobiology. Plenum Press, New York, pp 401–491

Correspondence: Dr. J. Zidar, Institute of Clinical Neurophysiology, University Medical Center, Zaloška cesta 7, 61105 Ljubljana, Yugoslavia

Quantification of spasticity and limb function (based on clinical examination, and directed to adult patients)

M. Sindou[1] and **M.F. Millet**[1,2]

[1]Hopital Neurologique, P. Wertheimer, and [2]Centre Germaine Revel, University of Lyon, France

Comparison of results, in different series treated by the same neurosurgical group, or from one team to another, needs reliable – but also simple and easily reproducible – clinical scales to quantify spasticity and limb functions.

The scales and scores presented here correspond to those used in our department in Lyon University. Some of them are classical and commonly used, others were developed to meet the requirements of the types of patients and pathologies we are dealing with: mainly adults affected with severe hemiplegia or paraplegia. Therefore this chapter does not concern quantification of spasticity and functions in children with cerebral palsy; they need specific tests and scoring systems which are the matter of the next chapter by Abbott et al.

Quantification of spasticity and spasms

Spasticity is determined by passively moving the limb segment and noting the resistance offered by the muscles. Only stretch at high velocity explores muscle tone. Limitation in passive mobilization at slow speed attests to the degree of capsular and/or tendino-muscular retraction, i.e., the so-called orthopaedic limitations.

The most sensitive scale for clinically quantifying spasticity is the Held's test, which measures the angle of appearance of the catch response to a high speed stretching, and its intensity and duration (Table 1).

In very severely affected patients, like those who are referred for functional neurosurgery, the Held's test proves to be too sophisticated. Therefore the most adequate tone scale is the five grade Ashworth's scale (Table 2).

Table 1. Evaluation of spasticity by measurement of the stretch-reflex (Held)

Studying:

1) Its angle of appearance from the usual reference positions.

2) Its intensity:
   - 0: no muscular contraction
   - 1: visible muscular contraction
   - 2: contraction with a short catch
   - 3: contraction lasting a few secondes (or with transient clonus)
   - 4: permanent clonus
   - 5: rigidity without any possible passive mobilization.

These measurements are performed at 3 different following velocities:
   - V1: slow stretching
   - V2: velocity of gravity
   - V3: *fast stretching*

Table 2. Tone scale (Ashworth)

Grade	Degree of muscle tone
1	No increase in tone
2	Slight increase in tone, giving a catch during stretch
3	More marked increase in tone; but affected part easily mobilized
4	Considerable increase in tone; passive movement difficult
5	Rigidity without any possible passive mobilization

Although not directly related to spasticity, *spasms* – which are more often encountered in patients with spinal cord lesions – can be quantified in parallel to muscular hypertonia, using Penn's scale of spasm frequency (Table 3).

Table 3. Spasm frequency scale (Penn)

Grade	Frequency of spasms
0	No spasms
1	Mild spasms induced by stimulation
2	Infrequent full spasms occurring less than once per hour
3	Spasms occurring more than once per hour
4	Spasms occurring more than ten times per hour

Table 4. Grading of abnormal postures and/or articular limitations during passive mobilization

Grade	Criteria
0	Normal
I	Flexion < 30°
II	Flexion between 30° and 60°
III	Flexion between 60° and 90°
IV	Flexion > 90°

Table 5. Normal amplitudes of passive articular movements in the lower limb

Hip	Extension	:	10° (with extended knee)
	Flexion	:	125° (with flexed knee)
	Abduction	:	45°
	Adduction	:	20°
	External rotation	:	45°
	Internal rotation	:	45°
Knee	Extension	:	0° (with extended hip)
	Flexion	:	140° (with flexed hip)
Foot	Dorsi-flexion of the ankle : 20° (with flexed knee)
	Plantar flexion of the ankle : 45°
	Supination-adduction (inversion) : 35°
	Pronation-abduction (eversion) : 20°
	Dorsal flexion of metatarsophalangeal joint : 40°
	Plantar flexion of metatarsophalangeal joint : 30°

Quantification of abnormal postures and articular limitations

The degree of *spontaneous abnormal posture*, for a given joint, can be quantified by calculating the angle between the abnormal posture and the reference position.

The lower limb reference position is the one in which the patient lay supine with the knees extended, the feet together, and the ankles positioned at 90°. Table 4 shows how these angles – for the hip and the knee – can be graded from 0 (normal situation) to IV (flexion greater than 90°). The score is established on the basis of the examination of the most limited articulation.

For the upper limb, the reference position corresponds to the arm and forearm along the trunk, the elbow extended, and the hand with its palmar aspect internally orientated, the wrist and fingers extended.

For each given movement, *articular passive mobility* is estimated by performing angular measurements of both extreme positions during passive forced mobilization, in the awakened, and, sometimes if the test is necessary, in the anaesthetized and curarized patient. The grading – for the hip and the knee – is the same as for spontaneous abnormal postures (Table 4).

The normal amplitudes of articular movements are listed in Table 5 for the lower limb and in Table 6 for the upper limb.

Quantification of voluntary motor activity

Mobility is classically evaluated using the five grade Lovett's scale (Table 7).

Table 6. Normal amplitudes of passive articular movements in the upper limb

Shoulder :	Abduction	: 160°	*Elbow* :	Extension	:	0°
	Antepulsion	: 160°		Flexion	:	145°
	Retropulsion	: 40°				
	External rotation	: 40°				
	Internal rotation	: 95°				
Wrist :	Extension	: 70°	*Hand* :	*Metacarpophalangeal joint		
	Flexion	: 80°		Extension	:	30°
	Radial inclination	: 20°		Flexion	:	90°
	(abduction)			*Proximal interphalangeal joint		
	Cubital inclination	: 45°		Extension	:	0°
	(adduction)			Flexion	:	100°
	Supination	: 80°		*Distal interphalangeal joint		
	Pronation	: 70°		Extension	:	30°
				Flexion	:	70°

Table 7. Motor scale (Lovett)

Grade	Muscular strength
0	No muscular contraction
1	Muscular contraction, no movement
2	Possible movement without gravity
3	Movement against gravity
4	Movement against strength superior to gravity
5	Normal motor strength

In case of severe deficits, it can be convenient to simply classify motor function as absent, non functional, and functional.

Functional disability scores

Besides an analytical assessment of the neurological status and a quantification of its components, there is a need for an evaluation of the disability in relation to the patient's functional status.

1) With this practical purpose, a global functional score was developed for *paraplegic patients* by Millet and Beneton at the Germaine Revel Center in Lyon. The evaluation can be performed easily by any member of the team. It quantifies five components that are directly influenced by spasticity, abnormal postures and articular limitations, and are part of the patient's every day life. These five components are: a) pain, b) spasms, c) sitting position, d) body transfers and e) ability for washing and dressing. The score goes from 0 to 4 for each component (Table 8), with a total of 20/20 qualifying a bedridden and totally dependent

Table 9. Functional disability score for the upper limb in hemiplegic patients

Grade	Description
I	Good active mobility with the possibility of prehension in the hand and fingers
II	Slight, but useful voluntary motor function
III	Easy passive mobilization, but without any useful voluntary movements
IV	Absence of useful active mobility; uneasy and painful passive mobilization, making it difficult to dress and wash

Table 8. Functional disability score for spastic lower limbs in paraplegic patients

Pain	0	No pain
		Unfrequent pain and of minor intensity; the patient does not complain spontaneously; without any consequence on daily life
	2	Frequent pain and of moderate intensity; the patient complains spontaneously; but without any practical consequence on daily life
	3	Very frequent pain and/or severe intensity; with practical consequence on daily life
	4	Permanent and unbearable pain.
Spasms	0	No spasm
	1	Unfrequent spasms and of minor intensity; only provoked by mobilization; without any functional consequence
	2	Frequent spasms and of moderate intensity; occurring at mobilization and also spontaneously, but without impairing the patients' comfort in sitting and lying position.
	3	Very frequent spasms and/or severe intensity; impairing the sitting and the lying position (awaking patient at night)
	4	Almost constant spasms; making impossible any correct sitting position and even lying position.
Wheel chair	0	No discomfort
	1	Minor discomfort, not reducing significantly sitting time in wheelchair
	2	Moderate disconfort, reducing sitting time in wheelchair
	3	Strapping is required to maintain correct sitting position
	4	Wheelchair impossible.
Transfers	0	Easy, alone
	1	Possible alone, but difficult
	2	Need for one person helping
	3	Possible but difficult with one person helping
	4	Need for two persons helping
Washing and dressing	0	Easy, alone
	1	Possible alone, but difficult
	2	Need for one person helping
	3	Possible but difficult with one person helping
	4	Need for two persons helping

patient. A score of 10/20 corresponds reproducibly to the threshold between a decent and an unacceptable condition, and thus as a minimal indication for surgery.

2) For *hemiplegic patients* with hyperspasticity in the upper limb, we have developed an appropriate personal functional scoring system (Table 9).

Conclusion

These proposals of quantification of spasticity and limb function are based on clinical examination, and are preferentially directed to adults. They have no other goal than to serve as guidelines for helping clinicians who are dealing with patients affected with severe hemiplegia or paraplegia. Of course many other scales and scoring systems could have been added to the present list. In addition it must be recalled that complete quantification of spasticity needs laboratory investigations, especially those based on H-reflex measurements and poly-electromyography (see chapter by Zidar and Dimitrijevic).

Correspondence: Prof. M. Sindou, M.D., D.Sc. Biol., Hopital Neurologique, University of Lyon, 59 Boulevard Pinel, F-69003 Lyon, France

Childhood spasticity assessment

R. Abbott and **M. Johann-Murphy** with the collaboration of **S.L. Forem**

Division of Pediatric Neurosurgery, New York University Medical Center, New York, U.S.A.

Increasingly the medical community is being called upon to treat children who, having sustained an acute neurologic injury and, surviving it, are left with a fixed functional handicap.

Etiology of dysfunction (Table 1)

The majority of hypertonic children have as the etiology cerebral palsy (CP) (Bleck 1987a, Ingram 1984, Siegfried 1985). It can be due to an injury occurring prenatally, at term or postnatally. Broadly, this disorder is of four types, dyskinetic, ataxic, spastic, or mixed, cerebral palsy (Ingram 1984). The *dyskinetic group* is divided according to the type of movement disorder manifest (e.g., athetoid CP, dystonic or tension athetosis CP) and is typically due to either perinatal kernicterus or asphyxia (Bleck 1987a). The *ataxic group* is subdivided into a 'congenital' subgroup (a autosomal recessive disease frequently associated with mental retardation) and a "ataxic diplegia" subgroup (usually associated with either a pre- or perinatal event such as hemorrhage or asphyxia or postnatal hydrocephalus) (Bleck 1987a, Ingram 1984). The *spastic group* is subdivided according to the pattern of spasticity hence spastic diplegia (involvement in all four limbs, legs ≫ than arms), spastic paraplegia (involvement in just the legs), spastic hemiplegia (asymmetric involvement frequently manifested as a bilateral hemiplegia) and spastic quadriplegia (involvement in all four extremities with the arm involvement meeting or exceeding the leg involvement) (Ingram 1984). While spastic diplegia is frequently associated with premature birth, all of the spastic subgroups are associated with births of low weight. The spastic hemiplegic also have an increased incidence of intraventricular hemorrhage. The *mixed*

group is, as its name implies, made up of individuals exhibiting features of more than one of the above described groups (Bleck 1987a). Typically, it is a mixture of the features of the spastic and dyskinetic groups and is due to a perinatal event such as asphyxia.

The risk factors vary according to the level of development of the infant's or child's nervous system. In the case of the *"very" preterm infant (< 32 weeks gestation)*, the major risk factor appears to be the immaturity of the nervous system (Stanley 1984a). The germinal matrix of the cerebrum is prone to injury in the premature infant and subsequent alterations in cerebral blood flow may lead to hemorrhage in the matrix with extravasation into the ventricular system or surrounding brain (Duncan et al. 1989, Wigglesworth 1984). During this period in the development of the nervous system the fiber tracts of the corticospinal system within the cerebrum pass through watershed areas of vascular profusion. Transient episodes of decreased blood flow as can occur during maternal hypoxia, hypotension or placental infarct can result in cerebral infarcts and injury to the corticospinal system (Wigglesworth 1984). *As the fetus matures past 32 weeks*, other risk factors become more important (Stanley 1984b, Wigglesworth 1984). These risks include such maternal problems as a surgery with general anesthesia, maternal diabetes, chronic infection in the mother, or toxemia. Deprivation in the supply of nutrition to the fetus can be the result of multiple fetuses, placental dysfunction which can occur during a partial separation from the uterine wall or with toxemia and a resultant infarct in the placenta. Infection of the fetus (especially toxoplasmosis and cytomegalovirus) and genetic syndromes are also important etiologies of the cerebral palsy. *Perinatally*, extrauterine asphyxia occurring due to the lack of respiration within the first minutes of life, hypoxia occurring subsequently and hyperbilirubinemia become increasingly important as causes of CP. The term cerebral palsy can also be used to describe disabilities due to *injuries occurring after birth and throughout childhood* (Stanley and Blair 1984). Key here is that the clinical state not be progressive and that the site of injury be within the brain. These injuries are typically caused by infections (>50%) with the next most common being accidents and blows to the head (20%). Other causes are suffocation/near drowning, post epileptic anoxia, post-operative complications resulting in anoxia, cerebral hemorrhages and strokes, malnutrition, heavy metal ingestion and approximately 2–3% will be idiopathic. All total, children with postnatal cerebral palsies comprise 11–14% of the total cerebral palsy population and they are relatively more involved with most exhibiting a pure spastic type of cerebral palsy.

There are *several diseases which do not fall under the grouping of cerebral palsy but which can also create*

Table 1. Etiology of cerebral palsy

Prenatal
   Prior to 32 weeks
      Maternal hypoxic/hypotensive event
      Placental infarct
   After 32 weeks gestation
      Maternal retardation, seizures, proteinuria or
        Hyperthyroidism
      Poor nutrition from placenta
        Multiple fetuses
        Placenta previa
        Placentae abruptia
        Marginal sinus rupture
        Toxemia
      Intrauterine infection
      Genetic syndromes
Perinatal
   Premature birth
      Intraventricular hemorrhage
   Breech presentation
   Extrauterine asphyxia/hypoxia
   Kernicterius
Postnatal/childhood
   Infections
      Meningoencephalitis
   Accidents/head injuries
   Anoxic episode
      Suffocation/near drowning
      Post epileptic anoxia
      Operative complication
   Cerebral vascular accident
   Malnutrition
   Heavy metal ingestion
   Idiopathic

functional disabilities of a degree which require treatment. Demyelinating diseases such as multiple sclerosis can result in spasticity during childhood or adolescence. Spinal dysraphisms can, on occasion, have an isolated cord segment below the cord lesion with resultant spasticity (Storrs and McLone 1989). As treatment of CNS neoplasms improves, event free survival time is increasing and functional deficits due to the original lesion and its treatment become of increasing concern. Finally, there are degenerative neurologic conditions (e.g., the leukodystrophies) with a very indolent course resulting in prolonged periods of stability with functional disabilities.

Examination

The thrust of the examination is to determine the degree to which the spasticity is affecting the individuals function, and to predict what the child's functional abilities will be after the spasticity is eliminated. The examiner must first question *what is disabling or preventing the child from developing normal limb function.* Poor limb function can result from orthopedic deformities such as torsion deformities or contractures, poor patterns of coordination and control of joint musculature, or abnormal tone in the muscles (either hyper- or hypotonia) (Bleck 1987b). Hypertonicity can be due not only to spasticity but also to rigidity, or tension athetosis (a hypertonicity usually involving the entire body and typified by an examiner being able to 'shake it out' by rapidly shaking or moving a limb) (Bleck 1987a). Resistance to movement in a limb can be due to hypertonia within the muscles, contracture of muscles or to a joint subluxation/dislocation.

Next, the examiner must consider *if the child is deriving any functional benefit from the spasticity* and, if so, will postoperative physiotherapy offset the loss in function which will occur with the diminution in spasticity (Abbott et al. 1990). Some individuals require the spasticity in their extensor muscle groups in order to bear weight and assist in transfer maneuvers or walk (Elk 1980). This may be increasingly significant as an individual ages. Thus one must attempt to evaluate the individual's underlying strength isolated from the spasticity. Since spasticity is an increase in tone resulting from a muscle stretch, one effective means to evaluate strength isolated from spasticity is to ask the individual to grade through a strength maneuver such as rising from a squat to standing position and then to go back down (Elk et al. 1985). This maneuver requires the leg's postural musculature to change its mode of contraction from a concentric one (muscle shortening contributing to movement of a limb) to an eccentric one (a controlled muscle lengthening which resists or breaks the limb's movement). It also is a clinical evaluation of the muscle length-tension ratio throughout the limb's excursion. Spastic children often can only control mid ranges of limb excursion (Bobath and Bobath 1982), thus it has observed that they frequently cannot grade through their full available range when moving from a squat to a standing position. Also, difficulties may be observed in the smoothness of this maneuver in the spastic population which could imply poor control of musculature during its changing from a concentric to eccentric mode of contraction. In children whose postural muscles are weak, the upper extremities are used to assist in moving from the squat to stand position or the child may thrust back into the examiner in order to accomplish the maneuver. We suggest that the child repat the maneuver several (e.g., seven) times to access the endurance of the postural muscles.

Having decided that the child's functional disabilities are due to the spasticity and that any loss in function in the perioperative period will be recovered with physiotherapy, the next question becomes *which procedure will best address the functional disabilities.* The goal of treatment is to improve function, not to "cure" the spasticity. There are cases when it is desirable to preserve spasticity in a muscle group (e.g., quadriceps spasticity in an individual with inadequate underlying strength to weight bear without it). In these cases selected tennotomies, nerve blocks or selective neurectomy may be preferred. In cases characterized by more diffuse spasticity, a more central lesion (e.g., rhizotomy, drezotomy) disrupting the afferent limbs of the reflex arcs causing this spread in activity may be more effective in globally reducing the spasticity.

The *assessment of tone* is difficult owing to its dynamic nature which reflects the multitude of its modulators (Ashby et al. 1974, Dimitrijević and Nathan 1967, Dimitrijević 1985, Lundberg 1964, 1969) and can be very difficult to "standardize". One approach is attempting to isolate the limb being tested by asking the individual to lay quietly, with its head looking straight up and arms resting adducted at their side (Bleck 1987a). The type of hypertonicity present is defined by rigidly adhering to the descriptive definitions for its various types. Spasticity is a velocity

Table 2. NYUMC muscle tone scale

−1	*Hypotonic* muscle floppy with less than normal tone
0	*Normal* muscle offers normal resistance to passive movement
1	*Mildly increased* muscle offers minimal resistance to passive movement but there is not impairment of active limb function
2	*Moderately increased* muscle offers moderate resistance to passive movement but examiner can move through muscle's full range. Active function is impaired by the hypertonicity
3	*Severely increased* muscle offers severe resistance to passive movement. Function is severely impaired

dependent resistance to stretching which increases as the velocity of stretching increases while rigidity gives way with repeated stretching of the involved muscle. Hypertonicity due to tension athetosis can be diminished by shaking the limb (Dimitrijević 1985, Bleck 1987a). The examination should first evaluate the degree of range loss in a muscle due to contracture by slowly stretching the muscle through its range (Baird and Gordon 1983). The maneuver is then repeated with velocity to evaluate for spasticity (Baird and Gorden 1983). Tone is graded on a 5 point scale (Table 2).

Contracture is evaluated as the number of degrees missing on goniometric examination (Stubero et al. 1988). Muscle groups tested include the hip flexors (using the Thomas test position), hip adductors, the knee flexors (tested with the hips flexed to 90° the knee is extended to measure the popliteal angle) and ankle plantar flexors (tested with the subtalar joint held in neutral).

Reflex testing, both deep tendon and postural, should be carried out in these children to better understand to what degree cocontraction and dysequilbrium are affecting function (Elk 1980). When performing deep tendon reflexes, one should note the pattern of muscle contraction elicited. Frequently, one will see not only activation of muscles within the myotome of the reflex arch being tested but also contraction of antagonist muscles and muscles in other limbs. Not infrequently, in the more severely affected children, one will see activation of a "startle reflex" with percussion of a tendon. This may mimic patterns of muscle contraction which occur in these children in response to environmental events with subsequent impairment of limb function.

Protective reactions are also tested, as they are

essential to maintain the upright position (Fiorentins 1973). If the individual is unable to reach out with the arms or legs to prevent a fall then the individual will not have the postural ability to maintain and protect him-/herself in the higher level positions of the motor developmental sequence (i.e., standing and walking). Often these individuals are very fearful of movement and prefer staying close to the ground. Protective abilities are an important consideration when evaluating a child for surgery and setting his/her postoperative goals.

When considering function, the evaluation must focus on *how well the child can get into and function in the seated and standing positions*. For any motor developmental position where the trunk is vertical, trunkal stability is of primary import. Evaluation of trunk control is necessary to predict function in unsupported positions such as sitting, half kneeling and standing (Bobath and Bobath 1982). Next the examiner determines how successful the child is in getting into and maintaining several functionally important seated positions (the long sit, short sit and side sit positions). The long sit position (sitting flat on the floor with the legs extended in front), while not especially functional, helps in determining to what degree hamstring tone is affecting the alignment of the pelvis and knees. The short sit position (the position one assumes in a chair) is probably the most important functional position for these children. This position also reveals the quality of trunkal control since it must be maintained with a relatively small base of support and the stability of the pelvis is not being assisted by the hamstring muscles. The side sit position (sitting with one's weight centered over one of the hips) is the position of function which should be encouraged when these children are on the floor. It can also be used to evaluate the child's ability to maintain control in a asymmetrical position. With regard to standing, one needs to assess the child's abilities in getting into that position as well as how well he/she functions in it (Bobath and Bobath 1982). Consequently, the transitional position of half kneeling is evaluated. The half kneeling position also gives an indication of the child's ability to dissociate his/her lower extremities, as required for reciprocal activities such as quadraped crawling and walking. Lastly, each of the positions is examined qualitatively and a grade is given reflecting how cosmetic or appropriately aligned the major joints are. This assesses the functional balance of body muscle activity around the joint.

Treatment goals

Having defined the child's functional abilities and disabilities, the examiner is now in a position to set forth the goals of the surgery as well as the anticipated needs of therapy post-operatively. It is important that these impressions be shared with the child and his/her family on several occasions prior to surgery as there are frequently hidden and falsely elevated expectations of the intended surgery.

At NYUMC we have defined five patient groups with regard to preoperative abilities/disabilities and to the functional goals of postoperative physical therapy (see Table 3). Overall goals for all groups are to increase strength and passive range of motion in the lower extremities.

Group I consists of individuals who use walking as their prime mode of locomotion and who do not require canes, crutches or walkers for assistance. The typical treatment goal is to improve the appearance and efficiency of their walking. Of prime importance in this group is the assessment of standing protective reactions, trunk control and hip stability while standing and walking. Essential to the examination is to determine whether the child's spasticity is important in the performance of standing and walking (Elk 1980). Typically these "independent" ambulators have adequate underlying strength and can easily repeat the squat to stand test 5–7 times. This group of children can perform the maneuver in a slow, controlled manner demostrating good control through the entire range of movement. Trunkal stability is assessed as are protective reactions. Ataxia will severely impair postoperative gains in this group. Protective reactions have been discussed earlier and their importance cannot be overly stressed in predicting postoperative gains. Typically this group will have only mildly compromised protective reactions.

Group II individuals are functional ambulators who require canes, crutches or walkers to assist in their

Table 3. Patient groups

Group 1	Independent ambulators
Group 2	Ambulators dependent on assistive devices (canes, crutches, walkers)
Group 3	Quadraped crawlers (either reciprocal or nonreciprocal; i.e., bunny hoppers)
Group 4	Commando or belly crawlers
Group 5	Totally dependent, no locomotive abilities

walking. The treatment goal for this group is to improve the quality of ambulation and, if appropriate, to decrease the amount of assistance required to ambulate. It is vital to acertain why these children require the assistive devices to ambulate. Children who use the assistive device to offset severe leg weakness may be deriving a functional benefit from spasticity in the antigravity muscles of the leg, particularly the quadriceps. A global reduction of tone in a weak child may cause the loss of functional ambulation. Careful evaluation of the squat to stand test is critical in the population. A weak child will often use the arms to pull up or may extend his or her back into the examiner in order to stand. Eccentric control (control over graded relaxation of a muscle) will be lacking, especially at the end ranges of movement. Also, concentric control, when the muscle is at its full length, will be poor or even absent. Other tests which give an indication of lower extremity strength are the transitional ability from 1/2 kneeling to standing and standing on a single leg.

While strength is a major factor to consider in assessing children in group II, trunkal control, protective reactions and the influence of spasticity on movement patterns must be examined. Poor trunk control or trunkal ataxia may cause dependence on an assistive device. Individuals in group II who have weakness or imbalance of the trunk and hip musculature would probably not be well served by a procedure which would decrease muscle tone being used functionally to splint a joint. This is especially the case if leg weakness is present. Children who are strong but rely on the assistive device due to impaired protective reactions will most likely remain dependent on the assistive device after a procedure which decreases the leg tone. The child with good strength and trunk control and who possesses good protective reactions is the optimal candidate for treatment in this group. If the child's leg tone can be normalized, he or she will often require less assistance in ambulation.

The children in Group III do not use walking as their prime mode of locomotion. Although they frequently can stand with an assistive device and take a few steps, *they reciprocally crawl, bunny hop or use a wheelchair to get about.* The goal for this group is to improve their ability to move through the motor developmental sequence which culminates in ambulation with an assistive device. Children of this group who are strong, have protective reactions in the sitting position, and have good trunk control but who are functionally limited by spasticity in the hip adductors, hamstrings and gastrocnemius muscles are greatly benefited by procedures which normalize the muscle tone. This is because the spasticity present in these muscles is disturbing the standing posture and precluding the development of ambulation. With normalization in muscle tone these children will often be able to ambulate with a rollator walker and can sometimes progress to using crutches or other less assistive devices. The key to this progression is the presence of protective reactions in the standing position. Children in this group who are weak or have poor trunk control may require higher bracing after surgery until strength and/or control develops.

A critical issue in the children in group III is the degree of range limitation. While range limitations are important considerations in all of the groups, range limitation appears to play a larger role in the loss of functional abilities in the group III children. We have found that in children under the age of six, range limitations can be stretched out with an aggressive stretching program. Ranging must be continued daily once full range has been achieved to avoid the recurrence of limitation in range which can occur with growth or illness. When children are older (> than 7 or 8 years) it becomes more difficult to stretch out the muscle to achieve its full function range. A older child with severe range limitation is usually better served by a tendon lengthening than a tone reducing procedure. We are on occasion called upon to perform rhizotomies in older children when, in the opinion of the orthopedist, a tendon lengthening procedure would rapidly be defeated due to underlying spasticity in the muscle whose tendon is to be lengthened.

Group IV is composed of individuals who are wheelchair bound and whose only mode of locomotion is commando crawling. Strength and protective reactions in this group of children are most often so compromised that functional ambulation is not a feasible goal. The initial goal in this group is to ease their care taking. Long range goals include better function in the sitting position. Key points in the evaluation of this patient group are the degree of head and trunk control, protective reactions and primitive reflexes present. Children with severe impairment in head and trunk control, in protective reactions and with strong primitive reflexes (e.g., asymmetric tonic neck reflexes or hyperstartle reactions) will have limited functional gains after procedures which decrease muscle tone.

The last group of children (group V) are unable to locomote. Very often these children have severely compromised cognition. Protective reactions as well as head righting are so impaired that functional gains will be minimal at best. The goal for this group is to improve the caretaker's ability to handle the child during the daily activities and to improve his or her ability to position the child in adaptive equipment. Of primary import in the evaluation of these children is the determination of the major cause of the handling and positioning difficulties for the child for they can be due not only to hypertonicity but also to the child's weight or to orthopedic deformities.

Conclusion

There will be an increasing demand for the evaluation and treatment of children who have a residual functional disability as our skills in treating the diseases of the nervous system increase. Only by clearly defining the clinical symptoms causing the disability and quantifying the disability can we hope to understand each individual patient and to further the treatment of his or her functional disabilities.

References

Abbott R, Forem S, Johann M (1990) Selective posterior rhizotomy for the treatment of spasticity, a review. Childs Nerv Syst S: 337–346

Ashby P, Verrier M, Lightfoot E (1974) Segmental reflex pathways in spinal shock and spinal spasticity in man. J Neurol Neurosurg Psychiatry 37: 1352–1360

Baird HW, Gordon EC (1983) Neurological evaluation of infants and children. JB Lippincott, Philadelphia, pp 60–63

Bleck EE (1987a) Orthopaedic management in cerebral palsy. JB Lippincott, Philadelphia, pp 1–65

Bleck EE (1987b) Orthopaedic management in cerebral palsy. JB Lippincott, Philadelphia, pp 121–142

Bobath B, Bobath K (1982) Motor development in the different types of cerebral palsy. W Heinemann, London, pp 1–100

Dimitrijevic MR, Nathan PW (1967) Studies of spasticity in man. 1. Some features of spasticity. Brain 90: 1–31

Dimitrijevic MR (1985) Spasticity. In: Swash M, Kennard C (eds) Scientific basis of clinical neurology. Churchill Livingstone, Edinburgh, pp 108–115

Duncan CC, Ment LR, Ogle E (1989) Acquired problems of the newborn. In: McLaurin RL, Venes JL, Shut L, Epstein F (eds) Pediatric neurosurgery. Saunders, Philadelphia, pp 230–238

Elk B (1980) Preoperative assessment and postoperative surgical occupational therapy for children who have undergone a selective posterior rhizotomy. South African J Occ Ther 14: 49–50

Elk B, Morgan N, Peacock WJ (1985) The importance of teamwork in the treatment of spastic cerebral palsied children undergoing selective posterior rhizotomy. South African Cereb Palsy J: 9–12

Fiorentino MR (1973) Reflex testing methods for evaluating cns development. CC Thomas, Springfield, pp 5–49

Ingram TTS (1984) A historical view of the definition and classification of the cerebral palsies. In: Stanley F, Alberman E (eds) The epidemiology of the cerebral palsies. JB Lippincott, Philadelphia, pp 1–12

Lundberg A (1964) Supraspinal control of transmission in reflex paths to motoneurons and primary afferents. In: Eccles JC, Schade JP (eds) Physiology of spinal neurons. Elsevier, Amsterdam, pp 197–221

Lundberg A (1969) Convergence of excitatory and inhibitory action on interneurons in the spinal cord. In: Brazier MAB (ed) The interneuron. Univ Calif Press, Los Angles, pp 231–265

Siegfried J, Lazorthes Y (1985) L2 neurochirurgie fonctionnelle de l'infirmité motrice d'origine cérébrale. Neurochirurgion 31 [Suppl 1]: 1–118

Stanley F (1984a) Prenatal risk factors in the study of the cerebral palsies. In: Stanley F, Alderman E (eds) The epidemiology of the cerebral palsies. JB Lippincott, Philadelphia, pp 87–97

Stanley F (1984b) Perinatal risk factors in the cerebral palsies. In: Stanley F, Alderman E (eds) The epidemiology of the cerebral palsies. JB Lippincott, Philadelphia, pp 98–115

Stanley F, Alberman E (1984) Birthweight, gestational age and the cerebral plasies. In: Stanley F, Alberman E (eds) The epidemiology of the cerebral palsies. JB Lippincott, Philadelphia, pp 57–69

Stanley F, Blair E (1984) Postnatal risk factors in the cerebral palsies. In: Stanley F, Alberman E (eds) The epidemiology of the cerebral palsies. JB Lippincott, Philadelphia, pp 135–149

Storrs BB, McLone DG (1989) Selective posterior rhizotomy in the treatment of spasticity associated with myelomengocele. In: Marlin A (ed) Current concepts in pediatric neurosurgery, vol 9. Karger, Basel, pp 173–177

Stuberg WA, Fuchs RH, Miedaner JA (1988) Reliability of goniometric measurements of children with cerebral palsy. Dev Med Child Neurol 30: 657–666

Wigglesworth J (1984) Brain development and its modification by adverse influences. In: Stanley F, Alderman E (eds) The epidemiology of the cerebral palsies. JB Lippincott, Philadelphia, pp 12–26

Correspondence: Prof. R. Abbott, M.D., Division of Pediatric Neurosurgery, New York University Medical Center, 550 First Avenue, New York, NY 10016, U.S.A.

Nonsurgical treatment of spasticity

Medical treatment of spasticity

D. Boisson[1] and **M. Eyssette**[2]

[1]Hôpital Neurologique, Lyon, and [2]Hôpital Henry Gabrielle, Saint Genis Laval, France

Introduction

According to the *definition* by Lance, spasticity is: "a motor disorder characterized by a velocity-dependent increase of tonic stretch reflexes with exaggerated tendon jerks, resulting from hyperexcitability of the stretch reflex, as one component of the upper motor neuron syndrome". Spasticity is obviously a heterogenous set of clinical states. As a matter of fact the release of the proprioceptive reflex can be the consequence of a lesion of the corticofugal pathways at any level of Central Nervous System (C.N.S).

Although unanimously accepted since 1981, this definition – both clinical and physiopathological – does not take into account the time elapsed since the onset of the injury, the extent of the lesion and the nature of CNS reaction. Spasticity is only one component of the upper motor syndrome and it may contribute only in a limited way to the total handicap. In some cases it is even more properly viewed as a beneficial side effect. Besides paresis, a wide variety of problems can be associated with spasticity and interfere with treatment decisions: flexor spasms in the spinal patient, dystonic posturing and synkinetic movements in the hemiplegic... For all these reasons, *treatment is often difficult.*

Spasticity can be useful as a sort of endogenous crutch; but it also can impede residal voluntary movements, participating in making the patient functionally disabled. Therefore its *treatment may be essential,* the more so since the negative features of the upper motor neuron syndrome: weakness and loss of dexterity are not accessible to any pharmacological treatment.

General principles

Whatever the drug used, (except for one, Dantrolene), the treatment induces, in various ways, a decrease of the excitability of spinal reflexes. Therefore, most of the studies (H reflex measurements) about antispastic drugs emphasize *the pharmacological effects of antispastic drugs on the spinal neurons and the segmental reflexes.* Among such tests, the H max/M max ratio is stable and sensitive; but it is a global measure. The vibratory inhibition of H reflex, thought to reflect presynaptic inhibition, is reproducible in a single subject. It is lessened in spasticity and reinforced by benzodiazepines but not by all musclerelaxants (Delwaide and Dresse 1984). The basic principle in applying these tests is to first study the electrophysiological modifications due to the neurological disease. Then, it becomes possible to explore the respective actions of the different drugs using these tests, and to select the most effective one.

Recent developments in techniques have led to spectacular *advances in the knowledge of distribution of neurotransmitters in the spinal cord.* (Betz 1987, Davidoff 1985, Delwaide and Dresse 1984, Hughes and Phil 1989, Katz 1988, Young and Delwaide 1981). Glycine and gamma-aminobutyric acid (GABA) are the major inhibitory transmitters in the spinal cord. (Figs. 1 and 2). Pharmacological properties of *Glycine,* the transmitter of the Renshaw system and of some reciprocal inhibitory interneurons, are selectively antagonized by strychnine. They have up till now been poorly investigated. Conversely, the knowledge above *GABA* receptors has progressed quickly over the last few years, due to the numerous studies about anti-

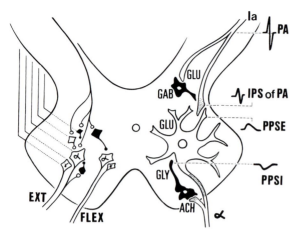

Fig. 1. Spinal organization of monosynaptic and oligosynaptic reflex pathways. *PA* action potential; *IPS* presynaptic inhibition potential; *PPSE* post-synaptic excitatory potential; *PPSI* post-synaptic inhibitory potential

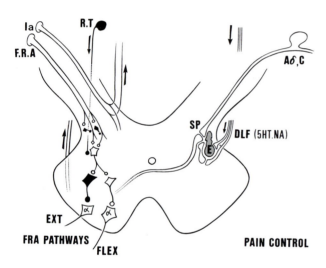

Fig. 2. Spinal organization of polysynaptic reflex pathways and pain control. *RT* reticulospinal tract; *DLF* dorsolateral funiculus; *FRA* flexor reflex afferents

spastic drugs. GABA receptors are complex supra-molecular structure of at least two major types. 1) GABA A receptors are blocked by bicuculline, their specific antagonist. Their activation leads to a net efflux of chloride ion that produces a depolarization of Ia afferents. This seems to be the causal event in presynaptic inhibition. 2) GABA B receptors are not affected by bicuculline, and are present on the same terminals of primary afferents in the spinal cord. Their activation leads to a blockage of calcium influx. Also to be considered is the possibility of central

actions so these too must be assessed in clinical practice.

Neurophysiological exploration is essential during the development phase of a new drug. In complementary animal studies, it can specify the mode of action at the spinal level. Then, for each new drug, clinical investigations are essential (Corston et al. 1981). Neurophysiological explorations are widely carried out to elucidate and specify each indication, and to study evolution with treatment. But any drug has potential side-effects, sometimes serious ones. Obviously long term use, at the lowest dosage, must be correlated to a real beneficial effect, and this has to be regularly checked.

The main antispasticity agents

Dantrolene

Dantrolene is unique among antispasticity agents: its therapeutic effect is peripheral, directly on contractile mechanisms within muscle. It has no action on reflex pathways. It inhibits the release of calcium ions from the sarcoplasmic reticulum. In doing this it prevents activation of the contractile apparatus and reduces the mechanical force produced by the contracting muscle (Pinder et al. 1977, van Winkle 1976, Joynt 1976). The blockage of calcium release is never complete and contraction is never abolished. "Fast units", able to produce rapid increase in tension, are the most affected. Although the effect of Dantrolene upon muscle spindle has already been described, its contribution to decreasing spasticity action is not known. Inspite of some side effects such as drowsiness and dizziness, no central antispastic effect has been proved (Meyler et al. 1981).

Initially, the dosage must be the low (one 25 mg tablet a day) then very gradually increased. The half life is 8–10 hours. The risk of a muscular weakness must be pointed out to the patient, and maximum doses (300 to 400 mg) must be avoided. The hepatotoxic effect is classic (1%) (Wilkinson et al. 1979), and has perhaps been overstated. It is increased by high doses and with additional other drugs. Liver function should be tested before starting treatment and periodically during therapy. Its use should be discontinued if benefits are not obviously confirmed by the patient.

Dantrolene is sometimes particularly useful in patients in whom there is no voluntary power left and spasticity predominates.

Medical treatment of spasticity

Benzodiazepines

Benzodiazepines can be used alone or as adjuvant therapy for all forms of spasticity. They have no direct GABA-mimetic effect, though they heighten the affinity of the binding of GABA, to GABA A receptors, on CNS membranes (Costa and Guidotti 1979). Their effectiveness at the spinal level is demonstrated in patients with total spinal cord trans-section. An amplification of presynaptic inhibition in GABA mediated inhibitory pathways where physiological release is already occuring, seems to be the most prominent and specific effect (Lossius et al. 1980, Delwaide 1985). Obviously Benzodiazepines are effective at many other levels and produce tranquillizing, sedative and anticonvulsant effects which can reduce their utility in brain injured patients. If the dosage is right and progressively reached, the tranquillizing properties are sometimes helpful and the side-effects are minimized.

The benzodiazepines are slowly metabolized and their half-lifes vary from about 15 hours for Tetrazepam (Myolastan *) to about 32 hours for Diazepam (Valium *) and to about 65 hours for Prazepam (Lysanxia *). Synergistic depression of the CNS, when other drugs or alcohol are consumed, must be avoided. Withdrawal of the treatment must be carefully and done gradually.

Baclofen

Baclofen, an analogue of GABA-para-chlorophenyl gamma-amino butyric acid, is not antagonized by bicuculline and is not strongly bound to classis GABA "A" receptors. Its (−) isomer is specifically bound to the recently discovered GABA "B" receptors, present on brain and spinal synaptic membranes. As with Benzodiazepine, Baclofen acts at the spinal level on the terminals of primary afferents. (Curtis et al. 1981, Duncan et al. 1976, Hassan and McLellan 1980, Lance 1980). When in the therapeutic range, the presynaptic effects of Baclofen prevail and suppress release of excitatory transmitters for both mono-synaptic and polysynaptic pathways. Baclofen is particularly effective against flexor spasms. It is often considered the drug of choice in spinal forms of spasticity. With higher concentration, post-synaptic effects are seen and Baclofen becomes a widespread neuronal depressant, but less sedative than diazepam. An analgesic effect of (−) Baclofen, with decrease of

response to noxious stimuli, has been demonstrated in experimental animals. Baclofen occasionally provides analgesia in some spastic patients. The hypothesis of a direct and specific interaction of Baclofen with substance P receptors has been explored (Wilson and Yaksh 1978) and the evidence for this is not persuasive.

Baclofen's half-life is around 8 hours. It must always be slowly introduced and 80 mg to 100 mg a day is usually therapeutic. Higher doses may be tolerated and are sometimes effective. The central side-effects, essentially hallucinations, confusion and drowsiness are not frequent. Combined drug therapy is possible, with care. Sudden withdrawal of the drug must be avoided.

Tizanidine

Tizanidine is an imidazoline derivative, closely related to Clonidine. It was initially believed to facilitate the action of glycine but this has not been confirmed. In fact, this potent agonistic action upon central alpha-2-adrenergic receptors prevents the release of excitatory aminoacids (L glutamate, Aspartate) from spinal interneurons (Davies and Quinlan 1985). More recently an action upon the alpha-2-adrenergic neurons of the Locus Coeruleus, which probably modulates the tonic reflex activity, has been stressed. Although Tizanidine now has been used for more than 10 years, with confirmed efficacy, it is not universally available. Clinical results and electrophysiologic studies have shown selective effects upon polysynaptic pathways with inhibition of their response to nociceptive stimuli. This central effect of depressing the reticulo-spinal excitatory pathways is probably also linked to the analgesic action of Tizanidine. (Nabeshima et al. 1987). Therapy begins very gently with a 4 mg tablet the first day, and gradually increasing up to a maximum of 24 mg a day, given in divided doses.

Tizanidine is usually well tolerated with only moderate side-effects despite some decrease of the diastolic pressure. Drowsiness is less common than with other central antispastic drugs and there is no decrease in the remaining muscular strength (Knutsson et al. 1982). Tizanidine seems particularly useful in spasticity associated with multiple sclerosis, where it can be used in association with other antispastic drugs.

Conclusions

Medical treatment of spasticity is not always easy.
Spastic patients present with polymorphic clinical
conditions and the spasticity can be widely variable
in the same patient. It seems clear. that medical
treatment cannot be completely satisfactory in spite
of the expansion in pharmacological research, while
many medications are able to effectively reduce reflex
activity, their action must be carefully questioned,
especially in patients who are struggling to regain
locomotion. All the drugs have potentially genuine
side-effects which restrict their long term administration.

A *combination of antispasticity drugs* is sometimes
beneficial for the patient's comfort, provided, they act
distinctly. In the near future, *new drugs will probably
appear* based on a better knowledge of pharmacological neurotransmitters, and the pathophysiology of
upper motor neurone control.

In all cases, *the medical treatment is only a part of
the management of spasticity and handicap.* It is never
a definitive one and must be carefully re-evaluated
regularly, in terms of the functional result achieved.

References

Betz H (1987) Biology and structure of the mamalian glycine
receptor. TINS 10: 113–117

Costa E, Guidotti A (1979) Molecular mechanisms in the receptor
action of benzodiazepines. Annu Rev Pharmacol Toxicol 19:
531–545

Curtis DR, Lodge D, Borstein JC, Peet MJ (1981) Selective effect
of (−) Baclofen on spinal synaptic transmission in the cat. Exp
Brain Res 42: 158–170

Corston RN, Johnson F, Godwin-Austen RB (1981) The assessment
of drug treatment of spastic gait. J Neurol Neurosurg Psychiatry
44: 1035–1039

Davidoff A (1985) Antispasticity drugs: mechanisms of action. Ann
Neurol 17: 107–116

Davies J, Quinlan JE (1985) Selective inhibition of responses of
feline dorsal horn neurones to noxious cutaneous stimuli by
Tizanidine (DS103-282) and Noradrenaline: involvement of alpha
2-adrenoceptors. Neuroscience 16(3): 673–682

Delwaide JP, Dresse A (1984) Les myorelaxants. Sem Hop Paris
60(40): 2897–2929

Delwaide JP (1985) Electrophysiological analysis of the mode of
action of muscle relaxants in spasticity. Ann Neurol 17: 90–5

Duncan GW, Shahani BT, Young RR (1976) An evaluation of
baclofen treatment for certain symptoms in patients with spinal
cord lesions: a double-blind cross-over study. Neurology 26:
441–6

Eyssette M, Rohmer F, Serratrice G, Warter JM, Boisson D (1988)
Multi-centrer, double-blind trial of a novel antispastic agent,
Tizanidine, in spasticity associated with multiple sclerosis. Curr
Med Res Opin 10(10)

Gonsette RE, Desmet Y, Demonty L (1984) Tizanidine, a new
antispastic agent: 6 years clinical experience in 152 MS sclerosis.
MTD Press Ltd, Lancaster Boston The Hauge Dordrecht,
pp 219–225

Hassan N, McLellan DL (1980) Double-blind comparison of single
doses of DS-103-282, Baclofen and placebo for suppression of
spasticity. J Neurol Neurosurg Psychiatry 43: 1132–6

Hughes JT, Phil D (1989) The new neuro-anatomy of the spinal
cord. Paraplegia 27: 90–98

Joynt RL (1976) Dantrolene sodium: long-term effects in patients
with muscle spasticity. Arch Phys Med Rehabil 57: 212–217

Katz RT (1988) Management of spasticity. Am J Phys Med Rehabil
67(3)

Knutsson E, Martensson A, Gransberg L (1982) Antiparetic and
antispastic effects induced by Tizanidine in patients with spastic
paresis. J Neurol Sci 53: 187–204

Lance JW (1980) Pathophysiology of spasticity and clinical
experience with Baclofen. In: Feldman RG, Young RR, Koella
WP (eds) Spasticity: disordered motor control. Year book,
Chicago, pp 185–203

Lossius R, Dietrichson P, Lunde PKM (1980) Effect of Diazepam
and desmethyldiazepan in spasticity and rigidity. A quantitative
study of reflexes and plasma concentrations. Acta Neurol Scand
61: 378–388

Meyler WJ, Bakker H, Kok JJ, Agoston S, Wesseling H (1981) The
effect of Dantrolene sodium in relation to blood levels in spastic
patients after prolonged administration. J Neurol Neurosurg
Psychiatry 44: 334–339

Nabeshima T, Matsuno K, Sugimoto A, Kameyama T (1987)
Antinociceptive activity induced by Tizanidine and Alpha-2
adrenoreceptors. Neuropharmacology 26: 1453–1455

Newman PM, Nogues M, Newman PK, Weightman D, Hudgson
P (1982) Tizanidine in the treatment of spasticity. Eur J Clin
Pharmacol 23: 31–35

Pinder RM, Brogden RN, Speight TM, Avery GS (1977) Dantrolene
sodium: a review of its pharmacological properties and
therapeutic efficacy in spasticity. Drugs 13: 3–23

van Winkle WB (1976) Calcium release from skeletal muscle
sarcoplasmic reticulum: site of action of dantrolene sodium?
Science 193: 1130–1131

Wilkinson SP, Portman B, Williams R (1979) Hepatitis from
dantrolene sodium. Gut 20: 33–36

Wilson PR, Yaksh TL (1978) Baclofen is antinociceptive in the
spinal intrathecal space of animals. Eur J Pharmacol 51: 323–330

Young RR, Delwaide PJ (1981) Drug therapy in spasticity. N Engl
J Med 304: 28–33, 96–99

Correspondence: Prof. D. Boisson, Hôpital Neurologique, 59 boulevard Pinel, F-69003 Lyon, France

Physical treatments of spasticity and chemical blocks

J.F. Mathé and **I. Richard**

Service de Rééducation Fonctionnelle, Hôpital Saint-Jacques, Nantes, France

Introduction

The lesions responsible for spasticity may be of various *importance*, *location* and *etiology*, leading to a number of different "spastic syndromes".

Considering the *importance* of the lesion, one may simply distinguish complete lesions, allowing only involuntary reflex motor expression, from incomplete lesions. In complete lesions, three "positive" clinical features characterize the motor disorder (Burke 1988): abnormal dystonic posture in a flexion or extension pattern, abnormal exaggeration of proprioceptive reflexes, and abnormal reflexes elicited by exteroceptive or even interoceptive stimuli, especially flexion or extension limb spasms. In incomplete lesions, voluntary motor control persists or reappears, but its expression is modified in a context dominated by the resistance of antagonists and the occurrence of cocontractions.

Depending on the lesion *location*, the spatial distribution of spasticity is different; it involves mainly upper limb flexors and lower limb extensors in hemiplegia, lower limb flexors and extensors in paraplegia, urethral striated sphincter – a particular but indeed important muscle – in spinal cord lesions, and all four limbs in some sequelae of head injury.

Beside lesion location, the *etiology* of the disease also plays a role in the clinical presentation and also the modalities of care, as, for example, in multiple sclerosis.

Clinical examination should not only focus on the diagnosis of spasticity, but also evaluate its disabling and harmful consequences, especially when only a few muscles are involved.

At this point, one has to consider the role of physical therapy in the treatment of spasticity. Whatever the internal mechanisms of spasticity may be, physical therapy may exercise influence in its clinical manifestation in a specific way. On the other hand everyday clinical experience shows that spasticity is influenced by peripheral or physical forces. Environmental conditions, such as cold or warmth, particular physiological situations, sometimes even psychological situations may interfere with spasticity. Spasticity is thus a dual phenomenon, with an endogenous component, concerning information processing, and an exogenous one, depending on the quantity and quality of the information input. This latter component may be especially modified by the physical therapy in order to prevent or control spasticity.

Prevention

During the acute period (Katz 1988) the first rule is to preserve perfect physiological homeostasis and satisfactory trophic conditions, even if the main concern at this time is treatment of the cause. The first days, if not the first hours, are crucial in the outcome of a hemiplegic, or even more a paraplegic patient.

Different techniques, simple although often fastidious, will prevent *cutaneous lesions*. Paraplegic patients must be turned every three hours, day and night. Gentle massage of pressure points are performed at the same time. Personal hygiene (including nails) should be perfect. The bed and later the clothes and shoes should be regularly checked, since they may threaten anaesthetic skin. Later, self-care is the only chance of success. Choosing the right wheelchair and the right cushion, instruction in regular self-raising from the wheelchair to relieve pressure zones are not mere details (Mathé 1989).

Blood circulation, particularly in the lower limbs, requires specific attention. Circulatory massage, regular mobilisation, and, above all, preventive medication of venous thrombosis are necessary.

Muscular retraction and articular ankylosis may be prevented by gentle mobilisation of all limb segments several times a day. Posturing must be performed as well for several reasons. The muscles rapidly loose sarcomeres, when left in a shorten position, especially if contracted with spasms in neglected patients (Tardieu et al. 1973). These therapeutic measures are useful in avoiding heterotopic ossification and algodystrophy particularly in the hemiplegic shoulder.

Intestinal passage should be rapidly stimulated by enteral feeding and an appropriate diet (for example addition of wheatbread and olive oil). Abdominal massage and daily anal stimulation ensure progression of fecaes and the defecation reflex.

Balanced bladder and renal function require special attention. The aim is to keep urine sterile and prevent lithiasis. This will be achieved if micturition is complete and the daily amount of urine passed is above two liters. If micturition cannot be obtained, sterile intermittent catheterisation, followed by clean intermittent catheterisation and clean self-catheterisation (Labat et al. 1985) are the techniques of choice that have few side-effects if performed six times a day.

Finally *standing*, performed as soon as possible either on a rotative bed or a stand-up device, is very helpful in preventing lower limb spasms in paraplegics.

Everyone knows how important these measures are and how complications may play a major role in the occurence or persistence of spasticity.

Motor schemes

In hemiplegia, extension of the lower limb and flexion of the arm, hand and fingers usually appear sooner or later. Bobath (1981) relying on the hypothesis of reciprocal innervation disturbance, first considered using inhibiting postures in the early stages in the evolution of spasticity inhibition postures (Fig. 1a). According to the principle that "proprioceptive systems determine motor output, i.e. responses originating from the central nervous system", she proposed specific postures which should be accomplished several times a day: 1) arm, wrist and fingers extension; 2) flexion and moderate abduction of the thigh, flexion of the knee. Later, thigh extension with the leg hanging flexed out of bed also provides

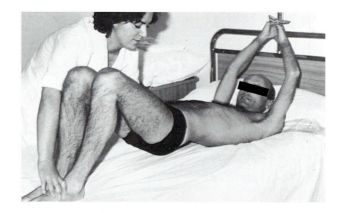

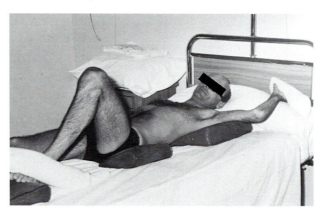

Fig. 1. a (bottom) Postures for inhibition of the spasticity in left upper and lower limbs. **b** (top) Specific training for hip control against syncinesia of the upper limb

abduction. These different postures are performed with the patient lying supine or on his side. Passive mobilisation by the physiotherapist will be included in these inhibition patterns. Hazardous mobilisation during dressing or nursing should be avoided.

Abnormal tonic reflexes, originating from cervical afferents may also be elicited. Active head rotation leads to ipsilateral upper limb flexion and contralateral upper limb extension. Finally the occurrence of associated reactions (co-contractions or syncinesis) due to uncontrolled spreading of facilitatory influences requires specific measures. The patient will for example, be asked to extend his hemiplegic arm, using his other (Fig. 1b), during active postural or balance exercises (Eggers 1988).

Spasticity and voluntary motor control

Motor control is affected in central nervous system disease. Although muscle weakness does exist, the main problem is "not the lack of force but the inability

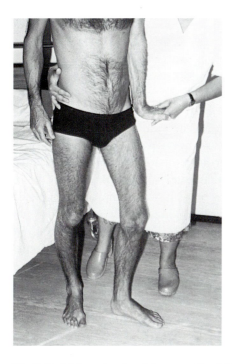

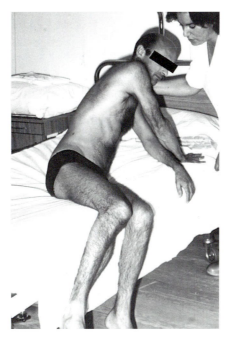

Fig. 2. (right) Learning for sitting up with a left hemiplegia. (left) Tonus control in stand up

to dispatch in several different ways, and several different kinetic combinations the motor output" (Bobath 1981). We have gradually learned that strengthening exercises are not only unsuccessful in such a complex disorder, but are also harmful, since they definitely increase spasticity and result in automatic, stereotyped motor patterns which will turn out to be useless. Similarly, any re-education program, if unduly long or intensive, will increase spasticity, even in muscle groups apparently at rest. A well known example is that of the reinforcement of upper limb spasticity during lower limb activity (Fig. 2).

Neuromotor facilitation techniques take advantage of body positions in which spasticity is minimized such as lying supine. This underlines the necessity of mat work. Motor control is developed following a proximo-distal progression. Movements will be assisted manually and performed without resistance (Fig. 3). For the lower limb, voluntary contraction is encouraged but movement should avoid the angle of threshold eliciting the stretch reflex in antagonic muscles. Further exercises are then introduced, favouring patterns opposite to spontaneous patterns such as knee flexion to counter spastic thigh extension. Concerning the upper limb, gross movements will be obtained, but only a few patients will achieve precise, fine motor movements.

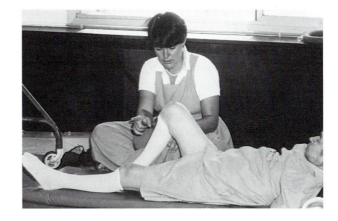

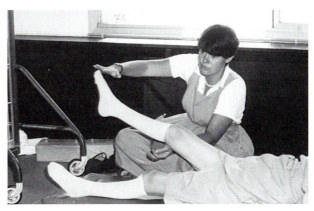

Fig. 3. Active contraction of quadriceps without any external resistance

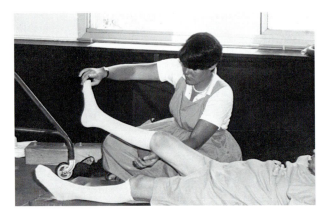

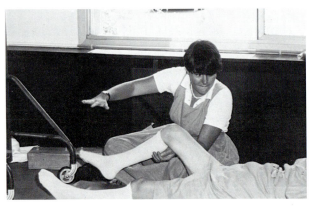

Fig. 4. Control of muscular relaxation

A sensory-motor approach has been recently proposed (Perfetti 1979). The aim is to allow progressive, voluntary motor control by inhibiting the basic motor disorders characteristic of hemiplegia (Fig. 4). Sensory information is elicited by tactile exploration. The exploration is first performed passively, then assisted and finally performed independently by the patient own, with and then without visual control. The patient therefore needs to organize this sensory information and compare it with his previous visual experience so as to identify the object or shape he has touched. Objects used are of increasing size so that distal articulations are involved before proximal ones. This type of exercise prevents stretch reflex exaggeration and later the occurrence of co-ordination syncinesia (Lion 1987).

Physical agents

Cold baths (Lion and Mathé 1985) may be very effective in reducing spasticity in multiple sclerosis. First based upon empirical statements, this technique

has physiological support (Waxman 1982) since nerve conduction may be improved by the cold. The patient's central temperature should be reduced by 1°C. The water is progressively cooled. The bath's duration depends on its effect on the patient's temperature. The benefit may last for several hours and be significant for the patient's everyday activity.

Functional electric stimulation, used to reactivate deficient muscle groups (Liberson 1961) is also effective in reducing spasticity and spasms (Bajd et al. 1985). This technique has been shown to improve hemiplegic gait during the early re-education period, but its long term effects deserve further discussion. Multiple output stimulation has both an efferent effect (agonist contraction) and an afferent effect by relaxing spastic muscles (Benezet 1988). Muscle or nerve (N. peroneus) stimulation may be used. The different stimulation parameters are adjusted for maximal effect. The onset of the stimulation is triggered either by a contact located in the heel of the sole (van Laere 1988) or manually by the patient (Brugerolle et al. 1988). In these cases the physiological rationale for the effect on spasticity remains unclear. Functional electric stimulation reduces upper limb spasticity in hemiplegia in a very indirect way by reducing during acute period, scapulo-humeral wasting (Eyssette and Boisson 1988).

Bio-feedback (Andre et al. 1986) is a re-education technique in which external, instrumental information provides insight on internal features of abnormal patterns of movement and allows learning of appropriate behaviour. This requires sensors to sample and encode relevant informations, a central processing unit, and an optic, auditive or sensory communication unit to provide quantitative and qualitative information back to the patient. In treatment of spasticity, negative biofeedback is used to encourage antagonist relaxation during agonist contraction.

Chemical blocks

Motor point infiltration has been proposed by Tardieu and Hariga (1964) and Tardieu et al. (1971, 1975) relying on the preferential activity of 45° or pure alcohol on gamma fusimotor fibers. 5% phenol solution has the same effect. This action decreases or suppresses the tonic stretch reflex without provoking paralysis (Katz 1989). The motor points that should be infiltrated are located on a reference map or determined after surface electric stimulation. 1.5 to 2 ml alcohol or 2 ml phenol are injected in the muscle

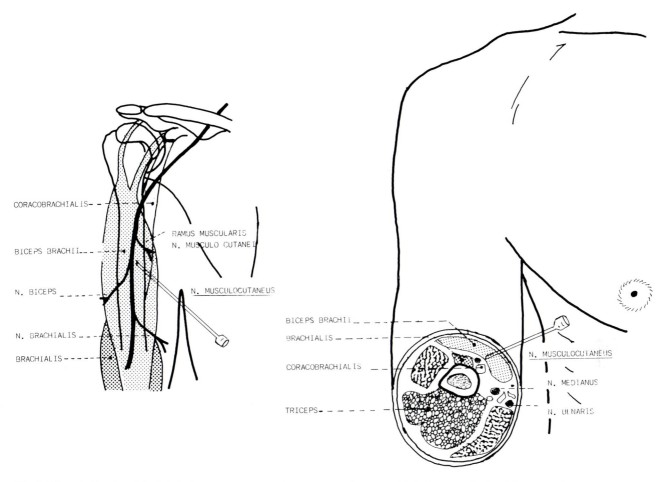

Fig. 5. Nerve infiltration (Alcohol–Xylocaïne) – N. Musculocutaneus at the upper third of the arm behind biceps muscle

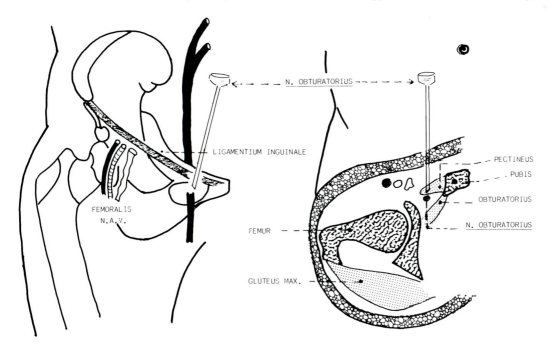

Fig. 6. Nerve infiltration (Alcohol–Xylocaïne) – N. Obturatorius in front of the unguinal ligament, 1 cm out of the pubis, perpendicularly to the skin, until 3 cm deep

at each motor point. Xylocaine may be added to reduce immediate pain. Painful reactions may appear later due to inflammation or haematoma. The limits of the method are related to the small number of muscles that can be stimultaneously infiltrated. Patients with spasticity in triceps suralis, and wrist and finger flexors, are the best candidates (Lion and Mathé 1985). Considering the limited and variable duration of the effects of the technique, we have progressively reduced its indications and now use it mainly as a test before neurological surgery.

Infiltration of a nerve or its branches causes chemical neurolysis. It has a wider action on a group of muscles, than motor point infiltration. This technique requires locating of the nerve, either by using precise anatomic data, percutaneous stimulation with a teflon sheathed electrode, or, if necessary surgical exposure of the nerve.

For the upper limb, biceps and brachialis spasticity (Fig. 5) may be treated by a percutaneous block of the N. musculo-cutaneus, the thenar muscles by block of the N. digitalis palmoris proprii.

For the lower limb the block may involve 1) N. obturatorius (Fig. 6) just lateral and below the pubic tubercle so as to infiltrate the anterior branch and thus lessen spasticity in the adductor brevis, adductor longus and part of adductor magnus; 2) N. tibialis (Fig. 7) at the fossa poplitea to relieve spasticity of the triceps suralis, tibialis posterioris, flexor digitorum longus; 3) N. plantaris medialis, behind the medial malleolus for flexor hallucis brevis spasticity.

Implantable reservoirs (Keenan 1988) may be used for severe spasticity in the upper limb, if limb mobilisation remains impossible inspite of all other treatments. A catheter, connected to a subcutaneous reservoir located in the chest is introduced into the axillary sheath. The reservoir is filled three times a week with anaesthesic solution (bupivacain). The

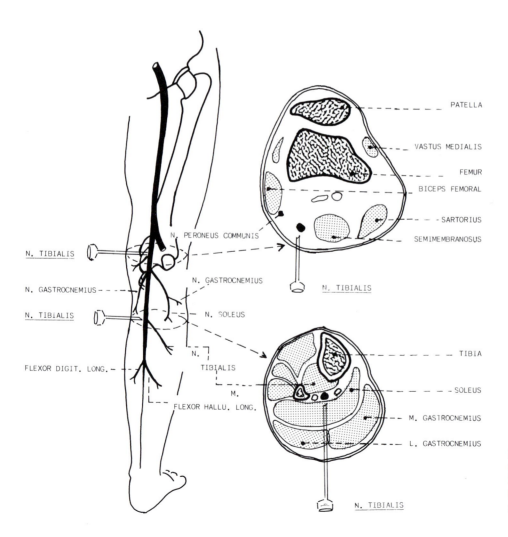

Fig. 7. Nerve infiltration (Alcohol–Xylocaïne) – N. Tibial behind the leg – at the poplitea fossa – and at the soleus arcade at the upper third of the calf

reduction of spasticity and the anaesthetic effect progressively allow efficient mobilisation of the upper limb.

Conclusion

Physical treatment is worthwhile in all patients in whom spasticity exists or may develop. It will prove sufficient in most cases, occasionally requiring concomitant pharmacological treatment, and should be systematically undertaken at an early stage and throughout recovery after a central nervous system lesion. Other treatments should be strictly reserved for the resistant cases and must always be preceded and followed with a program of physical treatment.

References

Andre JM, Brugerolle de Fraissinette B, Chellig L (1986) Le biofeedback en rééducation motrice. Ann Readapt Med Phys 29: 289–310

Bajd T, Gregoric M, Vodovnic L, Benko H (1985) Electrical stimulation in treating spasticity resulting from spinal cord injury. Arch Phys Med Rehabil 66: 515–517

Benezet P (1988) Rééducation de la marche de l'hémiplégie vasculaire de l'adulte. In: Hémiplégie vasculaire de l'adulte et médecine de Rééducation. Masson, Paris, pp 177–185

Bobath B (1981) Hémiplégie de l'adulte, bilans et traitement, 2nd edn. Masson, Paris

Brugerolle B, Albert A, Chomiki R, Thisse MO, Andre JM (1988) La stimulation électrique fonctionnelle pour l'utilisation de la main de l'hémiplégique. Ann Réadapt Med Phys 31(1): 63–68

Burke D (1988) Spasticity as an adaptation to pyramidal tract injury. In: Waxman SG (ed) Functional recovery in neurological disease. Raven Press, New York (Adv Neurol 47: 401–423)

Eggers O (1988) Traitement de l'adulte hémiplégique en ergothérapie par la méthode de Bobath, vol 1. Springer, France

Eyssette M, Boisson D (1988) La stimulation électrique fonctionnelle dans la prévention de l'algodystrophie réflexe de l'hémiplégique. In: Hémiplégie vasculaire de l'adulte et Médecine de Rééducation. Masson, Paris, pp 140–144

Katz RT (1988) Management of spasticity. Am J Phys Med Rehabil 67(3): 108–116

Katz RT (1989) Spastic hypertonia: mechanisms and measurement. Arch Phys Med Rehabil 70: 144–155

Keenam MAE (1988) Management of the spasticity of the upper extremity in the neurologically impaired adult. Clin Orthop 233: 116–125

Labat JJ, Perrouin-Verbe B, Lanoiselée JM, Mathé JF, Buzelin JM (1985) L'auto-sondage intermittent propre dans la rééducation des blessés médullaires et de la queue de cheval. Ann Réadapt Med Phys 28: 111–123; 125–136

Liberson NT (1961) Functional electrotherapy: stimulation of the peroneal nerve synchronized with the swing phase of the gait of hemiplegic patients. Arch Phys Med Rehabil 42: 101–105

Lion J (1987) L'approche sensori-motrice de la rééducation de l'hémiplégique. Concilia Medica Cedem Edit. France Tome 1(6): 159–166

Lion J, Mathé JF (1985) La Sclérose en plaques: mieux comprendre au quotidien, vol 1. Simep Villeurbanne France. Masson, Paris

Mathé JF (1989) Les contractures du paraplégique: Prevention des contractures. Ann Readapt Med Phys 32: 439–444

Perfetti C (1982) Condotte terapeutiche per la reeducazione motoria dell'emiplegico, vol 1. Ghedini, Milano

Tardieu G, Hariga J (1964) Traitement des raideurs musculaires d'origine centrale par infiltration d'alcool dilué (résultats de 500 injections). Arch Franc Péd 21(1): 25–41

Tardieu G, Tardieu C, Hariga J (1971) Infiltrations par l'alcool à 45° des points moteurs, des racines par voie épidurale ou du nerf tibial postérieur. Leurs indications dans les divers modes de "spasticité" (expérience de 10 ans). Rev Neurol 125(1): 63–68

Tardieu G, Tabary JC, Tardieu C, Tabary C, Gangnard L, Lombard M (1973) L'ajustement du nombre des sarcomères de la fibre musculaire à la longueur qui lui est imposée. Conséquences de cette régulation et de ses troubles pour les rétractions observées en Neurologie. Rev Neurol 129(1): 21–42

Tardieu G, Got C, Lespargot A (1975) Indications d'un nouveau type d'infiltrations au point moteur (alcool à 96°). Applications cliniques d'une étude expérimentale. Ann Med Phys 18(4): 539–557

van Laere M, Blonde W (1988) Valeur de la stimulation électrique fonctionnelle chez des hémiplégiques ayant un pied équin. Ann Réadapt Med Phys 31(1): 55–61

Waxman SG (1982) Current concepts in neurology: membranes, myelin and the pathophysiology of multiple sclerosis. N Engl J Med 306: 1529–1533

Correspondence: Prof. J.F. Mathé, Service de Rééducation Fonctionnelle, Hôpital Saint-Jacques, C.H.U., F-44035 Nantes, France

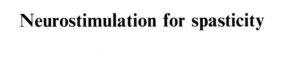

Neurostimulation for spasticity

Spinal cord stimulation for spasticity

J. Gybels[1] and **D. Van Roost**[2]

[1] Kliniek voor Neurologie en Neurochirurgie, Universitair Ziekenhuis "Gasthuisberg", Leuven, Belgium
[2] Neurochirurgische Universitätsklinik, Bonn-Venusberg, Federal Republic of Germany

Introduction

After the dramatic improvement of multiple sclerosis patients reported by Cook and Weinstein (1973), spinal cord stimulation (SCS) for the relief of spasticity and motor dyskinesias has been applied to a large number of patients. However, the overall effectiveness of this treatment has been a subject of considerable debate, some authors even reaching the conclusion that the observed results can be explained in terms of a placebo effect (Rosen and Barsoum 1979). In this review we will try to answer the question which is most important from the patient's point of view: (1) What is the effect of SCS on spasticity and accompanying motor impairment? We will also examine the data which are available with respect to the following questions which are important for the physician: (2) Is there a difference between the effect of SCS in MS patients, who have a fluctuating clinical course, and patients with other conditions, such as cerebral palsy, trauma, and cerebellar atrophies, in which the clinical course is either stabilized or progressive? (3) Does SCS at low (≤ 150 cs) and high (≥ 1.000 cs) frequencies produce different results? (4) Should the stimulating electrodes be placed rostral or caudal to the spasticity provoking lesion? (5) What can be learned from the clinical results of SCS about the possible mechanisms underlying the modifications it produces?

Definitions

When we use the term SCS we mean spinal cord stimulation with one or more electrodes or electrode contacts, positioned in the midline of the epidural (or endodural or subdural) space, posteriory either at the cervical, thoracic or lumbar level. Many authors use the term "dorsal column stimulation" to describe SCS.

The voltage, frequency, and pulse width parameters used in the early work for the modification of dystonic and hyperkinetic conditions (MDHC) were those used with SCS for pain therapy, namely 1–10 V, 2–200 Hz, and 100–500 μs. Cook, the initiator of SCS in MDHC for controlling ataxia, however, mentioned in 1976 the usefulness of higher frequency stimulation without further specifications. In the treatment of spasmodic torticollis, Gildenberg reported in 1978 and in 1981 better responses provided by frequencies in the range of 1000–1500 Hz, although the characteristic tingling sensations in the limbs was often absent. On the other hand, Waltz et al. emphasized in 1981 the necessity of extending the frequencies from 100 to 1400 Hz.

Technical developments

In the early years, a laminectomy in the thoracic area was needed in order to place bipolar electrodes extra-, endo- or intradurally over the midline of the spinal cord. Connections were made with a device implanted subcutaneously, usually in the subcostal or subclavicular region. The first, and most widely used, radiofrequency-linked arrangement allowed the electric power supply to be transmitted to the electrodes externally, by placing the coil antenna of a transmitter device over the skin covering the implanted receiver. The external miniaturized battery-powered transmitter generated the rectangular electric pulses and permitted variation in different parameters within certain ranges.

The reasons for uncoupling the electrodes from the supply and control are to be found in the high power requirements of SCS, about 2 orders of magnitude greater than those for cardiac pacing, and, moreover, in a demand for maximal adjustability of stimulation parameters.

Since 1973, the less invasive percutaneous installation of wire leads into the epidural space by means of a puncture needle (type "Tuohy-Huber" or "Hustead") has found wide acceptance especially as a preliminary selection procedure. It can be performed under local anaesthesia and fluoroscopic control. The percutaneously implanted wire electrode is not primarily attached to any intraspinal structure and is only subsequently held in place by adhesions due to minor local tissue reactions. This technique is therefore associated with a higher incidence of electrode displacements as compared with an open surgical implantation, which, for this reason, retains its value.

Wire electrodes for percutaneous insertion have been used in various forms: one single-lead electrode acting as a cathode in a monopolar arrangement, the device case serving as the anode; two single-lead electrodes in a bipolar arrangement; and one multiple-lead electrode using bipolar stimulation with many combination possibilities. The latter electrode type for multilevel trials over the upper cervical segment, together with stimulation frequencies from 100 to 1.400 Hz, was recommended by Waltz et al. for the treatment of dystonic and dyskinetic disorders (Waltz and Andreesen 1981, Waltz et al. 1981). The early stimulator implants had been an assembly composed of 4 disc electrodes in linear array, spaced 1 cm apart, molded in Dacron mesh and silicone rubber connected to a plug housing and had required a partial laminectomy of C4 to be inserted followed by a percutaneous testing prior to permanent receiver implantation. A newer 4-electrode catheter assembly can now be installed through an epidural needle and is connected with a computerized receiver which allows the lead combinations to be monitored on a continual basis through an external transmitter (Fig. 1). In spite of the higher energy requirements as compared with cardiac pacemakers, totally implantable and programmable systems for neurostimulation have been produced, employing lithium batteries that provide several years of service. The stimulator and electrode system can be interrogated for impedance and parameters stimulation in use. The patient's compliance for the totally implantable system is reported to be much better than for the radiofrequency-linked systems (with external parts), the inconvenience of the former being the

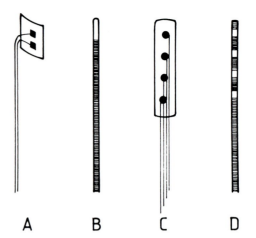

Fig. 1. Different types of electrodes for epidural stimulation (see text)

dependence on an attending doctor for reprogramming. Details of surgical technique can be found in Gybels and Van Roost (1987).

What is the effect of SCS on spasticity and other motor abnormalities?

In 1982 we reviewed the literature on the results of SCS for the modification of dystonic and hyperkinetic conditions (Gybels and Van Roost 1985). The effect of SCS on spasticity was included in this study which scrutinizes 39 papers from 19 authors or teams, describing about 1000 patients treated (Campos et al. 1981, Cook et al. 1981, Davis et al. 1981, Dooley 1977, Dooley and Nisonson 1981, Dooley and Sharkey 1981, Gildenberg 1981, Hawkes et al. 1981, Illis et al. 1980, Ketelaer et al. 1979, Klinger and Kepplinger 1982, Lazorthes et al. 1981, Plotkin 1980, Read et al. 1980, Reynolds and Oakley 1982, Richardson et al. 1979, Rosen and Barsoum 1979, Scerrati et al. 1982, Siegfried 1980, Waltz 1982, Waltz and Andreesen 1981, Young and Goodmann 1979).

We had difficulties in this review in differentiating spasticity from other motor impairments and in filtering the respective results, because many times these disorders – undoubtedly interconnected – were dealt with interchangeably. We thus experienced the advantage and the further need for describing results in terms of reproducible tests, using well-defined characteristics of motor function such as muscle strength, muscle tone and coordination. In the above-mentioned material, we grouped the percentage in each improvement category (no – fair – good – very

Table 1. Mean improvement, expressed as percentages of numbers of patients, derived from the most critically analyzed series only, from the largest series only, and from all series (material 1973–1982)

	Spasticity				Motor				Bladder				Overall			
	No	F	G	VG	No	F	G	VG	No	F	G	VG	No	F	G	VG
Critical	44	35	0	21	68	16	16	0	36	17	21	26	60	12	18	10
Large	39	21	22	18	44	18	20	18	37	25	12	27	40	14	26	19
Total	36	24	25	15	49	14	20	17	35	17	20	28	38	15	30	17

good) for just the most critically analyzed series, just the largest series and for all series (see Table 1). We considered a series to have been critically analyzed if it presented data from at least four tests in addition to a clinical examination. Series containing at least 30 patients were considered large.

"No" stands for no improvement at all, or deterioration; "fair" (F) for a slight improvement that does not change the pre-existing level of functioning and which often can only be perceived by neurological assessment; "good" (G) for an improvement that raises the pre-existing level of functioning in a way that it is useful in activities of the daily life and can be perceived by untrained eyes; "very good" (VG) for an improvement that leads to an spectacular gain of function.

The "overall" evaluation ranges from global functional amelioration irrespective of spasticity, motor or bladder function, to improvement of otherwise, mentioned impairments as, for instance, torticollis.

In Table 1, the figures for spasticity and especially those for bladder function improvement are noteworthy because of the high percentages in the "very good" column, even when the critically assessed series alone are considered.

Within each improvement category, we then searched for statistical agreement among the "critical", "large" and "total" populations, and found it significant only for bladder function (X^2-test, contingency tables: $\alpha = 0.10$).

We think that this statistical analysis rules out a false positive result due to data compilation artefacts as far as the bladder is concerned. For spasticity, better figures than for other motor improvement, may be statistically retrievable ($\alpha = 0.05$ in the Mann-Whitney test), but convincing unanimity is not present.

Using not too stringent standards, we concluded that with SCS a useful relief of disability in terms of bladder function was obtained in 40–50% of cases, a

useful spasticity amelioration in, maximally, 20–40% of cases, and a useful "overall" functional gain in 10 to 45% of cases.

In Table 2 we have listed the data from the literature from 1983 to 1988 inclusive. This table comprises 16 papers, describing about 340 patients. In view of the rather small number of patients in this material, we have not attempted to perform a statistical analysis. This material however shows an increase of critical analysis, by the use of standardized established rating scales, the use of quantitative technical tests and an attempt towards a double-blind experimental design.

A coarse comparison with Table 1, that displays the averages of the previously compiled material from 1973 to 1982, tallies as far as the scores for spasticity and motor performance are concerned. The figures of bladder improvement, in more recent studies, however, seem to be shifted away from the "very good" grade. The corresponding authors moreover emphasize the poorly objectifiable (Berg et al. 1982) and/or long-lasting (Hawkes et al. 1983, Illis et al. 1983) benefit of SCS in the treatment of bladder function impairment (in MS). One team concludes that they cannot recommend it for routine management (Hawkes et al. 1983).

Concerning spasticity, it is striking that equally well analyzed series of patients show completely different outcomes (Gottlieb et al. 1985, Dimitrijevic et al. 1986a). Two extensive studies have made an attempt to meet the crucial test of double-blind experimental design. The summaries of these studies read as follows:

– "SCS to reduce spasticity was evaluated in 7 patients (6 cerebral palsy, 1 trauma) who, along with their physicians, perceived significant and prompt benefit from stimulation. In two 24-hour test periods, on or off stimulation, we used quantitative measures of joint

Table 2. Improvement of spasticity, motor performance and bladder function, expressed as percentages of numbers of patients, resulting from spinal cord stimulation (material 1983–1988)

Authors, year pathology treated	Stimulation parameters	Spasticity				Motor performance				Bladder				Additional tests
		No	F	G	VG	No	F	G	VG	No	F	G	VG	
Hawkes et al. (1983)[a] stable MS	Th1–Th9 33 Hz 4–5 yrs follow-up									33 (n = 15)	67			4
Illis et al. (1983)[b] MS	1 year follow-up									58 (n = 12)	8	33		3
Tallis et al. (1983) stable MS	upper of mid-thoracic 33 Hz 200 µs					70 (n = 23)	17	9	4					
Waltz and Davis (1983) cerebral palsy	C2–C4 100–1400 Hz 6–64 mths follow-up					15 (n = 90)	12	41	32					
dystonia	previous thalamic surg. in 37/55 patients					31 (n = 55)	7	31	31					
Barolat-Romana et al. (1985) cervical injury	upper thoracic 75–100 Hz 100–250 µs several hours/day	(n = 6)		50	50									4
Gottlieb et al. (1985) cerebral palsy	C2–C4 1–1400 Hz 8–23 mths stimulation	(n = 6)												3
Nakamura and Tsubokawa (1985)[c] sequel of apoplexia	C5; C7 100–350 Hz 300–500 µs 12–14 hours/day	(n = 3)	33	67										1
Barolat-Romana and Myklebust (1986) trauma and nontraumatic		12.5 (n = 16)		37.5	50									
Dimitrijevic et al. (1986) chronic spinal cord injury	C2–T12 30–50 Hz 200 µs 3–15 days	22 (n = 59)	15	34	29									
Dimitrijevic et al. (1986) chronic spinal cord injury	long term	of 15 implanted, 8 continue stimulation												3
Fredriksen et al. (1986)[d] MS	C2–T2 25–100 Hz 0,5–1 ms	after 1 month 54 ——35—— (n = 49) long term 60 ——27—— (n = 49)								after 1 month 9 ——76—— (n = 49) long term 12 ——73—— (n = 49)				2
Broseta et al. (1987) spasticity	C2–C3 200–1400 Hz 50–100 µs 38 mths follow-up	80 (n = 5)	20											
dystonia						67 (n = 3)	33							
torticollis						50 (n = 2)			50					
Cioni and Meglio (1987)[e] CVA	cervical 80 Hz 200 µs	20 (n = 10)	80			27 (n = 11)	9	64						4
Koulousakis et al. (1987) MS/myelopathy	cervical/lumbar resp. for tetra- and paraparesis	25 (n = 16)	25	44	6	100 (n = 16)				42 (n = 12)	25	33		
Barolat et al. (1988) spinal cord injury	T1–T7 50–100 Hz 200–300 µs long term	(n = 14)		43	57					——7—— (n = 14)				6

Table 2. (*Continued*)

Authors, year pathology treated	Stimulation parameters	Spasticity				Motor performance				Bladder				Additional tests
		No	F	G	VG	No	F	G	VG	No	F	G	VG	
Hugenholtz et al. (1988)[f] cerebral palsy	C2–C4 50–1500 Hz 200 μs	(n = 8)												6

Comments:
[a] Optimum response on day 6 or 7 of SCS. Only 3 out of 13 patients had lasting benefit. Complications in 9 out of 31 patients.
[b] In 3/4 of the patients the beneficial effect is lost in about 1 year, not only because of technical failure.
[c] Effect of SCS is delayed for 3–9 days; continuous improvement may be obtained for at least 4 months after the beginning of stimulation.
[d] Subjective improvement in bladder and motor symptoms, only substantiated by objective parameters for the bladder; same subjective improvement with TENS as with SCS.
[e] Especially efficacious during voluntary movements and gait.
[f] In this prospective double-blind study of high cervical spinal cord stimulation conducted in 8 moderately disabled, spastic, cerebral palsied children no significant improvement over base-line function during chronic SCS at either optimal stimulation parameters or random placebo parameters could be demonstrated

compliance and stretch reflexes, and a standardized neurological examination. Neither method did better than chance in determining whether SCS was actually being received" (Gottlieb et al. 1985).
– "A prospective double-blind study of high cervical SCS conducted in 8 moderately disabled, spastic CP children failed to demonstrate any significant improvement over base line function during chronic SCS at either optimal stimulation parameters or random placebo parameters" (Hugenholtz et al. 1988).

Is there a difference of SCS in MS patients versus patients with a stabilized or progressively deteriorating disorder?

What about the possibility of false positive interpretations arising from the interference of a spontaneously fluctuating course in MS? We believe we have ruled this out by separating and matching the results in MS patients to those in patients affected by disorders with a stabilized or progressively deter-

Table 3. Paired scores originating from observations of a common investigator of the effects of spinal cord stimulation on overall improvement, expressed as percentages

	MS				Stabilized or progressively deteriorating disorders			
	No	F	G	VG	No	F	G	VG
Dooley (1977)	36 (n = 42)	——64——			36 (n = 14)	——64——		
Siegfried (1980)	– (n = 7)	14	86	–	25 (n = 4)	50	25	–
Campos et al. (1981)	8 (n = 12)	33	42	17	– (n = 12)	8	75	17
Davis et al. (1981)	36 (n = 69)	–	57	7	16 (n = 32)	53	31	–
Dooley and Sharkey (1981)	36.2 (n = 69)	14.5	13	36.2	32 (n = 25)	–	12	56
Lazorthes et al. (1981)	67 (n = 111)	12	19	2	72 (n = 46)	——28——		
Reynolds and Oakley (1982)	50 (n = 2)	–	–	50	25 (n = 4)	–	50	25
Waltz (1982)	30 (n = 27)	——70——			23 (n = 193)	11	35	31

No no improvement; *F* fair; *G* good; *VG* very good

iorating clinical course. Table 3 lists these paired scores which originate from the observations of a common investigator. The average percentage of MS patients who experienced an amelioration to some degree, namely 67%, turns out to be slightly lower than the analogous average of stabilised or progressively deteriorating cases, which amounts to 71%. Their standard deviations, however, are equivalent and statistical analysis (X^2-test, nonparametric tests, and linear correlation) fails to discern, at a high level of significance, the scores of both groups as belonging to different populations.

Does SCS at low (≤ 150 cs) and high (≥ 1.000 cs) frequency produce different results?

Not much data is available to answer this question. From a physiological point of view, the rationale for high frequency stimulation does not exist, since dorsal column fibres will not follow high frequency stimulation. The result will be an out of phase firing of the stimulated fibres. Waltz has claimed that the high cervical location of the electrode and the specific polarity and frequency of stimulation could make the difference between success and failure in each patient (Waltz 1982). Hugenholtz et al. (1988) showed that 8 individuals with cerebral palsy had optimal relief using stimulation frequencies between 500 and 1450 hz. As noted by Dimitrijevic et al. (1986b) little has been written in the SCS literature regarding the importance of the intensity of the stimulus, but this may be an important parameter. High stimulation strength can enhance spasticity in patients in whom a lower stimulus strength suppressed spasticity.

Should the stimulating electrode be placed rostral or caudal to the spasticity provoking lesion?

This question has been addressed by Dimitrijevic et al. in careful studies of a great number of spinal cord injury patients (Dimitrijevic et al. 1986a, b, Campos et al. 1987). They concluded that the effect of SCS on spasticity had a more pronounced effect when stimulating occurred below the lesion rather than above in incomplete injuries, and that a maximum control of spasticity occurred with electrode placement in the thoraco-lumbar enlargement. This view is shared by some (Richardson et al. 1979) while refuted by others (Siegfried, Laitinen, personal communication).

Complications

Complications of SCS that have repeatedly been reported are: 1) lead break down, with eventual current leakage, in some 10% of the cases; 2) electrode displacement, also in some 10% of the cases and 3) infection, in some 5% of the cases. The two first complications are largely responsible for the fact that SCS is frequently not a single and simple, but a time-consuming and expensive technique (Illis 1983).

An exacerbation of MS within the first two weeks of stimulation has been reported in 5 out of 31 patients by Hawkes et al. (1981).

Other, more anecdotically reported complications were: pain at the stimulation site, CSF leakage, difficulties in keeping the electrodes buried under the skin, transient cord compression, epidural haematoma after laminectomy, haematoma at the receiver pocket, psychological difficulties in adjusting to the treatment program, a fibrotic reaction of the meninges presenting as pain or as reduction in effect for a given stimulus voltage, and a reversible aggravation of spasticity by excessive stimulation.

What can be learned from the clinical results of SCS about the possible mechanisms underlying the modifications it produces?

No real scientific or statistically significant data are available, but nevertheless, single but careful observations can provide clues as to the working mechanisms of SCS in spasticity and motor disorders.

The proposed hypotheses of the working mechanisms can be listed as follows:

Psychogenic

SCS has been reported to have a placebo effect (Rosen and Barsoum 1979). Conversely, clinical and physiological data discount a placebo effect (Illis et al. 1980, 1976, Sharkey et al. 1981, Berg et al. 1982). The laterality effect seems to rule out a global sedation factor (Walker 1982).

Biochemical

SCS stimulates synthesis and transport to synaptic terminals of new proteins or other macromolecules (Ketelaer et al. 1979). It encourages release of biochemical substances such as endorphins (Spiegel 1982). It stimulates release of long-lasting transmitter substances (Philips in Dimitrijevic et al. 1981). Based upon cerebrospinal fluid (CSF) peptide analysis, enkephalins are not involved (Hawkes et al. 1981). Central hypercholinergic state may arise from SCS in MS (Cook in Young and Goodman 1979).

Segmental

SCS increases the amount of background afferent activity in a partially deafferented neuronal system (Davis et al. 1981). It depolarizes/blocks the afferent limb of the reflex arc (Gildenberg 1981). It stimulates the descending inhibitory pathways below the level of maximum occurrence of MS plaques (Read et al. 1980). It reduces nociceptive input, which can aggravate spasticity (Read et al. 1980). It suppresses central over-reactivity to normal spindle input (Hagbarth in Dimitrijevic et al. 1981). Antidromic activation of residual structures of spinal cord results in moderation of segmental mechanisms of spasticity below the lesion (Dimitrijevic et al. 1986b). SCS may also activate local inhibitory processes or depolarizes local excitatory pathways (Maiman et al. 1987).

Suprasegmental

SCS influences the ascending/descending reticular system (Waltz et al. 1981). It has supraspinal involvement (Siegfried et al. 1978, Dimitrijevic et al. 1986a) acting at spinal and brainstem levels, but not by arousal (Sedgwick et al. 1980). It reaches higher brain centers orthodromically (Davis et al. 1981). It activates long-loop reflexes which have inhibitory action on the spinal cord (Delwaide in Dimitrijevic et al. 1981). SCS disrupts patterned activities (Phillips in Dimitrijevic et al. 1981). Largely common circuits for pain and spasticity might be the anatomical substratum of effects of SCS on both (Spiegel 1982).

Autonomic

SCS effects autonomic function (Read et al. 1980). It has a direct inhibitory effect on sympathetic tone (Richardson et al. 1979). and this might be the explanation for bladder improvement (Ojemann in Richardson et al. 1979). It alters non-adrenergic pathways, influencing the urinary tract (Dooley and Sharkey 1981), with a primary effect on smooth muscle (Hawkes et al. 1981).

Miscellaneous

SCS has both a direct and indirect (via released neurotransmittors) effect on nervous tissue (Waltz et al. 1981). It can result in a modification of functional and anatomical reorganization through synaptic facilitation or the plastic properties of the synaptic zone (Illis 1973, Illis et al. 1976): spinal cord "kindling" (Cook et al. 1981), permeability and ion fluxes (Cook 1976), and control of rhythmic neurons in an ephaptic transmission (Cook 1976). Recruitment of additional regional spinal cord activity (Sharkey et al. 1981) as well as spatial summation and recruitment in still-functioning motor units has been theorized. (Plotkin 1980). Increase of central excitatory state (Illis et al. 1976) as well as external initiation of presynaptic depolarization (Cook 1976) have also been advanced.

There are no data, either clinical or experimental (Wiesendanger 1985, Maiman et al. 1987) to indicate clearly what might be the working mechanisms of SCS in spasticity and motor disorders, and one still is left, more than a decade after the introduction of SCS for these disorders, with rather vague theories, which at best can be described as "good neurologizing".

Concluding remarks

The appreciation of the value of SCS in the treatment of spasticity remains difficult. Our own attitude has been defined by our review in 1982 which included personal experience (Ketelaer et al. 1979) and in which we estimated that SCS for spasticity has questionable clinical value, achieving a useful overall relief from disability in 10% of the cases when the literature is critically analyzed. We feel supported in this viewpoint by the present review, particularly when taking into account the results of prospective studies with a double-blind design (Hugenholtz et al. 1988). Not everybody will share this view. Where does this leave SCS for the treatment of spasticity and associated motor disorders, particularly since we now know that the intrathecal administration of small doses of baclofen has impressive effects on spasticity? It is perhaps wise to limit the exploration of this technique to a very selected group of patients, such as unilateral spasticity, spasticity of the upper limbs etc... where the value of intrathecal administration of baclofen has as yet not been established.

Acknowledgement

The authors are indebted to Mrs. M. Feytons–Heeren for expert technical assistance.

References

Barolat-Romana G, Myklebust JB (1986) Immediate effects of spinal cord stimulation on spinal spasticity. Presented at 7th Meeting ESSFN, Birmingham

Barolat-Romana G, Myklebust JB, Hemmy DC, Myklebust B, Wenninger W (1985) Immediate effects of spinal cord stimulation in spinal spasticity. J Neurosurg 62: 558–562

Barolat G, Myklebust JB, Wenninger W (1988) Effects of spinal cord stimulation in spasticity and spasms secondary to myelopathy. Appl Neurophysiol 51: 29–44

Berg V, Bergmann S, Hovdal H, Hunstad N, Johnsen HJ, Levin L, Sjaastad O (1982) The value of dorsal column stimulation in multiple sclerosis. Scand J Rehabil Med 14: 183–191

Broseta J, Garcia-March G, Sanchez-Ledesma MJ, Barbera J, Gonzalez-Darder J (1987) High-frequency cervical spinal cord stimulation in spasticity and motor disorders. Acta Neurochir [Suppl] 39: 112–116

Campos RJ, Dimitrijevic MM, Faganel J, Sharkey PC (1981) Clinical evaluation of the effect of spinal cord stimulation on motor performance in patients with upper motor neuron lesions. Appl Neurophysiol 44: 141–151

Campos RJ, Dimitrijevic MR, Sharkey PC, Sherwood AM (1987) Epidural spinal cord stimulation in spastic spinal cord injury patients. Appl Neurophysiol 50: 453–454

Cioni B, Meglio M (1987) Spinal cord stimulation improves motor performances in hemiplegics: clinical and neurophysiological study. Acta Neurochir [Suppl] 39: 103–105

Cook AW (1976) Electrical stimulation in multiple sclerosis. Hosp Pract 11: 51–58

Cook AW, Weinstein SP (1973) Chronic dorsal column stimulation in multiple sclerosis. NY St J Med 73: 2868–2872

Cook AW, Taylor JK, Nidzgorski F (1981) Results of spinal cord stimulation in multiple sclerosis. Appl Neurophysiol 44: 55–61

Davis R, Gray E, Kudzma J (1981) Beneficial augmentation following dorsal column stimulation in some neurological diseases. Appl Neurophysiol 44: 37–49

Dimitrijevic MR, Faganel J, Young RR (1981) Underlying mechanisms of the effects of spinal cord stimulation in motor disorders. Appl Neurophysiol 44: 133–140

Dimitrijevic MM, Dimitrijevic MR, Illis LS, Nakajima K, Sharkey PC, Sherwood AM (1986a) Spinal cord stimulation for the control of spasticity in patients with chronic spinal cord injury. I. Clinical observations. Central nervous system trauma 3: 129–144

Dimitrijevic MR, Illis LS, Nakajima K, Sharkey PC, Sherwood AM (1986b) Spinal cord stimulation for the control of spasticity in patients with chronic spinal cord injury. II. Neurophysiologic observations. Central nervous system trauma 3: 145–152

Dooley DM (1977) Demyelinating, degenerative and vascular disease. Neurosurgery 1: 220–224

Dooley DM, Nisonson I (1981) Treatment of patients with degenerative diseases of the central nervous system by electrical stimulation of the spinal cord. Appl Neurophysiol 44: 71–76

Dooley DM, Sharkey J (1981) Electrical stimulation of the spinal cord in patients with demyelinating and degenerative diseases of the central nervous system. Appl Neurophysiol 44: 218–224

Fredriksen TA, Bergmann S, Hesselberg JP, Stolt-Nielsen A, Ringkjob R, Sjaastad O (1986) Electrical stimulation in multiple sclerosis. Comparison of transcutaneous electrical stimulation and epidural spinal cord stimulation. Appl Neurophysiol 49: 4–24

Gildenberg PL (1978) Treatment of spasmodic torticollis by dorsal column stimulation. Appl Neurophysiol 41: 113–121

Gildenberg PL (1981) Comprehensive management of spasmodic torticollis. Appl Neurophysiol 44: 233–243

Gottlieb GL, Myklebust BM, Stefoski D, Groth K, Kroin J, Penn RD (1985) Evaluation of cervical stimulation for chronic treatment of spasticity. Neurology 35: 699–704

Gybels J, Van Roost D (1985) Spinal cord stimulation for the modification of dystonic and hyperkinetic conditions. A critical review. In: Eccles JC, Dimitrijevic ME (eds) Recent achievements in restorative neurology. 1. Upper motor neuron functions and dysfunctions. Karger, Basel, pp 56–70

Gybels J, Van Roost D (1987) Spinal cord stimulation for spasticity. In: Symon et al. (eds) Advances and technical standards in neurosurgery, vol 15. Springer, Wien, pp 63–96

Hawkes CH, Fawcett D, Cooke ED, Emson PC, Paul EA, Bowcock SA (1981) Dorsal column stimulation in multiple sclerosis: effects on bladder, e.g. blood flow and peptides. Appl Neurophysiol 44: 62–70

Hawkes CH, Beard R, Fawcett D, Paul EA, Thomas DGT (1983) Dorsal column stimulation in multiple sclerosis; effects on bladder and long term findings. Br Med J 287: 793–795

Hugenholtz H, Humphreys P, McIntyre WMJ, Spasoff RA, Steel K (1988) Cervical spinal cord stimulation for spasticity in cereral palsy. Neurosurgery 22: 707–714

Illis LS (1973) Regeneration in the central nervous system. Lancet i: 1035–1037

Illis LS (1983) Central nervous stimulation in neurological disease. J Roy Soc Med 76: 905–909

Illis LS, Sedgwick EM, Oygar AE, Sabbahi Awadalla MA (1976) Dorsal column stimulation in the rehabilitation of patients with multiple sclerosis. Lancet i: 1383–1386

Illis LS, Sedgwick EM, Tallis RC (1980) Spinal cord stimulation in multiple sclerosis: clinical results. J Neurol Neurosurg Psychiatry 43: 1–14

Illis LS, Read DJ, Sedgwick EM, Tallis RC (1983) Spinal cord stimulation in the United Kingdom. J Neurol Neurosurg Psychiatry 46: 299–304

Ketelaer P, Swartenbroeckx G, Deltenre P, Carton H, Gybels J (1979) Percutaneous epidural dorsal cord stimulation in multiple sclerosis. Acta Neurochir (Wien) 49: 95–101

Klinger D, Kepplinger B (1982) Quantification of the effects to epidural spinal electrostimulation (ESES) in central motor disorders. Appl Neurophysiol 45: 221–224

Koulousakis A, Buchhaas U, Nittner K (1987) Application of SCS for movement disorders and spasticity. Acta Neurochir [Suppl] 39: 112–116

Lazorthes Y, Siegfried J, Broggi G (1981) Electrical spinal cord stimulation for spastic motor disorders in demyelinating diseases – a cooperative study. In: Hosobuchi Y, Corbin I (eds) Indications for spinal cord stimulation. Excerpta Medica, Princeton, pp 48–57

Maiman DJ, Myklebust JB, Barolat-Romana G (1987) Spinal cord stimulation for amelioration of spasticity: experimental results. Neurosurgery 21: 331–333

Nakamura S, Tsubokawa T (1985) Evaluation of spinal cord stimulation for postapoplectic spastic hemiplegia. Neurosurgery 17: 253–259

Plotkin R (1980) Pisces stimulation for motor neurone disease. Acta Neurochir [Suppl] 30: 429–433

Read DJ, Matthews WB, Higson RH (1980) The effect of spinal cord stimulation on function in patients with multiple sclerosis. Brain 103: 803–833

Reynolds AF, Oakley JC (1982) High frequency cervical epidural stimulation for spasticity. Appl Neurophysiol 45: 93–97

Richardson RR, Cerullo LJ, McLone DG, Gutierrez FA, Lewis V (1979) Percutaneous epidural neurostimulation in modulation of paraplegic spasticity. Six case reports. Acta Neurochir (Wien) 49: 235–243

Rosen JA, Barsoum AH (1979) Failure of chronic dorsal column stimulation in multiple sclerosis. Ann Neurol 6: 66–67

Scerrati M, Onofrio J, Pola P (1982) Effects of spinal cord stimulation on spasticity. H-reflex study. Appl Neurophysiol 45: 62–67

Sedgwick EM, Illis LS, Tallis RC, Thornton ARD, Abraham P, El-Negamy E, Docherty TB, Soar JS, Spencer SC, Taylor FM (1980) Evoked potentials and contingent negative variation during treatment of multiple sclerosis with spinal cord stimulation. J Neurol Neurosurg Psychiatry 43: 15–24

Sharkey PC, Dimitrijevic MM, Campos RJ, Dimitrijevic MR (1981) Remarks on spinal cord stimulation and the placebo effect. Appl Neurophysiol 44: 119–125

Siegfried J (1980) Treatment of spasticity by dorsal cord stimulation. Int Rehab Med 2: 31–34

Siegfried J, Krainick JU, Haas H, Adorjani C, Meyer M, Thoden U (1978) Electrical spinal cord stimulation for spastic movement disorders. Appl Neurophysiol 41: 134–141

Spiegel EA (1982) Relief of pain and spasticity by posterior column stimulation. A proposed mechanism. Archs Neurol (Chicago) 39: 184–185

Tallis RC, Illis LS, Smedgwick EM (1983) The quantitative assessment of the influence of spinal cord stimulation on motor function in patients with multiple sclerosis. Int Rehab Med 5: 10–16

Walker JB (1982) Modulation of spasticity: prolonged suppression of a spinal reflex by electrical stimulation. Science 216: 203–204

Waltz JM (1982) Computerized percutaneous multi-level spinal cord stimulation in motor disorders. Appl Neurophysiol 45: 73–92

Waltz JM, Andreesen WH (1981) Multiple-lead spinal cord stimulation: technique. Appl Neurophysiol 44: 30–36

Waltz JM, Davis JA (1983) Cervical cord stimulation in the treatment of athetosis and dystonia. Adv Neurol 37: 225–237

Waltz JM, Reynolds LO, Riklan M (1981) Multi-lead spinal cord stimulation for control of motor disorders. Appl Neurophysiol 44: 244–257

Wiesendanger M, Chapman CE, Marini G, Schorderet D (1985) Experimental studies of dorsal cord stimulation in animal models of spasticity. In: Delwaide PJ, Young RR (eds) Clinical neurophysiology in spasticity. Elsevier Science Publishers BV, Amsterdam, pp 205–219

Young RF, Goodman SJ (1979) Dorsal spinal cord stimulation in the treatment of multiple sclerosis. Neurosurgery 5: 225–230

Correspondence: Prof. J. Gybels, Department of Neurology and Neurosurgery, UZ Gasthuisberg, Herestraat 49, B-3000 Leuven, Belgium

Deep brain and cerebellar stimulation for spasticity

J. Siegfried

AMI Klinik Im Park, Zürich, Switzerland

Since the introduction of stereotactic brain operations in humans by Spiegel and Wycis in 1947 (Spiegel et al. 1947), most surgical efforts to improve dystonic conditions and abnormal movements have focused on localized destruction of various parts of the thalamus, mesencephalon, and cerebellar nuclei. Many types of movement disorders were treated by this technique, which allows the destruction of more or less specific subcortical parts of the brain without damaging the overlying brain structures, and thus ameliorate diseases which had previously been difficult or impossible to treat. For the physiological localization of the target to be destroyed, electrical stimulation has been always used, but the application of this method for therapeutic use was only introduced in 1962. At that time Mazars implanted electrodes in the sensory thalamic nuclei for pain relief (Mazars et al. 1973) and Cooper in the same year described chronic cerebellar stimulation for motor movements disorders (Cooper 1973). However, while pain treatment by chronic brain stimulation has become a method of treatment which has clear applications and usefulness with very satisfactory results in the majority of cases, the treatment of spasticity with cerebral and cerebellar stimulation is still controversial and is today not really an alternative of great interest.

Cerebral stimulation

Mundinger was the first to report the implantation of chronic electrodes in the thalamus, pulvinar, and dentate nucleus for movement disorders, particularly spasmodic torticollis (Mundinger 1977). Good results in (a) facial dyskinesias in a series of torsion dystonia, (b) double athetosis, and (c) arm dystonia in a case of traumatic spasticity were reported in his last paper,

apparently using stimulation of the *ventrolateral part of the thalamus* and/or the *zona incerta*. However, in a 1982 review of patients, Mundinger emphasized the importance of stimulation-induced paresthesias overlying the affected area (Mundinger and Neumüller 1982), so that the *sensory thalamic nuclei* were certainly involved. Mazars, who first stimulated sensory thalamic nuclei to alleviate deafferentation pain, found also that associated abnormal movements were controlled (Mazars et al. 1980). He stressed the importance of stimulation paresthesias over the affected part of the body. He also felt that for stimulation to be successful, the dyskinesias had to be associated with a sensory deafferentation, and that stimulation acted as a substitute for sensory information delivered to the nucleus ventroposterolateralis. The effect on spasticity in these patients suffering from so-called thalamic pain syndrome with sensory and motor deficit has been not mentioned. The largest series of patients with involuntary movement disorders being treated by deep brain stimulation is the one of Cooper et al. (1980). To improve the efficacy, thalamic somato-sensory responses were recorded to aid in electrode placement and in obtaining optimal stimulation parameters; effects on related spasticity are not reported.

In 1982 we implanted two sensory thalamic nuclei electrodes, one on each side, in a 41 years old patient suffering from deafferentation pain in the legs after traumatic paraplegia and an associated, severe spasticity. There was virtually immediate control of pain and clonus with bilateral ventroposterolateral thalamic stimulation. After stimulation was stopped, the clonus reappeared within 2 minutes. These bilateral systems were also programmed for 1 minute of stimulation each 2 minutes. An additional case has been operated on a couple of years later with the same effect (Siegfried 1986).

Cohadon has experience of chronic stimulation of the non specific sensory thalamic system (*centrum medianum*) in the treatment of prolonged posttraumatic unconsciousness (Cohadon et al. 1985). If, in some cases, clear improvement of the overall situation was observed, motor functions were much less affected and axial tonic disturbances were at best only slightly modified.

Method

Only stereotactic techniques allow exact placement of deep brain electrodes. Many stereotactic frames can be used for this purpose. The thalamic target is calculated radiologically after ventriculography. The two main criteria necessary to achieve a correct and chronic placement of a stimulation system in the brain are a very flexible, non-traumatic electrode and a water-tight reversible electrode anchoring device; a system that achieved these goals has been developed by us (Siegfried et al. 1983). After the clinical effect is observed during a test period of a few days, the electrode will be connected to a programmable neuropacemaker implanted subcutaneously in the infraclavicular region.

Discussion

Only the stimulation of the sensory nuclei of the thalamus seems to improve the spasticity. Some of the mechanism, which may be involved, will be mentioned. There are two broad theory categories; (1) the stimulation inhibits sensory activity, and (2) the stimulation supplies or augments sensory activity. Although these theories admittedly ignore some of the complexities involved, they do provide a simple beginning upon which to add further information (Siegfried 1987). Cooper (1982) and Andy (1983) ascribed the beneficial effects of thalamic stimulation to a functional ablation of the discharging systems. Cooper supported this argument with early experimental work and theorized that motor symptoms may be the result of an inhibitory–facilitatory imbalance. He stated that lesions or stimulation in the posterior VL suppresses a posterior VL sensory funnel and moves the balance more toward normal. On the other hand, it has been demonstrated by DeLong that a significant proportion of neurons in the putamen,

globus pallidus, and thalamic/subthalamic region that are related to active movements of specific body parts also respond to somatosensory stimulation of the same body part; thus, abnormal modulation of pallidal output may lead to motor movement disorders (DeLong and Georgopoulos 1979). Consequently, somatosensory inputs of a specific and restricted nature may be used to control or monitor movements. The clinical examples of cutaneous input modifying motor activity are the "geste antagoniste" (putting the index finger on the chin), which is in some cases sufficient to control spasmodic torticollis, and the inability of athetotic patients to control their movements without the help of sensory input. The theory that the stimulation of sensory thalamic nuclei supplies absent or decreased "sensory input" is thus very attractive. This input is to the thalamus which then relays it on to the motor cortex, or perhaps the input is directly to the motor cortex. The importance of VL and especially the VPL input to the motor cortex is indicated by the fact that 70% of all thalamo-cortical connections are from VPL, and 95% are from VLc, VLo, and VPLo (Porter 1984). The physiological importance of the thalamus as a receiver of information from the basal ganglia and a projector of revised information onto the motor and premotor cortex has been emphasized (DeLong et al. 1984, Evarts and Wise 1984).

Since the initial report of Cook and Weinstein (1973) on the improvement of spasticity in patients affected by multiple sclerosis and who were treated by spinal dorsal cord stimulation system for pain, many reports have confirmed these observations, although the appreciation of the value of this method in the treatment of spasticity remains difficult (see Chapter 11). The mechanisms by which spinal cord stimulation may improve spasticity have never been clearly demonstrated; they can be purely spinal (propriospinal) or through suprasegmental influences. However, when we stimulate the sensory thalamic nuclei, we are acting on the same system as stimulation on the dorsal cord. That improvement in motor movement disorders is obtained by electrical stimulation of the ventrolateral thalamus, the pulvinar, the zona incerta and the non specific sensory system may suggest that the results are not related to a specific nucleus. Since all these structures are near the sensory thalamic nuclei, it has been suggested that the sensory inputs were facilitated by the stimulation (Siegfried and Pamir 1987). It can also be argued that spread of the stimulating current can excite the reticular nucleus and the zona incerta, which belong to the reticular formation; the latter has a well-recognized inhibitory function (Jasper 1961).

Cerebellar stimulation

Chronic stimulation of the cerebellar cortex was introduced by Cooper in 1973 (Cooper 1973, Cooper et al. 1973). In 1976 he reported the results of cerebellar stimulation for fifty patients with cerebral palsy (Cooper et al. 1976). This group was enlarged to 141 patients in a subsequent report in 1978 (Cooper et al. 1978). In the later group 41% of the patients were rated having moderate to marked improvement of their spasticity, 32% demonstrated mild improvement and 24% had no clinical change. After these publications other centers initially reported similar results, with moderate to marked improvemnt of spasticity in 85% of the cases (Davis et al. 1982), or only in 15% (Ivan and Ventureyra 1982). However, as more neurosurgeons adopted the technique, papers began to report that the effects of cerebellar stimulation were unpredictable. Intelligent patients with similar clinical spasticity had dramatic differences in the postoperative changes in spasticity according to Penn et al. (1980). Our limited experience was not convincing, as far as the spasticity alone is concerned (Siegfried and Hood 1985), even if some improvement of the general condition in cases of cerebral palsy can be reported (Siegfried and Lazorthes 1985). In addition to the uncertainty of results, neurotoxicity with demonstrated pyramidal cell drop-out, even though disputed, also detracted from the procedure (Babb et al. 1977, Brown et al. 1977, Dauth et al. 1977, Larson et al. 1978). Its popularity waned.

Chronic stimulation of the dentate nucleus has been applied successfully by Schvarcz et al. since 1978 to relieve spasticity and to improve function in patients with cerebral palsy (Schvarcz et al. 1980, 1982). Relief of spasticity and improvement in performing complex voluntary movements as well as improvement of speech, balance and gait were reported. No other experiences with chronic stimulation of the dentate nucleus have been mentioned in detail to our knowledge.

Method

The surgical placement of small silicone mesh plates bearing electrodes on the cortex of the anterior or posterior lobe of the cerebellum is performed under general anaesthesia, with the patient in the sitting position. Small craniectomies, approximately 3 cm in diameter, are made bilaterally, positioned to expose the upper portion of the posterior lobe of the cerebellum and allow access to the upper surface or cortex of the anterior lobe of the cerebellum on each side. The electrodes will then be connected to a receiver or a programmable neuropacemaker implanted in a subcutaneous pocket in the infraclavicular region.

The stereotactic approach to the dentate nucleus is performed with the stereotactic frame mounted upside down. A visualization of the fourth ventricle is obtained by fractional pneumoencephalography, allowing the drawing of a base line passing through the fastigium of the fourth ventricle. The target point is 10 mm behind the floor of the fourth ventricle, 5 mm below the base line and 14 mm lateral to the midline. The electrode is connected, in a second stage, with a receiver or a programmable neuropacemaker implanted subcutaneously in the infraclavicular region.

Discussion

The role of motor activity regulation of the cerebellum was mentioned as early as the 18th century by von Haller (1766) and later by Flourens (1824). Almost 100 years ago, Sherrington (1898) as well as Lowenthal and Horsley (1897) demonstrated that stimulation of the cerebellum produced a reduction in the extensor tone of decerebrate animals. Dow (1938) showed that, following prolonged stimulation, slow fluctuation in the spontaneous electrical activity of the cerebellum occurred for several minutes and that the level of this activity was inversely related to extensor tone in the decerebrate cat. With repetitive stimulation there follows a period of electrical silence if the period of stimulation has been short, or a period of convulsive after-discharge (represented by an increase in amplitude and frequency of background activity) if the stimuli are more intense or the train is slightly prolonged. After the convulsive pattern, a period of reduced activity or electrical silence follows and then the normal electrogram once again appears. This sequence of electrical changes has been shown to be accompanied by alterations of spinal cord function and, therefore, must be related to alterations in cerebellar neuronal discharge.

Cerebellar stimulation has been demonstrated,

particularly by Brenner (1935), to influence motor function of the cerebral cortex. The threshold of motor cortex to electrical excitation is lowered during stimulation of various parts of cerebellum, but a somatotopic arrangement was not detected. It was also demonstrated by Moruzzi (1950) that both facilitatory and inhibitory effects result from stimulation of the cerebellum.

Facilitation and increase of excitability as well as inhibition may be a cortical or a brain stem function. However, Snider (1974) proposed that the well-known inhibitory functions of the cerebellum can be obtained by electrical stimulation for the control of abnormal cerebral and thalamic paroxysms. Cerebellar cortical stimulation can inhibit the deep cerebellar nuclei by activating the Purkinje cells. The antidromic activation of cerebellar afferents, the synaptic activation of neurons of the dentate nucleus, and the trans-synaptic activation of neurons of the reticular formation by cerebellar cortical stimulation has been experimentally demonstrated by Bantli et al. (1976).

There is no doubt that the primary function of the cerebellum is the regulation or control of movements, posture, and tone. It may be that it exerts some control over many other functions of the nervous system, since it has extensive fiber connections with other parts of the brain and spinal cord. The rationale for increasing the inhibitory effect of the cerebellum by electrical stimulation can be supported; however, the clinical results are thus far disputed, and its application has progressively decreased. Better clinical evaluation, better studies of different stimulation parameters and more precise indications could renew interest in this method.

Conclusion

Cerebral and cerebellar stimulations seem to be promising therapies in the treatment of dystonic, hypertonic, dyskinetic and hyperkinetic conditions. Spasticity can be certainly influenced. However, we need a rational and careful approach to resolve the compelling uncertainties about these techniques as well as further endeavours to ascertain the effectiveness of these procedures. A conclusive evaluation would avoid the problems of overapplication followed by disrepute; at this time we cannot recommend the widespread application of cerebral and cerebellar electrical stimulation for spasticity.

References

Andy DJ (1983) Thalamic stimulation for control of movement disorders. Appl Neurophysiol 46: 107–111

Babb TL, Soper HV, Lieb JR, Brown WJ, Ottino CA, Crandall PH (1977) Electrophysiological studies of long-term electrical stimulation of the cerebellum in monkeys. J Neurosurg 47: 353–365

Bantli H, Bloedel JR, Tolbert D (1976) Activation of neurons in the cerebellar nuclei and ascending ventricular formation by stimulating of the cerebellar surface. J Neurosurg 45: 539–554

Bremer F (1935) Traité de physiologie normale et pathologique, vol 1. Roger, Binet, Le Cervelet Masson, Paris

Brown WJ, Babb TL, Soper HV, Lieb JP, Ottino CA, Crandall PH (1977) Tissue reactions to long-term electrical stimulation of the cerebellum in monkeys. J Neurosurg 47: 366–379

Cohadon F, Richer E, Bougier A, Deliac P, Loiseau H (1985) Deep brain stimulation in cases of prolonged post-traumatic unconsciousness. In: Lazorthes Y, Upton ARM (eds) Neurostimulation: an overview. Mt Kisco Futura, New York, pp 247–250

Cook AW, Weinstein SP (1973) Chronic dorsal column stimulation in multiple sclerosis. N Y State J Med 73: 2868–2872

Cooper IS (1973) Effect of chronic stimulation of anterior cerebellum on neurological diseases. Lancet i: 131

Cooper IS (1982) A general theory of causation and reversibility of involuntary movement disorders. Appl Neurophysiol 45: 317–323

Cooper IS, Crighel E, Amin I (1973) Clinical and physiological effects of stimulation of the paleocerebellum in humans. J Am Geriatr Soc 21: 40–43

Cooper IS, Riklan M, Amin I, Waltz JM, Cullinan T (1976) Chronic cerebellum stimulation in cerebral palsy. Neurology 26: 744–753

Cooper IS, Riklan M, Tabaddor K, Cullinan T, Amin I, Watkins ES (1978) A long-term follow-up study of chronic cerebellar stimulation for cerebral palsy. In: Cooper IS (ed) Cerebellar stimulation in man. Raven Press, New York, pp 59–99

Cooper IS, Upton ARM, Amin I (1980) Reversibility of chronic neuralgic deficits: some effects of electrical stimulation of the thalamus and internal capsule in man. Appl Neurophysiol 43: 244–258

Dauth GW, Defendini R, Gilman S, Tennyson K, Krezmer L (1977) Long-term surface stimulation of the cerebellum in monkey. Surg Neurol 7: 377–384

Davis R, Engle H, Kudzma J, Gray E, Ryan T, Dusnak A (1982) Update of chronic cerebellar stimulation for spasticity and epilepsy. Appl Neurophysiol 45: 44–50

DeLong MR, Georgopoulos A (1979) Motor functions of the basal ganglia. In: Brookhard JM, et al (eds) Handbook of physiology. The nervous system. American Physiological Society, Bethesda, pp 1017–1061

DeLong MR, Georgopoulos AP, Crutcher MD, Mitchell SS, Richardson RT, Alexander GE (1984) Functional organisation of the basal ganglia: contributions of single cell recording studies. Functions of the basal ganglia. Ciba Foundation Symposium 107. Pitman, London, pp 64–82

Dow RS (1938) The electrical activities of the cerebellum and its functional significance. J Physiol (Lond) 94: 67–84

Evarts EV, Wise SP (1984) Basal ganglia outputs and motor control. Functions of the basal ganglia. Ciba Foundation Symposium 107. Pitman, London, pp 83–102

Flourens P (1824) Recherches expérimentales sur les propriétés et les functions du système nerveux dans les animaux vertébrés. Crerot, Paris

Gybels J, Van Roost D (1987) Spinal cord stimulation for spasticity. Adv Tech Stand Neurosurg 15: 63–96

Ivan LP, Ventureyra ECG (1982) Chronic cerebellar stimulation in cerebral palsy. Appl Neurophysiol 45: 51–54

Jasper HH (1961) Thalamic reticular system. In: Sheer DE (ed) Electrical stimulation of the brain. University of Texas Press, Austin, pp 277–287

Larson SJ, Sances A, Hemmy DC, Millar ZA (1978) Physiological and histological effect of cerebellar stimulation. Neurosurgery 1: 212–213

Lowenthal M, Horsely V (1897) On the relation between the cerebellar and other centers (namely cerebral and spinal) with special reference to the action of antagonistic muscles. Proc R Soc Lond 61: 20–25

Mazars G, Merienne L, Cioloca G (1973) Stimulations thalamiques intermittentes. Rev Neurol 128: 273–279

Mazars G, Merienne L, Cioloca G (1980) Control of dyskinesias due to sensory deafferentation by means of thalamic stimulation. Acta Neurochir [Suppl] 30: 239–243

Moruzzi G (1950) Problems in cerebellar physiology, Thomas, Springfield

Mundinger F (1977) Neue stereotaktisch-funktionelle Behandlungsmethode des Torticollis spasmodicus mit Hirnstimulatoren. Med Klin 72: 1982–1986

Mundinger F, Neumüller H (1982) Programmed stimulation for control of chronic pain and motor disease. Appl Neurophysiol 45: 102–111

Penn RD, Myklebust B, Gottlieb FL, Agarwal GC, Etzel M (1980) Chronic cerebellar stimulation for cerebral palsy. Prospective and double-blind studies. J Neurosurg 53: 160–165

Porter R (1984) Basal ganglia links for movement mood and memory (general discussion). Functions of the basal ganglia. Ciba Foundation Symposium 107. Pitman, London, pp 3–29

Schvarcz JR, Sica R, Morita E (1980) Chronic self-stimulation of the dentate nucleus for the relief of spasticity. Acta Neurochir 30 [Suppl]: 351–359

Schvarcz JR, Sica R, Morita E, Bronstein A, Sanz O (1982) Electrophysiological changes induced by chronic stimulation of the dentate nucleus for cerebral palsy. Appl Neurophysiol 45: 55–61

Sherrington CS (1898) Decerebrate rigidity and reflex coordination of movement. J Physiol (Lond) 22: 319–332

Siegfried J (1986) Effets de la stimulation du noyau sensitif du thalamus sur les dyskinesies et la spasticité. Rev Neurol (Paris) 142: 380–383

Siegfried J (1987) Stimulation of thalamic nuclei in human: sensory and therapeutical aspects. In: Besson JM, Guilbaud G, Peschanski M (eds) Thalamus and pain. Elsevier, Amsterdam New York Oxford, pp 271–278

Siegfried J, Comte P, Meier R (1983) Intracerebral electrode implantation system. J Neurosurg 59: 356–359

Siegfried J, Hood T (1985) Brain stimulation procedures in dystonic, hypertonic, dyskinetic and hyperkinetic conditions. In: Eccles J, Dimitrijevic M (eds) Recent achievements in restorative neurology. 1. Upper motor neuron functions and dysfunctions. Karger, Basel, pp 79–90

Siegfried J, Lazorthes Y (1985) La neurochirurgie fonctionnelle de l'infirmité motrice d'origine cérébrale. Neurochirurgie 31 [Suppl 1]: 1–118

Siegfried J, Pamir MN (1987) Electrical stimulation in human of the sensory thalamic nuclei and effects on dyskinesias and spasticity. In: Struppler A, Weindl A (eds) Clinical aspects of sensory motor integration. Springer, Berlin Heidelberg New York, pp 283–288

Snider RS (1974) Cerebellar modifications of abnormal discharges in cerebral sensory and motor areas. In: Cooper, Riklan, Snider (eds) The cerebellum, epilepsy and behavior. Plenum Publishing, New York, pp 3–18

Spiegel EA, Wycis HT, Marks M, Lee AJ (1947) Stereotaxic apparatus for operating on the human brain. Science 106: 349–350

Von Haller A (1766) Elementa physiologiae corporis humanis. In: Tomus quartus: cerebrum, nervi, musculi. Francisci Grasser, Lausanne

Correspondence: Prof. Dr. J. Siegfried, AMI Klinik Im Park, Seestrasse 220, CH-8002 Zürich, Switzerland

Intrathecal Baclofen administration for spasticity using implantable pumps

Pharmacological bases of intrathecal Baclofen administration

Ph. Decq and **Y. Keravel**

Hôpital Henri Mondor, Creteil, France

In 1912, Babinski wrote "I had often wondered, when faced with patients stricken by paraplegia with severe spasms, who seemed to have kept their full muscular strength, if it would not be feasible to try to eliminate the spasms by means of a surgical procedure directed at the posterior root; yet the fear of complications had always prevented me from carrying out this theory. Two years later, in 1908, Foerster was credited with the realization and implementation of the technique of the operation that now carries his name. This operation has been used mostly for the treatment of Little's disease and has quite often been successful. But this operation includes risks; *it would be abandoned without hesitation if some day a new substance were found capable of abolishing or diminishing the tendinous reflexia without side effects*" (Babinski 1912).

A specific GABA-B agonist (Jerusalem 1968): Baclofen, one of the most effective substance in the treatment of spasticity, was introduced in 1967 (Birkmayer et al. 1967) in the medical therapeutic armamentarium. Concerning severe spasticity, oral administration of Baclofen can lead to high doses with important side-effects. The reason is *the poor crossing of Baclofen through the blood-brain-barrier*. To get round this obstacle, R. Penn, in collaboration with J.S. Kroin, is proposed in 1984 a new treatment of spasticity by direct spinal intrathecal administration of Baclofen (Penn and Kroin 1985). The effectiveness of the method is linked with the presence of high concentration of GABA-B binding sites in the superficial layers of the posterior horn (Price et al. 1987). Moreover, it allows a dramatic decrease of the dose, from an average of 60 milligrammes/day in oral administration to an average of 100 microgrammes/day intrathecally. To avoid daily intrathecal injection by lumbar puncture, this method requires help from pump devices which have been previously used for regional chemotherapy. These devices are made up of a reservoir, which contains the drug and a propellant which provides the desired flow.

Plasma and CSF levels

It is known from animal experiments and studies in healthy volunteers that Baclofen given orally is rapidly and virtually completely absorbed from the gastro-intestinal tract. The plasma concentration in man reaches a peak level in about 2 hours, the half-life is 3–4 hours; most of the drug is excreted unchanged. The passage of the drug into the brain is very restricted. After an intra-venous bolus injection of 10 mg/kg of Baclofen, Faigle and Keberle found only a mean concentration of 0.5 µg/g (fresh weight) in the brain of different animals (Faigle and Keberle 1972).

Knutsson et al. (1974) presented in 1974 the first clinical pharmacokinetic study of Baclofen treatment in eleven spastic patients.

– At 10 mg given at 8, 12 and 18 h each day, four hours after the noon dose the mean plasma concentration was 102 ng/ml (50 to 203). The levels in CSF were below 12 ng/ml (the lowest concentration allowing quantitative determination) in 3 cases and between 13 to 27 ng/ml in others.

– At 20 mg × 3 per day, the average plasma level was 275 ng/ml (151 to 445). The concentration in CSF was below 12 ng/ml in 3 cases and in the remaining two, it was 20 and 64 ng/ml.

– 14 hours after the last dose, in patients with 10 mg × 3 per day, concentration was below 12 ng/ml in both plasma and CSF. In patients with 20 mg × 3 per day, levels were below 12 ng/ml in CSF and 19 to 143 ng/ml in the plasma.

Kroin and Penn (1988) performed a CSF pharmacokinetic study. Seven patients were given an intrathecal Baclofen bolus of 50 or 100 μg, depending upon how much effect the drug had on spastic problems. CSF samples were drawn at 30 min, 1 h, 2 h, 3 h and 4 h. After centrifugation, samples were directly injected into a HPLC (High Performance Liquid Chromatography) system. The quantitative analysis was by peak height with a detection limit in this assay of 30 ng/ml. The mean elimination half-life was about 90 min, the mean lumbar clearance was 39.2 ml/h and the mean volume of distribution was 85.6 ml. An additional bolus study included two patients that had incorrectly received a large bolus (2 and 4 mg) due to malfunction of a prototype pump. In this case, the mean elimination half-life was 4–6 h. In ten other patients who had been receiving continuous intrathecal Baclofen infusion for at least 48 h, simultaneous lumbar and cisternal CSF drug level in the spinal subarachnoïd space showed a 4-fold decrease as Baclofen ascends from the lower spinal region to the rostral limit of the spinal cord.

GABA-B receptors

A clear separation exists between receptors which recognize the antagonist Bicuculline and those that do not. These two classes have been designated GABA-A and GABA-B sites, respectively (Bormann 1988, Bowery et al. 1984). Baclofen has been shown to be a selective ligand for the bicuculline-insensitive GABA receptors (GABA-B) (Bowery et al. 1980).

The original idea of intrathecal administration of Baclofen was proposed by Penn before knowing the exact localization of GABA-B receptors in the spinal cord. The efficacy of the method is now better understood by the superficial localization of these receptors in the dorsal horn, quickly reached by the drug after a very short distance of tissue diffusion. GABA-B receptors, located by autoradiography, are present in high concentrations in laminae I, II, III and IV of the dorsal horn (Bowery et al. 1987), with a maximum concentration occurring in laminae II (Price et al. 1987). Much lower levels were detected in the ventral horns. GABA-A sites are more uniformly distributed throughout the dorsal and ventral horns (Bowery et al. 1984, 1987) (Table 1). Neonatal administration of

Table 1. GABA-A and GABA-B binding site distribution in the rat spinal cord p mol/g wet wt

Spinal cord region	GABA-A	GABA-B
Marginal layer	0.81 + 0.13	2.22 + 0.34
Substantia gelatinosa	0.94 + 0.20	12.13 + 0.14
Lamina x and intermediate larger	5.36 + 1.88	5.43 + 0.74
Ventral horn	2.23 + 0.74	2.15 + 0.35

Bowery et al. (1987)

Capsaicin reduces, by 40–50%, the GABA-B binding sites (Price et al. 1984). Unilateral rhizotomy reduces the number of GABA-B sites in the dorsal horn without affecting levels in the ventral horn. The greatest reduction occurred in lamina II with 18% loss 2 days after surgery, 23% after 4 days, 25% after 6 days and 48% after 15 days. This change after 15 days is comparable to that produced 4 months after neonatal capsaicin treatment. The only apparent difference between rhizotomy and capsaicin treatment occurred is lamina IV where rhizotomy produced a greater reduction than capsaicin (Price et al. 1987). This would support the view that up to 50% of GABA-B binding sites are located on nerve terminals.

Chronic, high-level exposure to Baclofen led to a down-regulation of GABA-B receptor numbers in the rat spinal cord (Kroin et al. 1989). Using osmotic minipumps, normal rats were infused intrathecally with Baclofen (0.5 μg/h) for four weeks. In the substantia gelatinosa, the number of sites was reduced by 36% in the Baclofen infused animals as compared to the control group.

GABA-B receptors have been linked to the blockage of voltage-gated Ca^{++} channels (Bormann 1988, Dolphin and Scott 1987) or increase in K^+ conductance (Grahwiler and Brown 1985). The coupling to either K^+ or Ca^{++} ionophores is mediated by pertussis toxin-sensitive G proteins (Bormann 1988, Innis et al. 1988).

Baclofen antagonism

One major concern in intrathecal Baclofen use is pharmacological complication, and thus specific treatment for an inadvertent overdose.

Intravenous Physostigmine (2 mg) was reported to reverse the respiratory depression and somnolence due to Baclofen overdose in 3 patients (Müller-Schwefe and Penn 1989). In animal experiments, Physostigmine (0.1 mg/kg I.V.) maintained an adequate respiratory rate when given at 30 minutes intervals to dogs which had received 50–400 mg Baclofen intracisternally (Müller-Schwefe et al. 1989). Physostigmine has been proposed based upon its its clinical effect in opiates overdose, but it is not a specific GABA-B antagonist.

In 1987, a specific GABA-B receptor antagonist, Phaclofen, was made available (Kerr et al. 1987). Pre-administration of large doses of Phaclofen could block the effects of Baclofen on central respiratory activity of rabbits (Schmidet et al. 1989). One year later, a new antagonist, 2-Hydroxy-Saclofen was introduced and reported to be more effective than Phaclofen (Kerr et al. 1988). 2-Hydroxy-Saclofen reversibly reduced the Baclofen mediated presynaptic reduction of the monosynaptic excitation by impulses from primary afferent fibres of the rat (Curtis et al. 1988).

Recently, Benzofuran analogues of Baclofen have been reported as a new class of GABA-B receptor antagonist (Kerr et al. 1989).

References

See pages 115, 116

Correspondence: Dr. Ph. Decq, Service de Neurochirurgie Hôpital Henri Mondor, F-94010 Creteil, France

CSF pharmacokinetic of intrathecal Baclofen administration

B. Sallerin-Caute and **Y. Lazorthes** with the collaboration of **R. Bastide**

Department of Neurosurgery, Hôpital de Rangueil, Toulouse, France

For the achievement of an optimal pharmacotherapy with intrathecal Baclofen, an analysis of the relationships between therapeutic effects and frug concentration in CSF may be valuable. We had previously developed a sensitive method for the measurement of Baclofen concentration in human CSF (Sallerin-Caute et al. 1988). The present pharmacokinetic study was carried out within the framework of a clinical investigation (see chapter by Lazorthes and Verdié).

Four patients, with severe spasticity, were selected for this pharmacokinetic study. Baclofen was injected into the subarachnoïd space via the programmable pump and CSF samples (0, 5 ml) were collected via an implantable drug site at 0, 5; 1; 2; 2, 5; 3; 4; 5; 8; 11; 15; 18; 24 hours after administration. The samples were immediately frozen and kept in a deep-freeze at −20°C until analysis. Baclofen levels were determined by High Performance Liquid Chromatography (HPLC) as previously reported (Sallerin-Caute et al. 1988). HPLC analysis revealed the presence of a single peak which corresponded to the real Baclofen concentration without interference from any endogenous CSF material.

The time course of CSF Baclofen concentrations is given in Fig. 1.

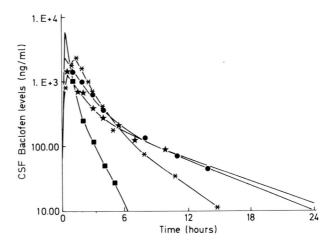

Fig. 1. Time course of CSF Baclofen concentrations. Baclofen CSF concentration falls in accordance with a bi-exponential model. During the first four hours, Baclofen decreased rapidly with distribution half-lives of 0.2, 0.8, 0.95 and 1 hours. The elimination half-lives are 0.9, 2.4, 4.7 and 5 hours. The clearances calculated from the area under the graph are 0.012 l/h to 0.08 l/h. The V.D. calculated from the elimination phase is variable from 0.05 to 0.16 liters. These results show that there is a great variability of kinetic parameters for each patient

References

See pages 115, 116

Correspondence: Dr. B. Sallerin-Caute, Centre Hospitalier de Rangueil, Av. Jean Poulhes, F-31054 Toulouse, France

Drug pump technical description, operative procedure and post-operative management

Ph. Decq and **Y. Keravel**

Hôpital Henri Mondor, Creteil, France

Implantable drug pumps: technical description

Results of publications describing intratechal administration of Baclofen emphasize that the most effective method of infusion is continuous rather than the bolus administration (Lazorthes 1988, Müller et al. 1987, Penn 1988). Two kinds of implantable drug pumps, permitting continuous infusion, are today available for Baclofen intra-thecal administration, a gas driven pump (Infusaid 400®)* and an electronic pump (Synchromed®)**.

1. The Infusaid 400 pump

The principles on which the pump works were devised by Blackshear et al. (1972). The pump is manufactured by Infusaid Inc. The first clinical trials were conducted in 1982 for regional chemotherapy of hepatic metastases (Colbert, et al. 1948, Ensminger et al. 1981).

The pump consists of a titanium reservoir which is divided into two chambers by an impermeable diaphragm and welded to a metal bellow (Fig. 1). The outer chamber contains a fluid such as Treon which can vaporize at body temperature. The inner chamber is an expandable drug chamber that can be filled through an inlet silicone septum by a trans-cutaneous injection. The silicone membrane should be punctered with a Huber needle to avoid damaging it. The volume change of the vaporizing fluid exerts a constant pressure on the inner chamber (whatever the inner chamber volume) and leads to a slow expulsion of the drug through a capillary tube rolled around the body of the pump. Its length (several meters) determines the flow rate.

The filling of the pump increases the volume of the inner chamber and decreases the volume of the outer one by a pressure induced phase shift back to the liquid state. The two phase changing fluid is thus compressed. The result is a constant pressure on the inner chamber by the gas which leads to a slow expulsion of the drug. The outflow is always constant because the decreasing of the outer chamber pressure is directly proportional to the decreasing of the inner chamber volume. This source of energy is theoretically inexhaustible.

The outflow is governed by Poiseuille law: $Q = \pi D^4 \Delta P / 128 \, \mu l$ ($\pi = 3, 14$, $D =$ inner diameter of the capillary catheter, $l =$ length of the capillary catheter, $P =$ differential pressure between the inner chamber and the tip of the catheter, $\mu =$ the drug viscosity).

The desired outflow (1 to 6 ml per day) is adjusted in the factory by varying the lengths of the capillary tubing, depending on the outside pressure (vein, artery, subarachnoïd space) and the drug viscosity. After implantation, outflow variations may occur in case of fever (modifications of body temperature) or high altitude [atmospheric pressure variations (Fig. 2)]. The drug dose is adjusted by modifying the drug concentration at the time of refilling.

Zierski and Müller (1988) reported 2 cases of pump failures in their experience of 73 pumps implanted for pain and spasticity. In both cases, their conclusion was that "the source of failure was obstruction of the outflow from the pump, caused probably by an obstruction within the resistance capillaries".

---

* Infusaid, 1400 Providence Highway, Norwood, MA 02062, USA

** Medtronic 7000 Central Avenue NE, Mineapolis, MN 55432, USA.

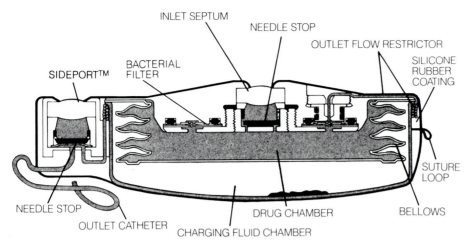

Fig. 1. The Infusaid implantable Pump contains an inexhaustible power supply. The desired drug is contained within an expandable titanium reservoir. During filling, the bellows expands compressing the two-phase charging fluid, then compresses the bellows forcing the drug through a membrane filter and preset flow restrictor. The cycle repeats itself each time the pump is refilled

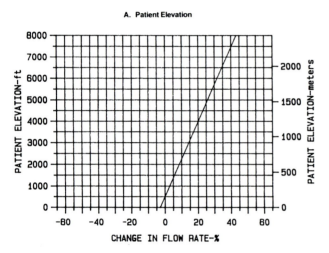

Fig. 2. Outflow variations with altitude

2. The Synchromed pump

This pump, manufactured by Medtronic Corp. is an implantable, battery-powered device that stores the drug and dispenses it according to instructions received from the programmer.

Each pump contains a collapsible 18 ml drug reservoir, microprocessor-based circuitry, lithium thionyl-chloride battery, antenna, acoustic transducer, peristaltic pump, bioretentive filter through which the drug passes as it leaves the drug reservoir and a fill port with a self-sealing septum and needle stop.

The pump has three sealed chambers: one contains the drug reservoir, the second an hybrid electronic module and battery, and the third a peristaltic pump. The peristaltic positive displacement pump forces the drug from the reservoir through a bacterial filter and

silicone rubber tubing into a catheter to the administration site. The pump is driven by an integral step motor which is controlled by pulses from a battery-powered hybrid electronic control. The electric circuitry adjusts the fluid delivery rate by altering the frequency of control pulses (Fig. 3).

This pump will provide chronic infusion for about four years at typical dosage regimens. Penn has changed one of his first pumps after five years. The pump utilizes a 0.22 micron bacterial retentive filter in the fluid pathway to prevent the transmission of contaminants.

The Synchromed pump utilizes a miniature peristaltic pump which provides a delivery accuracy of $+/- 15\%$. The flow accuracy measured at the catheter tip is $\pm 15\%$ under the following conditions: $35\,°C$ to $42\,°C$, with back pressure of 0 to 300 mm Hg, and 0 to approximately 1230 meters elevation. The freon-like gas within the outer chamber aids the emptying of the reservoir only as the volume approaches the 2 cc limit. In certain pumps the expansion of the gas causes a deflection of the back surface of the reservoir and as the reservoir volume approaches the last 2 cc's (only in these specific pumps) the flow rate and efficacy will appear to be reduced.

Five units were used to compare fluid output at different reservoir volumes (especially low volume). All pumps were kept at normal operating temperature $(37\,°C \pm 2°)$ and atmospheric pressure. The test was repeated three times. The results showed that the pumps stayed within the tolerance at reservoir volumes between 18 to 3.5 ml's. The pumps started to fail the 15% limit between 3.5 to 2 ml. The pump output dropped significantly below 2 ml volumes.

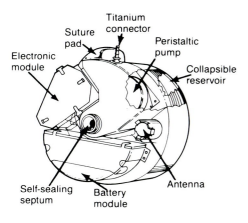

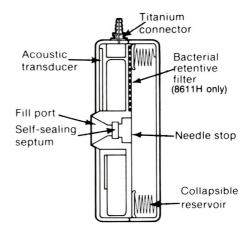

Fig. 3. The synchromed pump

Therefore, the patient may feel a diminished efficacy of the Baclofen treatment when the pump reservoir volume is below 3.5 ml but this is not inevitable for all pumps unless the volume is below 2 ml.

The minimum infusion rate of the device is of 0.096 ml per day (0.004 ml per hour). When the pump is in its "stop" mode, the rotor is still functioning at its mechanical and electrical minimum. In order to ensure that absolutely no drug is being delivered the pump reservoir must be emptied and eventually rinsed with saline solution. The reason for the pump's continuous function is to assure control of the leak rate, which under these conditions is never above a maximum of 5 mcl/hr (it is usually less than 1 mcl/hr).

Baclofen solutions have maintained > 90% stability (HPLC Analysis) following 16 weeks of exposure to Synchromed systems maintained under clinical conditions.

The programming feature allows the physician to achieve optimal spasticity relief and minimal side-effects without reformulating the drug concentration or changing the reservoir contents (Fig. 4).

3. Comparisons of specifications

	Synchromed	Infusaid
External properties:		
Material	Titanium	Titanium
Thickness	27.5 mm	28 mm
Weight (empty)	185 g	208 g
Diameter	70 mm	87 mm
Drug reservoir		
Material	Titanium	Titanium
Usable capacity	18 ml	47 ml
Dead space	2.4 ml (max.)	3.5 ml
Power source	Lithium thionyl-chloride battery	changing fluid
Flow rate	0.004 ml/hr (4 mcl/hr or 0.096 ml/day) to 0.9 ml/hr.	fixed between 1 and 6 ml/day
Device life	44 months (nominal) at a flow rate of 0.5 ml/day	limited only by puncture life of septum (~2000)

Infusion Mode	Drug is Dispensed	Graphic Representation of the Infusion Mode
Bolus	Once, at a prescribed dose for a specified time.	Bolus
Continuous	Continuously, at a specified rate.	Continuous
Continuous-Complex	Continuously, in a series of 2-10 steps for specified times. The example shows two five-step cycles.	Continuous-Complex
Bolus-Delay	Intermittently, at a prescribed dose and at specified intervals.	Bolus-Delay

Fig. 4. Graphic representation of infusion modes possible with the implanted Synchromed pump

4. Other implantable pumps in test phase

1) Minimed programmable pump (insulin).
2) Siemens programmable pump (insulin).

3) Infusaid model 1000 programmable pump (insulin, chemotherapy).
4) Cormed.
5) Travenol.

5. *Conclusion*

For numerous authors, a programmable implantable pump is the most convenient device for intrathecal Baclofen administration because of its ability to adjust as frequently as desired the flow rate non-invasively through programming.

In fact, after the pump implantation, it is not always so easy to immediatly find the right dose. We often have to look for it because the result of the initial trial with bolus doses is different from the result obtained with a continuous infusion. Moreover the dose increases with time and it is sometimes very useful to vary the dose during day and night, using a continuous complex infusion mode.

Operative procedure

Patients with severe, stabilized spasticity due to spinal cord injury or multiple sclerosis and refractory to orally administred Baclofen are candidates for intrathecal administration of Baclofen.

Patients with psychological disorder or who cannot understand this mode of treatment have to be excluded. Lastly, regular intervals of refilling and theoretical dangers of overdoses require a certain geographic dependance.

1. *Initial trial*

To evaluate the efficacy of intrathecal Baclofen infusion, pump implantation must be preceded by intrathecal lumbar injection of incremental bolus doses of Baclofen.

The screening doses range from an initial start dose of 25 mcg to 100 mcg with incremental steps of 25 mcg. This can be performed in the following three ways:
  – by direct lumbar puncture;
  – via an external intrathecal lumbar catheter; its main risk is meningitis, which increases with the trial duration;
  – by implantation of an intrathecal lumbar access site. This system lowers the risk of infection during a long trial period. It is better to wait for cicatrization to eliminate any interference with the trial. In addition,

the pump can be fixed direct to the access site avoiding the implantation of a new lumbar intrathecal catheter (This can also be done with the Infusaid pump system). However, an access site independent of the pump infusion system is also of interest, allowing subsequent sampling of cerebro-spinal fluid (CSF) for pharmacological evaluations.

The intrathecal catheter is positioned under fluoroscopic control. The distal end of the catheter should be placed at the level of the conus medullaris, between T10 and L2.

2. *Pump implantation*

After the trial, the selected patients have a pump implanted. Each kind of pump requires specific technical details for implantation which are explained in the technical manual delivered with each pump. The implantation can be performed under regional anaesthesia (regional block with local anaesthesia at the lumbar puncture point) or under general anaesthesia (on request of the patient or, above all, in case of excessive rigidity in flexion).

The pump is implanted subcutaneously in the right or left abdomen where there is sufficient skin and subcutaneous tissue to support the implanted system. The site of the pump is determined with consideration of skin integrity, cosmesis, patient activity, clothing and belt lines.

In lateral recumbent position the patient is prepped and draped, exposing both the pump site and the catheterization site. This allows for simultaneous pump pocket preparation and catheterization if desired.

The catheter is placed into the intrathecal space in the lumbar region with a Tuohy needle. The tip of the catheter must be placed under fluoroscopy. For spasticity of the lower limbs, the best level is between T10 and L2, at the level of the conus medullaris. During the entire procedure it is important to observe after each step a CSF back flow to confirm placement and patency of the catheter.

Some anchors have been designed to insure catheter fixation and to prevent excessive tension or angulation of the catheter. Absence of anchors may lead to catheter migration; but presence of anchors may lead to catheter kinking.

The catheter is then tunneled subcutaneously to the pocket site. A subcutaneous pocket is prepared in the abdomen in which the pump should fit snugly.

The pump must be implanted less than 2.5 cm from the surface of the skin. Pocket hematoma and extensive trauma and devitalization of subcutaneous tissue fat must be avoided. Careful attention must be paid to keep wound infection to a minimum. Short-term prophylactic antibiotics (used as for shunt procedures) can be useful.

Post-operative management

During the first week after implantation, the flow rate is adjusted through programming to achieve a optimal clinical response. Then the autonomy is calculated from knowing the daily dose and the drug concentration of the solution used. Two Baclofen concentrations are avaible: 500 and 2000 micro-grammes per ml. The choice depends on pump technical properties, pump accuracy and the pro-grammed daily dose. The need for refilling is a restriction for the patient and the medical team and this points to one of the limits of the method compared with the other surgical procedures.

Complications and failure of intrathecal adminis-tration of Baclofen are described with the results in the following two chapters (see chapters sixteen and seventeen).

One of the major technical problem is what to do when an abrupt increase of spasticity occurs during long-term intrathecal treatment:

1. X-ray controls look for mechanical catheter complications: migration or kinking.

2. Amplifier check will ensure that the pump works.

3. Programmer gives information about battery power.

4. Emptying the pump permits one to compare the real residual volume to the residual volume indicated by the programmer. This provides informations about pump accuracy.

5. Lumbar injection of a bolus (25 to 100 microgrammes) of Baclofen by direct lumbar puncture will lead to disappearance of spasticity in case of mechanical catheter complication. In that case, after a careful examination of X-rays, myelography can be performed. It assesses the permeability of the catheter and the sub-arachnoid space. It can be done by puncture at a site placed between the pump and its catheter. If there is no such site, it can be done operatively by disconnection of the pump catheter.

Another way is to fill the pump with a radio-isotope after it is first emptied of drug and the reservoir flushed with saline solution.

References
See pages 115, 116

Correspondence: Dr. Ph. Decq, Service de Neurochirurgie Hôpital Henri Mondor, F-94010 Creteil, France

Intrathecal infusion of baclofen for spasticity: the RUSH and the US multicenter studies

R.D. Penn

Department of Neurosurgery, Rush-Presbyterian-St. Luke's Medical Center, Chicago, Illinois, U.S.A.

The ideal treatment for spasticity should have the following characteristics. First, it should not damage any part of the nervous system which is functioning normally or has the potential for recovery. Thus, motor and sensory pathways would remain intact so that no further neurological loss would be inflicted by the treatment. Second, it should be reversible, so that as the degree of spasticity changes, the treatment could be adjusted appropriately. A corollary is that it should be effective with mild spasticity as well as the most severe. Third, it should involve as little surgical intervention as possible because of the already compromised medical status of the patient. Finally, there should be a way to test if it will work before employing the technique.

Seven years ago, the possibility of such a solution for spasticity seemed remote; complex destructive operations were the only alternative for patients who had failed to respond adequately to oral antispastic agents. Many patients were left untreated because the operations available seemed too major for their debilitated state or the expertise for doing such operations was not available. Today, the situation has changed dramatically. Introduced in 1984 (Penn et al. 1985), intrathecal baclofen infused by implanted drug pump has now been proven to be safe and effective, and meet the criteria for the ideal treatment just outlined. It was apparent from the first intrathecal injection of microgram quantities of baclofen, that this $GABA_B$ agonist has profound effects on the spinal cord circuits underlying the spastic state (Penn et al. 1984). Unlike oral administration which may improve spasticity by at most two points on the Ashworth scale, intrathecal baclofen was found to reduce muscle tone to normal in patients with even the worst rigidity. In fact, the worse the initial rigidity the more dramatic the effect (Penn et al. 1987). After working with implanted drug pumps, it also became clear that the amount of rigidity needed for function could be obtained by precise adjustment of dose. Furthermore, in some patients reducing spasticity unmasked normal patterns of voluntary motor control.

These assertions about the effects of intrathecal baclofen are based on experience treating patients in the US and in Europe. This article will present the US results.

I. The Rush clinical trial of intrathecal baclofen*

Once the effectiveness of bolus intrathecal baclofen had been demonstrated, the suitability of implanted drug pumps for long-term treatment had to be established. We initiated such an open prospective study in 1984 and have entered twenty nine patients each of whom has been followed at least 12 months. A well defined patient population was chosen because many different types of spasticity exist and for a beginning study we wanted to limit the variables caused by widely differing pathology. Thus, the patients had spinal cord injury (SCI) or multiple sclerosis (MS) primarily with cord involvement; severe spasms and rigidity; and the signs of spasticity which included hyperactive phasic reflexes, clonus and/or Babinski signs. All had failed to improve significantly on maximum tolerated doses of oral antispastic agents including baclofen. Patients had to be willing to return

---

* *The Rush Spasticity Project*: D. Corcos, Ph.D.; G. Gottlieb, Ph.D.; J.S. Kroin, Ph.D.; S.A. Kroin, Can. Phil.; M. Latash, M.S.; J.M. Magolan, M.N.S.; B. Parke, M.D.; S.M. Savoy, M.N.S.

to Rush regularly for refills of the pump and evaluations. Twenty patients also volunteered for the randomized double-blind trial. The investigational plan was as follows:

Patient selection

1. Criteria for inclusion:
   a. Males and females between 18 and 65 years of age.
   b. A patient diagnosis of severe chronic spasticity due to a cord trauma or multiple sclerosis.
   c. The patient's spasticity has been refractory to orally administered baclofen or side-effects have been unacceptable at an effective dose.
   d. The patient's spasticity has stabilized.
   e. The patient has adequate CSF flow as determined by myelogram or other studies.
   f. Prior to implantation of the SynchroMed™ pump, the patient must have responded to a single dose of 100 μg or less of intrathecal baclofen.
   g. The patient has voluntarily signed the Informed Consent Form after its contents have been fully explained.
2. Criteria for exclusion:
   a. The patient has an implanted programmable medical device; e.g. cardiac pacemaker.
   b. The patient is pregnat or is not using an adequate method of birth control (if not menopausal).
   c. The patient has a psychological disorder which may interfere with the collection or interpretation of the study data.
   d. The patient is unable to give informed consent or understand this mode of treatment.
   e. The patient has a history of hypersensitivity to baclofen.
   f. The patient has a history of impaired renal function, severe hepatic or gastrointestinal disease.
   g. The patient has had a cerebral stroke.

Patient population

Thirty-one patients with severe disabling spasms entered the study. Two of the patients who were screened with bolus intrathecal baclofen and responded, declined a pump implant because baclofen did not change their deafferentation pain due to the spinal injury, which was their primary concern. Of the remaining twenty-nine long term patients, fifteen had spinal cord injuries and fourteen multiple sclerosis (Table 1). All patients had long-standing spasticity which significantly interfered with their activities of daily living and could not be controlled by oral doses of antispastic medications. They had marked rigidity (Ashworth $\bar{x} = 3.9$) and frequent, severe muscle spasms (spasm score $\bar{x} = 3.3$) despite oral baclofen doses averaging 83 mg/day (range 15–200). Higher doses were not tolerated because of drowsiness or confusion. The multiple sclerosis patients primarily had spinal involvement with, at most, mild cerebellar or cognitive deficits. One of these patients was ambulatory for short distances with crutches, while the rest were wheelchair bound. The spinal cord trauma patients had injuries in the midcervical to midthoracic levels. While one patient was ambulatory for short distances with crutches, the remainder were wheelchair bound with minimal voluntary motor control in lower extremities. All study patients were functionally dependent, unable to dress themselves or provide other self-care.

Screening phase

Each patient was screened with lumbar intrathecal bolus doses of baclofen beginning with 50 μg. If there was no response to this dose, 75 μg was administered, and if no response 100 μg, the maximum screening dose, was administered. Patients who did not respond or had any adverse reactions were to be removed from the study. Those responding with no untoward effects were offered the opportunity of having a SynchroMed™ pump implanted. All patients who were screened responded. As mentioned above, two elected not to participate in the study because pain was not relieved.

Implantation

The pump was implanted in the abdominal wall and attached to a lumbar subarachnoid catheter planted under fluoroscopic control. All operations were done under local or regional anaesthesia. Details of the operation are provided in previous publications.

Dose finding

Following implantation, the pump was filled with baclofen and programmed to deliver a continuous

Table 1. RUSH – patient characteristics

Pt	Dx	Age/Sex	Max Oral mg/d Baclofen	Initial Ashworth	Initial Spasm	Ash.	Last Fill Spasm	Up Months
1	SCI	42/F	15	5	5	1	1	58
2	SCI	19/F	80	5	5	3.25	4	58
3	MS	53/F	60	4.4	3	1.75	1	58
4	MS	35/F	100	4	4	1	0	56
5	MS	39/F	80	4.1	0	1.0	1	55
6	SCI	22/F	100	4.6	5	1	1.5	50
7	SCI	NA/M	80	1.3	4	1	0	43
8	SCI	40/F	40	1.3	4	1	0	38
9	MS	53/M	80	4.75	4	1	0	34
10	MS	60/F	60	4.25	4	1	0	30
11	MS	39/F	80	5	0	1	0	25
12	MS	40/F	80	4.4	2	1	0	24
13	MS	44/F	60	4.75	3	1.37	2	25
14	SCI	42/M	160	5	4	1	1	23
15	SCI	25/M	80	2.1	3	1	0	23
16	SCI	36/F	120	5	3	1	0	22
17	SCI	41/F	80	5	3	1	0	20
18	SCI	37/M	80	2.25	3	1	0	19
19	SCI	45/M	80	4.4	2	1.5	0	18
20	SCI	49/M	200	2.4	2	1	0	17
21	MS	42/M	60	4.75	4	1	0	16
22	MS	40/M	100	2.8	4	1.25	1	17
23	MS	48/F	40	4.8	4	1.12	0	15
24	SCI	22/M	80	2.8	4	1	0	15
25	MS	59/M	80	4.1	4	1	1	12
26	SCI	29/M	160	4.4	4	1	2	12
27	MS	31/F	65	3.5	3	1	0	11
28	SCI	25/M	150	4.5	3.5	1	1	5
29	MS	45/F	120	4	1	1	0	0

daily dose equivalent to one and one-half to two times the bolus dose. During the immediate post-operative period this dose was gradually adjusted until muscle tone was brought to normal and spasms stopped. Steps of 20 to 30% were made every 24 hours as needed. After discharge, patients returned at three to six week intervals for pump refills, dose adjustments and safety and efficacy ratings. A subset of 20 patients from this study consented to participate in a double-blind crossover study that was conducted during the interval between screening and discharge.

Test materials and protocol approval

Baclofen U.S.P. was supplied in powder form by CIBA-GEIGY Corporation, Summit, New Jersey. Baclofen (1 mg/ml) solutions in 0.9% sodium chloride injection were prepared in the hospital pharmacy at Rush-Presbyterian- St. Luke's Medical Center using aseptic technique. The 1 mg/ml solution was further diluted to appropriate volume with normal saline. The protocol was approved by both the Human Investigation Committe at Rush and the FDA. Each patient signed an informed consent form.

Table 2. Ashworth scale for measuring muscle tone

Grade	Degree of muscle tone
1	No increase in tone
2	Slight increase in tone, giving a "catch" when affected part is moved in flexion or extension
3	More marked increase in tone, but affected part easily flexed
4	Considerable increase in tone; passive movement difficult
5	Affected part rigid in flexion or extension

Spasm frequency scale

Grade	frequency of spasms
0	No spasms
1	Mild spasms induced by stimulation
2	Infrequent full spasms occurring less than once per hour
3	Spasms occurring more than once per hour
4	Spasms occurring more than ten times per hour

Efficacy measurements

Efficacy assessments consisted of examinations to gauge rigidity using the five-point Ashworth scale and spasms using a five-point spasm scale (Table 2). The Ashworth score was taken as the sum of scores at the hip (abduction and flexion), knee and ankle joint on both sides, divided by eight since in some patients the spasticity was not equal to both sides or at all three joints.

Patient disposition

All but one patient is still being followed at the present time. He died six months ago of aspiration pneumonia due to the progress of his multiple sclerosis. This respiratory problem was unrelated to his baclofen treatment.

Efficacy results

As a group, rigidity was reduced to normal after baclofen initiation and has been maintained in the normal range throughout the study. The MS patients had a pre-study average Ashworth score of 4.3 and an average score of 1.5 at the three month follow-up and an average 1.1 at their last follow-up. SCI patients had an initial average Ashworth score of 3.6 which was followed by a similar reduction in score subsequent to baclofen administration (Fig. 1).

In MS patients who were symptomatic, spasms were reduced from a mean of 3.0 to 1.0 or less. A similar pattern was observed for SCI patients, falling from 3.4 initially to 1.0 or lower at the last follow-up (Fig. 2).

Uniformly, patients have reported better sleeping patterns because of reduced spasms (Penn 1988). Improvements in activities of daily living have been described in detail elsewhere (Parke et al. 1989).

Dose adjustments

Over the first twelve months the dosage necessary to maintain normal tone and reduced spasms has gradually increased. Overall, the dosage then remained constant (Fig. 3). However, in four patients the dosage continued to increase to the 600–800 µg/day range. This required inconvenient, frequent refills. To manage this problem "drug holidays" were used. Morphine was substituted for baclofen for several weeks, and the baclofen restarted (Table 3). This strategy was used

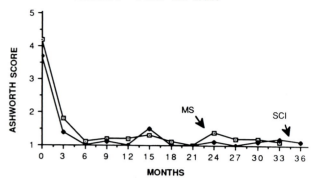

Fig. 1. Graph of the average reduction in muscle tone over 36 months of baclofen infusion in two patient groups, MS and SCI. Time O represents the value prior to baclofen treatment

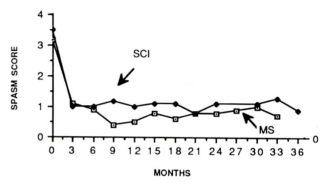

Fig. 2. Graph of the average reduction in spasms over 36 months of baclofen infusion in two patient groups, MS and SCI. Time O represents the value prior to baclofen treatment

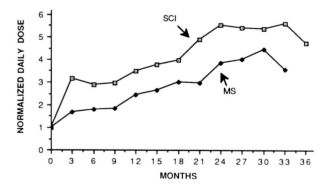

Fig. 3. Normalized dosage for the combined MS and SCI groups

six times in the four patients and in three patients it was successful. The last patient was unusual in that his spasticity pre-operatively showed wide fluctuations. Attempting to control him with a steady dose

Table 3. Baclofen "holidays"

Pt. No.	Duration (Weeks)	Pre-Holiday			Post-Holiday		
		Dose	Ashworth	Spasms	Dose	Ashworth	Spasm
1	7	836	1	2	310	1	1
1	8	588	1	2	251	1	2
2	2	757	1	5	340	1	2
2	1*	659	3.3	3	497	1	2
3	3	848	4.75	2.5	406	1.5	0
15	12	698	1	3	300	1	0

* Dilaudid

Table 4. Adverse drug reactions

Pt	Date	Dose (μg)	Description	Resolution
1	4/18/86	717	Mild light headedness Occasional blurred vision Nystagmus with lateral gaze	Decrease dose to 622 μg
17	6/19/87 (within 1 hr of implant)	Bolus dose unknown	Nystagmus Double vision Light-headedness Orthostatic hypotension Cerebellar dysmetria	Resolved without intervention
		335	Drowsiness Dry Mouth	Dose reduced to 306 μg
19	8/27/87 (within 1 hr of implant)	Bolus dose unknown	Double vision	Resolved without intervention
23	11/20/87	253	Drowsiness	Reduced to 215 μg
26	4/29/88	252	Dry Mouth	No attempt to resolve

of baclofen was difficult and lead to a high daily rate. He was provided with a programmer and instructed to give himself baclofen only when the spasms or rigidity occurred. With this flexibility he has achieved good control at lower dosages, ranging from 400 to 600 μg per day.

Half of our patients employ the complex mode of delivery. Lower rates are used during the day so that more muscle tone is preserved for motor function. At night the dose is increased to reduce muscle spasms which might otherwise interfere with sleep. The ability to titrate dose precisely and vary it in a circadian rhythm may account for the excellent control we have achieved and why baclofen has not interrupted functional activities or created muscle weakness.

Adverse drug reactions and pump and catheter complications

Several minor adverse drug reactions were observed during the study (Table 4). These were either transient and resolved on their own, resolved with a dose reduction or no attempt was made to resolve them. Two drug overdoses occurred. Both patients became comatose and were hospitalized with respiratory support. They recovered without complications within 3 days and were restarted on baclofen once the source of the problem with the pumps was identified (Penn et al. 1987). At the time we did not realize that physostigmine might be helpful as an antidote, so it was not used (Müller-Schwefe et al. 1989). The original pump design was modified following the overdoses and no further serious medication problems have occurred.

System complications are listed in Table 5. Two pumps have stalled, one pump developed a telemetry failure and one pump had an alarm occurring intermittently. All were replaced under local anaesthesia without further complications. In two patients after 4.3 years the battery in the pump became depleted and the pumps were replaced with new ones. The expected battery life is between 4–5 years. Most of the

Table 5. Complications

I System	Frequency
a) catheter kink	4
b) catheter break	1
c) pump stall	2
d) pump overinfusion	2
e) intermittant alarming	1
f) pump telemetry failure	1
II Procedural complications	
a) catheter disconnection	2
b) catheter dislodgment	1
c) catheter cut	1
d) pocket revision	2
e) infection	0

pump failures were in earlier models; the new version appears to function with a very low failure rate, close to that of cardiac pacemakers. As would be anticipated, a number of catheter dislodgments and kinks have occurred. Three patients were doing strenuous stretching exercises including yoga, and wheelchair karate, when the catheters pulled out of the subarachnoid space. Better anchoring procedures have solved these problem and the patients remain active. Procedural complications due to surgery are also listed in Table 5. These occurred primarily in the earlier patients before the implant technique was fully developed.

Motor laboratory studies

Beside clinical evaluations of rigidity and spasms, quantitative testing of reflexes and voluntary motor control were performed. These results are detailed elsewhere (Latash et al. 1989) but should be mentioned briefly. In a number of patients we were able to demonstrate an improvement in the pattern of voluntary muscle activation when baclofen suppressed abnormal reflex activity. Figure 4 shows such a test. Prior to baclofen an attempt at movement produces marked coactivation of agonist and antagonist muscle groups. After baclofen selective muscle activation can occur. This unmasking of normal motor function by reducing spasticity has important implications for patient rehabilitation. In part, it explains the improvement in activities of daily living which has been achieved after the spasticity has been eliminated.

Double-blind study

Twenty of the patients entered a randomized balanced double-blind crossover study. The results of

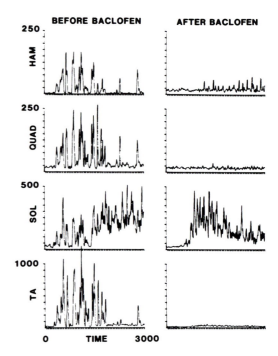

Fig. 4. EMG activity during voluntary activation of ankle extensors. Before intrathecal baclofen (left) all four muscle groups are coactivated. After baclofen (right) a more selective activation of the soleus muscle occurs

this trial have been recently published (Penn et al. 1989). Intrathecal baclofen infusion was compared to saline. The Ashworth and spasms scores were each reduced by 3 grades during the baclofen periods in both the multiple sclerosis and the spinal cord injury groups. The significance value for change was $P < 0.005$. This makes intrathecal baclofen the only surgical procedure which has been shown to be effective in blinded controlled tests with objective outcome measures.

II. The US multicenter studies

As it became apparent that intrathecal baclofen might be a useful treatment for spasticity, two multicenter studies were designed and initiated: an European one and an American one. The US study, due to a number of logistical problems, has only been in progress for less than a year. To date, thirteen patients have been screened and twelve implanted with an average follow up of 4 months. So far, the results seem similar to the Rush series. Figure 5 shows the screening results on all thirteen patients. A marked reduction in Ashworth and spasm scores is seen, the same magnitude as the Rush findings. If the Rush series, the two multicenter studies and Müller's series

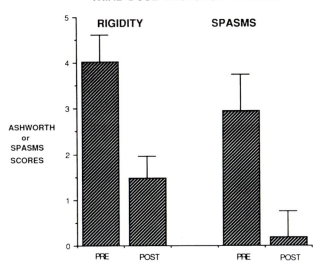

MULTICENTER STUDY

TRIAL DOSE RESPONSE -4 HOURS

Fig. 5. Ashworth and spasms scores of the thirteen patients in the U.S. multicenter study. Note dramatic decrease in rigidity and spasms 4 hours after bolus of 50–75 μg of intrathecal baclofen

with the nonprogrammable pump are combined, approximately three hundred patients have now been tested. In all of these, spasticity of spinal cord injury has responded well to baclofen.

Conclusions

The goals for treatment of spasticity which were enumerated at the beginning of this chapter have been met by the use of intrathecal baclofen for severe spinal spasticity. Because a drug is delivered by a programmable pump, dosage can be adjusted to precisely meet the patient's needs. No damage has occurred to the nervous system so motor and sensory function remain intact. If spasticity increases or decreases, even during daily cycles, baclofen infusion can be modulated accordingly. Prior to implantation, a test dose can be given to predict the response and to provide a trial so the patient can understand what can and cannot be achieved by the infusion. Finally, the implantation of the catheter and pump is done under local anaesthesia and is well tolerated even by severely debilitated patients.

Th drug pump and catheter systems have caused a number of difficulties. As experience has been gained the surgical complication rate has declined markedly and the implantation system has been improved. It is

noteworthy that all the Rush patients who have been implanted continue to be treated successfully. Even if a serious problem occurred they insisted on keeping the system so that treatment could be reinstated. The only "draw back" to the technique is that it has been so useful that the patients feel that they cannot do without it.

A number of important questions still remain to be answered. While intrathecal baclofen has proven effective for spasticity of spinal origin, it may not be as useful for spasticity due to different types of pathology. In our limited experience dystonia does not respond well, nor spasticity due to hereditary progressive lateral sclerosis. The degree of response in supraspinal causes of spasticity and in cerebral palsy patients remains to be determined. If we are to know the range of conditions and the types of spasticity that will respond to this technique, randomized blinded tests with each well defined patient group will have to be performed. This will require considerable effort, but such trials are certainly justified.

Another issue is whether or not baclofen is the best drug for spasticity. Morphine can be substituted for baclofen and one investigator has used it exclusively (Erickson et al. 1989). Both medications, or even others, may have important roles in the future. One disappointment has been that neither drug helps the disturbing dysaesthetic pain due to CNS injury. A useful drug for this problem is not yet available; the search for one should be a priority. Finally, other applications of drug pumps to treat CNS disease should be considered. The goal of restoration of function after injury could be addressed by infusion of neurotropic substances and replacement therapy for neurotransmitter deficiency disease needs to be investigated. The success of intrathecal baclofen for spinal spasticity which suppresses abnormal neural circuits and unmasks normal ones should be a stimulus for further experimentation.

Acknowledgements

We wish to acknowledge the National Institutes of Health and the Food and Drug Administration, Orphan Drug Division for their support of this study and Medtronic, Inc., for technical assistance.

References

See pages 115, 116

Correspondence: R. D. Penn, M.D., Department of Neurosurgery, Rush-Presbyterian-St. Luke's Medical Center, 1653 W. Congress Parkway, Chicago, Illinois 60612, U.S.A.

Intrathecal infusion of Baclofen for spasticity: the Toulouse and the French Multicenter Studies

Y. Lazorthes and **J.C. Verdié** with the collaboration of **B. Sallerin-Caute** and **R. Bastide**

Department of Neurosurgery, Hopital de Rangueil, Toulouse, France

I. The Toulouse experience

Since 1984, 20 patients were treated with chronic intrathecal administration of Baclofen.

The methodology followed 5 successive steps:

Material and method

1) First step: Clinical preselection was based on the following criteria:
– Severe debilitating spasticity secondary to a stable spinal cord or cerebral lesion, from a traumatic origin (para-, tetra- or hemiplegia), a demyelinating disease such as multiple sclerosis, or a motor disability of cerebral origin with spasticity predominating.
– Failure of medical treatment, including oral Baclofen administration (Lioresal R*), at high doses. In the present experiment all the patients had taken, on average, 60 to 100 mg (mean: 90 mg) of Baclofen per 24 hours in association with other antispastic drugs such as diazepam and sodium dantrolene.
– Absence of contra-indications, whatever they may be: pharmacological (concerning Baclofen), psychological or local, such as bedsores or skin lesions in the lumbo-abdomino-pelvic region which would preclude the percutaneous implantation of a catheter and even more the implantation of a drug-delivery system.
– Consent from the patient, clearly informed, as to the contraints imposed by the method and the therapeutic limits.
– Favourable environment for rigorous and regular follow-up as an outpatient.
2) Second step: Selection based on the lumbar intrathecal Baclofen administration test is an essential step before considering chronic intrathecal administration of Baclofen. Its aim was to test individual tolerance, to judge the efficacy of intrathecal administration and to fix the dose of Baclofen effective for 8 to 12 hours in order to rapidly optimize the prescription for chronic treatment.

This requires a test period lasting several days and sometimes several weeks. Therefore we stopped using an externalized lumbar sub-arachnoid catheter for an implant lumbar intrathecal access site (Cordis Multi-purpose Access Port, MPAP, or Miniport).

At the end of the trial, the lumbar intrathecal access port is left in position. This allows subsequent sampling of CSF not only for cytobacteriological examination but also for pharmacokinetic study (HPLC assay) (Sallerin-Caute 1988).

Out of 43 patients who were candidates for chronic intrathecal Baclofen administration, only 20 were selected, as described, for a pump implantation (Table 1). 23 patients with spastic and motor syndromes were tested with short-term intrathecal administration but were not selected for chronic administration. The exclusion factors were:
– significant ineffectiveness of intrathecal administration;
– over-effectiveness with loss of useful spasticity of the lower limbs enabling the patient to stand and walk or
– decrease of the remaining motor performance of the upper limbs, and also
– foreseeable difficulties with regularly follow up of the patient.

During the initial trial period with bolus intrathecal administration it was noticed that the effects of the drug were felt after a period latency period of 45 to 60 minutes.

Firstly, we observed a decrease of muscular hypertonia then the progressive disappearance of clonus, the monosynaptic tendon reflexes and finally Babinski's sign. The dose-dependent effect is considerable since muscle tone and reflexes can be entirely abolished. Similarly the distribution of Baclofen in the CSF must occur very rapidly but to a variable level with a metameric action, predominantly caudal, depending on the local concentration. The duration of the effect is variable, dose-dependent and the reappearance of the symptoms occurs in a reverse order and just as rapidly. The effect can be perfectly reproduced by another administration.
3) Third step: The implantable drug-release systems that we used changed with time. For the first 6 patients chronic administration was performed through the lumbar intrathecal access port used for the test. This required repeated daily injections leading to inaccuracy in the prescription and a not negligible risk of infection. Because of these restrictions and risks we now use only implantable, programmable drug-release systems that allow accurate administration of the individual doses of Baclofen. The last 12 patients have had the implantation of a "Synchromed" system. During the changeover period, 2 patients were implanted with a mechanical pump of the "Secor Cordis" type. Lack of sufficient accuracy in this delivery system led us to explant the two patients and replace them with Synchromed systems.
4) Fourth step: determination of the efficient daily dose or dose titration period

During the first weeks, doses were progressively increased, depending on their clinical and electrophysiological H reflex effects, by increments of the order of 10 to 20% of the daily dose.

The initial effective daily dose was extremely variable from one

Table 1. Patients treated with chronic intrathecal administration of baclofen (n = 20)

Cas	Age Sex	Aetiology	Previous treatment	Drug delivery systems	Baclofen I-TH mcg/24h	Follow-up (Months)
1	47,F	M.S.	S.C.S.* Baclofen: 80 mg	Access Port	200 – Bolus	27
2	30,M	Trauma Cr.	Baclofen: 100 mg	Access Port	45 – Bolus	9
3	70,M	Cer. Vasc.	Baclofen: 80 mg	Access Port	50 – Bolus	5
4	64,F	Trauma, Th4	Baclofen: 90 mg	Access Port	50 – Bolus	12
5	56,M	Trauma, C6	Baclofen: 90 mg	Access Port	200 – Bolus	26
6	37,M	Trauma, Th10	Baclofen: 90 mg	Access Port	210 – Bolus	3
7	29,M	Trauma, C5	S.C.S.* Baclofen: 80 mg	Synchromed	500 – Bolus	43
8	27,M	Cer. Palsy	S.C.S.* Baclofen: 90 mg	Synchromed	100 – Bolus	13
9	56,F	M.S.	Baclofen: 100 mg	Synchromed	100 – Bolus	18
10	26,M	Trauma, Th8	Baclofen: 80 mg	Synchromed	48 – Cont.	56
11	27,M	Trauma, Th4	Baclofen: 90 mg	Synchromed	312 – Cont.	42
12	37,F	M.S.	Baclofen: 60 mg	Synchromed	220 – Cont.	41
13	51,F	M.S.	Baclofen: 60 mg	Synchromed	218 – Cont.	33
14	43,M	Isch. Med.	Baclofen: 60 mg	Synchromed	131 – Cont.	33
15	30,M	Trauma, Th1	Baclofen: 100 mg	Synchromed	250 – Cont.	30
16	43,F	M.S.	Baclofen: 80 mg	Synchromed	180 – Bolus	30
17	14,M	Myelitis	Baclofen: 80 mg	Synchromed	168 – Cont.	33
18	40,M	M.S.	Baclofen: 100 mg	Synchromed	208 – Cont.	32
19	27,F	M.S.	Baclofen: 90 mg	Synchromed	300 – Cont.	8
20	49,M	M.S.	Baclofen: 90 mg	Synchromed	324 – Cont.	7

* *S.C.S.* Cervical Spinal Cord Stimulation

patient to another: it was on average 95 mcg/24 h, ranging from 15 to 250 mcg.

After determination of the effective daily dose, depending on clinical evaluation and side-effects, adjustments had to be made periodically.

5) Fifth step: Chronic ambulatory follow-up was done by a pharmacist from our team (B.S-C) who was responsible for maintaining a constant link between our laboratory, the patient and his family, and his medical environment.

With chronic treatment, the daily consumption increased moderately during the first months of treatment before becoming stable. It was, on average, 190 mcg/24 h, but the difference between individual daily doses was large, ranging from 48 to 500 mcg.

Results

20 patients were selected for implantation, during the period from May 1984 to December 1989. In September 1990 the mean follow-up was 28 months (range 6 to 56).

1) Results were evaluated as follows:

Spasticity was quantified using the Ashworth's score, and spasms according to their frequency (from 0 to + +). Functional improvement resulting from a reduction in spasticity was evaluated scoring the different motor performances with the scale proposed by R. Davis for cerebral palsy treated with electric neurostimulation of the cerebellum cortex. Having

already used this scoring system in the same conditions (Lazorthes 1985, 1990), we found it practical to transfer it to the present situation.

The clinical results on hypertonia were correlated with the H max/M max ratio. The Hoffman reflex measurement was carried out using different protocols according to the various clinical steps:
– during the test period, the H reflex was measured before and after a bolus intrathecal injection;
– after implantation and during the period of titration of therapeutic dose, the H reflex was monitored semi-continuously during perfusion of the effective therapeutic dose and correlated with the clinical modification of spasticity;
– finally, during out-patient follow-up, isolated measurements of the H reflex were carried out frequently in order to bring the ratio H max/M max to normal levels (value equal to or less than 0.5).

2) Results after chronic administration (n = 20):

In all the patients, reduction in spasticity was significant (Table 2) and remained stable over time.

Functional improvement varied greatly between patients; it was dependent on both the clinical stage and the aetiology. 4 patients showed a good and durable functional improvement (i.e., greater than + 3

Table 2. Results regarding spasticity and functional improvement (n = 20)

Cas	Spasticity Ashworth Scale before	after	Painful spasms before	after	Functional improvement (Davis Scale)	Complications	Therapy (September 89)
						Overdose	
1	5	1	+ +	0	+2	Cath displacement	Stop
						Evolutive M.S.	
2	5	3	+	0	+2	Cath displacement	Stop
						Local sepsis	
3	5	1	+ +	0	+3	Cath displacement + hypotonia	Stop
4	4	2	+ +	+ +	+3	/	Stop
5	4	2	+	0	+3	Sepsis, Meningitis	Stop
6	5	2	+	0	0	Sepsis	Stop
						Huntington's Disease	
7	5	2	+ +	0	0	Resp. infection +	Stop
8	4	2	+	0	+2	overdose	Stop
						Pump failure	
9	5	3	+ +	0	0	Sepsis + Meningitis	Stop
10	4	1	+	0	+7	/	Cont.
11	5	2	+	0	+2	/	Cont.
12	5	2	+ +	+	0	/	Cont.
13	5	2	+	0	0	/	Cont.
14	4	1	/	/	+1	Meningitis	Cont.
15	5	2	+	0	+2	/	Cont.
16	5	2	+	0	+4	/	Cont.
17	5	2	/	/	+4	/	Cont.
18	5	2	+	0	0	/	Cont.
19	5	2	+ +	0	0	/	Cont.
20	5	1	+	0	+5	/	Cont.

in the Davis scale). It was moderate (i.e. between 1 and 3) in 9 other patients and nil in the last 7 patients.

3) Results in relation to aetiologies

The most frequent aetiology was spinal trauma (8 patients) and by multiple sclerosis (8 patients). Comparing the results obtained in these two subgroups it has been observed that the best results were in the post-traumatic lesions, especially when the paraplegia was incomplete.

4) Complications:

– *Technical complications*

a. A displacement of the catheter from the subarachnoid space into the epidural or the more superficial layers occurred in 4 cases.

b. 2 patients who were initially treated with a mechanically activated "Secor" pump delivering isolated bolus doses, were explanted owing to the inaccuracy of the system of administration. In these 2 patients the system was replaced by a programmable Synchromed pump with which intrathecal treatment was successfully continued.

c. Lastly, one patient, the only motor invalid of cerebral origin in this series, received an overdose causing respiratory depression and temporary coma. The pump, which developed a defect, had to be stopped as an emergency and explanted. The pump was an implantable programmable first generation device (DAS system from Medtronic), implanted in September 1984; it had operated perfectly for more than a year, before failure.

– *Infectious and neurological complications*

Subcutaneous sepsis around the implanted device was observed in 4 cases, and meningitis in 3. All these infectious complications were observed in patients treated via access points.

No permanent nor transient neurological deficits occurred.

– *Pharmacological complications*

During the initial titration phase, muscular hypotonia was observed in 5 patients. Three of them had been treated via an access port; owing to the technique used, the exact dose administer was difficult to determine. In the two other patients-who were treated via a Synchromed system – hypotonia was rapidly counteracted during the titration period. One case was particularly sensitive to the antispastic effects of intrathecally administered Baclofen since the daily prescription reached a stabel 48 mcg/24 h at the time of writing this report. This stresses the necessity for a very exact individual prescription and that this accuracy can only be reached using programmable implantable pumps.

An incident of minor overdose causing diffuse muscular hypotonia and a state of temporary drowsiness was observed in 4 patients (3 of whom treated via an access port).

In 2 patients a serious overdose accident occurred causing progressive respiratory depression and transient coma. In the first patient, the accident arose from malfunction of the pump which supplied more than the required amount of drug. The coma and respiratory depression were progressively corrected by respiratory assistance with tracheal intubation, repeated lumbar puncture and i.v. hyper-rehydration to increase the renal elimination of Baclofen. The pump was then explanted and this type of treatment not resumed in this patient. In the other patient, suffering from advanced multiple sclerosis, the overdose occurred after a bolus administration of 200 mcg of Baclofen into the access port. The respiratory depression and coma, which were both much more moderate, reversed spontaneously without the need for respiratory resuscitation.

Discussion

In the present series (n = 20), the follow-up period (on average 18 months) and the long-term results are sufficient to conclude that maintenance of stable clinical effects without secondary acquired tolerance are achieved. However, in all the patients, the 24-hour doses had to be steadily increased over the first months so that the average effective dose rose by 90 to 190 mcg.

In order to optimise the prescription, we were guided, not only by clinical evaluation, but also by the quantitative modifications of Hoffmann's monosynaptic reflex (H reflex) as well as by assay of Baclofen levels in the CSF during treatment. The Hmax/Mmax ratio followed during clinic visits is an index of effectiveness which must also be considered in the light of the therapeutic aims. The very high efficacy of intrathecal Baclofen administration is confirmed by the fact that, not only can the ratio be normalized, it can also be reduced to zero with complete disappearance of the H reflex. This situation is, of course, not to be sought when useful spasticity is to

be maintained in a patient, in that case the ratio H max/M max should be maintained in a range between 50% (normal) and 30%.

II. The French Multicenter Study

Material and method

The French cooperative study as of mid 1989 consisted of 40 patients selected according to the criteria previously described and implanted with a "Synchromed" Medtronic device. 12 were from Toulouse (Pr. Lazorthes), 8 from Créteil (Pr. Keravel), 7 from Clermont-Ferrand (Dr. Colnet), 5 from Montpellier (Pr. Frerebeau), 4 from Lyon (Pr. M. Sindou) and 4 from Grenoble (Pr. A.L. Benabid).

As the series from Toulouse has already been studied – in the first part of this chapter –, only the 28 patients from other centers will be considered in the following section.

The majority of those selected (26/28) suffered from severe spasticity of spinal origin: 13 spinal cord trauma, 8 multiple sclerosis, and 5 other spinal diseases. The age of the patients ranged from 16 to 64 years (mean: 34). There were 17 men and 11 women. The daily doses of Baclofen are reported in Table 3.

Table 3. The daily doses (n = 28)

	Range	Mean
Oral (mg) before I–T administration	40–150	97
I–T (mcg)		
– Initial	2–100	52
– Chronic*	3–340	113

* Mode of administration: Bolus: 3; Infusion: 25

Results

The clinical results were analysed using the same criteria (Ashworth scale and Davis scale) and are summarized in Table 4.

Table 4. Clinical results follow-up: 1–19 months (mean: 8)]

* Hypertonia Ashworth scale	1	2	3	4	5
– before	/	1	6	13	8
– after	5	11	6	6	/

* Spasm improvement: 12/28	
* Functional gain	– Important	2
	– Moderate	12
	– Nil	14

The pharmacological and technical complications are reported in Table 5.

Table 5. Pharmacological and technical complications

* Undesired hypotonia	:	2
* Drowsiness	:	2
* Respiratory depression	:	0
* Catheter replacements	:	4
* Sepsis – Drug Delivery System explanted	:	1

Discussion

Total clinical results are similar, and complications are less than in the experience reported by Lazorthes' group. But the mean follow-up is less (8 versus 18 months). All the patients in this cooperative study have benefited from a "Synchromed" drug delivery system. The 5 authors of this multicentric study have observed the same variability in the individual daily doses of Baclofen (Table 3).

The present study confirms the efficacy of Baclofen administration in patients suffering from disabling spastic syndrome resistant to long-term oral antispastic therapy.

This phenomenon of pharmacological tolerance observed with oral administration was counteracted by the administration of very low doses of Baclofen intrathecally. The therapeutic effect was obtained, after the titration period, with an average dose of 90 mcg/day. We did however observe a very large variation in the efficacy threshold between patients.

References

Babinski J (1912) Réflexes tendineux et réflexes osseux. Bull Med

Birkmayer W, Danielczyk W, Weiler G (1967) Zur Objektivierbarkeit des myotonolytischen Effctes eines Aminobutter Säurederivates (CIBA). Wien Med Wschr 117: 7–9

Blackshear PJ, Dormon FD, Blackshear PJ Jr (1972) The design and initial testing of an implantable infusion pump. Surg Gynecol Obstet 134: 51–56

Bormann J (1988) Electrophysiology of GABA-A and GABA-B receptor sybtypes. TINS 11(3): 112–116

Bowery NG, Hill OR, Hudson AL, Doble A, Middlemiss DN, Shaw J, Turnbull M (1980) Baclofen decreases neurtransmitter release in the mammalian CNS by an action at a novel GABA receptor. Nature (Lond) 283: 92–94

Bowery NG, Price GW, Hudson AL, Hill DR, Wilkin GP, Turnbull MJ (1984) GABA receptor multiplicity. Visualization of different receptor types in the mammalian CNS. Neuropharmacology 23(2B): 219–231

Bowery NG, Hudson AL, Price GW (1987) GABA-A and GABA-B receptor site distribution in the rat central nervous system. Neuroscience 20(2): 365–383

Colbert N, Izrael V, Renaud J, Laugier A (1948) Chimiotherapie anti-cancéreuse et pompes implantables. Concours Med 106(25): 2376–2380

Curtis DR, Gynther BD, Beattie DT, Kerr DIB, Prager RH (1988) Baclofen antagonism by 2-hydroxy-Baclofen in the cat spinal cord. Neurosci Lett 92: 97–101

Dolphin AC, Scott RH (1987) Calcium channel currents and their inhibition by Baclofen in rat sensory neurons modulation by guanine nucleotides. J Physiol (Lond) 386: 1–17

Dunlap K (1986) Two types of gamma-aminobutyric acid receptor on embryonic sensory neurons. Br J Pharmacol 74: 579–585

Ensminger W, Niederhuber J, Dakhil S, Thrall J, Wheeler R (1981) Totally implanted drug delivery system for hepatic arterial chemotherapy. Cancer Treat Rep 65: 393–400

Erickson DL, LOJ, Michaelson M (1989) Control of intractable spasticity with intrathecal morphine sulfate. Neurosurgery 24(2): 236–238

Faigle JW, Keberle H (1972) The metabolism and pharmacokinetics of Lioresal. In: Birmayer W (ed) Spasticity – a topical survey. Huber, Bern, pp 94–100

Gahwiler BH, Brown DA (1985) GABA-B receptor activated K+ current in voltage-clamped CA3 pyramidal cells in hyppocampal cultures. Proc Natl Acad Sci USA 82: 1558–1562

Hankey GJ, Stewart-Wynne EG, Perlman D (1986) Intrathecal Baclofen for severe spasticity. Med J Aust 145(9): 465–466

Innis RB, Nestler EJ, Aghajanian GK (1988) Evidence for G protein mediation of serotonin- and GABA-B- induced hyperpolarization of rat dorsal raphe neurons. Brain Res 459: 27–36

Jerusalem F (1968) Doppelblindstudie über den antispastischen Effekt von ß-(4-Chlorophenyl)-aminobuttersäure (CIBA) bei multipler Sklerose. Nervenarzt 39: 515–517

Kerr BBI, Ong J, Prager RH, Gynther BD, Curtis DR (1987) Phaclofen: a peripheral and central Baclofen antagonist. Brain Res 405: 150–154

Kerr DIB, Ong J, Johnson GAR, Abbenante J, Prager RH (1988) 2-hydroxy-Saclofen: an improved antagonist at central and peripheral GABA-B receptors. Neurosci Lett 92: 92–96

Kerr DIB, Ong J, Johnston GAR, Berthelot P, Debaert M, Vaccher C (1989) Benzofuram analogues of Baclofen: a new class of central and peripheral GABA-B receptor antagonists. Eur J Pharmacol 164: 361–364

Knutsson E, Lindblom U, Martensson A (1974) Plasma and cerebrospinal fluid levels of Baclofen (Lioresal ®) at optimal therapeutic responses in spastic paresis. J Neurol Sci 23: 473–484

Kroin JS, Penn RD. Cerebrospinal fluid pharmacokinetics of lumbar intrathecal Baclofen. Personal communication

Kroin JS, Penn RD, Beissinger RL, et al. (1984) Reduced spinal reflexes following intrathecal baclofen in the rabbit. Exp Brain Res 54: 191–194

Kroin JS, Singh R, Penn RD, Bianchi GD (1989) Chronic intrathecal Baclofen reduces GABA-B binding in rat substantia gelatinosa. Receptor modulation: up and down regulation 1. Soc Neurosci Abstr 15: 975 (389.10)

Latach ML, Penn RD, Corcos DM, Gottlieb GL (1989) Short-term effects of intrathecal baclofen in spasticity. Exp Neurol 103: 165–172

Latash ML, Penn R, Corcos D, Gottlieb G (1990) Intrathecal Baclofen unmasks residual voluntary motor control in spasticity. J Neurosurg 72: 388–392

Lazorthes Y (1985) Neuropharmacologie en application intrathécale. In: Siegfried J, Lazorthes Y (eds) La neurochirurgie Fonctionnelle de l'Infirmité Motrice Cérébazle. Neurochirurgie 31 [Suppl 1]: 95–101

Lazorthes Y (1987) Chronic intrathecal administration of baclofen in severe spasticity. In: Ensminger WD, Selan JL (eds) Infusion systems in medecine. Futura Publishing, Mount Kisco NY, pp 327–336

Lazorthes Y (1988) Chronic intrathecal administration of

Baclofen in treatment of severe chronic spasticity. In: Muller H, Ziersky J, Penn R (eds) Local spinal therapy of spasticity. Springer, Berlin Heidelberg New York Tokio, pp 215–222

Lazorthes Y, Sallerin-Caute B, Verdié J-C, Bastide R, Carillo JP (1990) Chronic intra-thecal Baclofen administration for control of severe spasticity. J Neurosurg 72: 393–402

Müller H, Zierski J, Dralle D, Börner U, Hoffmann O (1987) The effect of intra-thecal Baclofen on electrical muscle activity in spasticity. J Neurol 234(5): 348–352

Müller H, Zierski J, Penn RD (1988) Local spinal therapy of spasticity. Springer, Berlin Heidelberg New York Tokio, pp 155–214

Müller H, Zierski J, Dralle D, Hoffmann O, Michaelis G (1988) Intrathecal baclofen in spasticity. In: Muller H, Zierski J, Penn RD (eds) Local spinal therapy of spasticity. Springer, Berlin Heidelberg, pp 155–214

Müller-Schwefe G, Penn RD (1989) Physostigmine in the treatment of intrathecal Baclofen overdose. J Neurosurg 71: 273–275

Müller-Schwefe G, Penn RD, Kroin JS. Physostigmine in the treatment of intrathecal Baclofen overdose. Personal communication

Parke B, Penn RD, Savoy SM, Corcos D (1989) Functional outcome following delivery of intrathecal baclofen in patients with multiple sclerosis and spinal cord injury. Arch Phys Med Rehab 70: 30–32

Penn RD (1988) Chronic intrathecal baclofen for severe rigidity and spasms. In: Muller H, Zierski J, Penn RD (eds) Local spinal therapy of spasticity. Springer, Berlin Heidelberg New York Tokio, pp 151–154

Penn RD, Kroin JS (1984) Intrathecal baclofen alleviates spinal cord spasticity. Lancet i: 1078

Penn RD, Kroin JS (1985) Continuous intrathecal baclofen for severe spasticity. Lancet ii: 125–127

Penn RD, Kroin JS (1987) Long-term intrathecal baclofen infusion for treatment of spasticity. J Neurosurg 66: 181–185

Penn RD, Savoy S, Corcos D, Latash M, Gottlieb T, Parke B, Kroin J (1989) Intrathecal Baclofen for severe spinal spasticity. N Engl J Med 320(23): 1517–1521

Price GWX, Wilkin GP, Turnbull MJ, Bowery NG (1984) Are Baclofen-sensitive GABA-B receptors present on primary apparent terminals of the spinal cord? Nature 307(5946): 71–74

Price GW, Kelly JS, Bowery NG (1987) The location of GABA-B receptor binding sites in mammalian spinal cord. Synapse 1(6): 530–538

Sallerin-Caute B, Monsarrat B, Lazorthes Y, Cros J, Bastide R (1980) A sensitive method for the determination of Baclofen in human CSF by high performance liquid chromatography. J Liquid Chromatogr 11(8): 1753–1761

Schmid K, Böhmer G, Gebauer K (1989) GABA-B receptor mediated effects on central respiratory system and their antagonism by Phaclofen. Neurosci Lett 99: 305–310

Siegfried J, Rea GL (1987) Intrathecal application of baclofen in the treatment of spasticity. Acta Neurochir 39: 121–123

Zierski J, Müller H (1988) Implantation of parts and pumps. Technique for intra-thecal administration of drugs. In: Müller H, Zierski J, Penn R (eds) Local spinal therapy of spasticity. Springer, Berlin Heidelberg New York Tokio, pp 215–222

Correspondence: Prof. Y. Lazorthes, M.D., Department of Neurosurgery, Hopital de Rangueil, Avenue Jean Poulhes, F-31054 Toulouse, France

Neuro-ablative procedures for spasticity

Selective peripheral neurotomies for the treatment of spasticity

P. Mertens and **M. Sindou**

Service de Neurochirurgie, Hopital Neurologique P. Wertheimer, Lyon, France

When an excess of a spasticity leads to disequilibrium in the tonic balance of a limb segment and if the concerned group of muscles is under the control of a single peripheral nerve, neurotomy at its level may be indicated. Neurotomies cut all types of sensory fibers as well as motor fibers: therefore they must be as selective as possible. Neurotomies reequilibrate the tonic balance between agonist and antagonist muscles. This results in reduction of abnormal joint postures and improvement in residual voluntary movement.

Peripheral neurotomies were first introduced by Lorenz in 1887 who sectioned the obturator nerve for adduction spasticity in the hip. Stoffel, in 1912, developed tibial neurectomy for the treatment of the spastic foot and median neurectomy for the spastic pronation of the forearm. Later, several authors periodically reported on their technical modalities and clinical indications (Banks and Green 1960, Keats 1957, Silfverskiold 1923). Recently, interest in neurotomies has been renewed by Gros et al. (1977), by introducing the use of intraoperative electrical stimulation to identify the constituent fascicles of the nerve, as well as microsurgical techniques, for neurotomy.

The site of the neurotomy must be peripheral enough so that the fascicles corresponding to the distal muscular nerve branches can be anatomically identified. Sectioning must be – as far as possible – limited to the fascicles innervating the hyperspastic muscles.

Neurotomies need also to be quantitatively selective, so as to suppress the excess of spasticity without impairing motor function or producing amyotrophy. To achieve this goal it is necessary to preserve at least one fifth of the motor fibers.

This chapter will describe the surgical techniques for the various neurotomies as well as preoperative assessment and post-operative care. Also, there will be a discussion of our post-operative results and of the literature data (Mertens 1987).

General principles

Preoperative assessment

Careful preoperative assessment is necessary to determine, first whether abnormal postures are only related to spasticity or complicated by additional orthopaedic factors. This can be answered on the basis of a clinical and radiological examination and, if necessary, by local, temporary anaesthetic blocks using bupivacaine. Such tests determine whether articular limitations are due to spasticity and/or muscular-tendinous contractures and/or articular ankyloses (only spasticity is influenced by the test). In addition, these tests give the patient a chance to appreciate what to expect from the operation.

The second step is to determine which nerves or fascicles are to be cut and to what degree.

Preoperatively, a multidisciplinary team analizes the patient's spasticity, articular limitations and residual voluntary mobility.

Surgical technique

The technical features common to all neurotomies will be developed in the following paragraphs.

The limb must be sterilized and draped in such a way that the surgeon can have view of all muscular responses.

The patient is operated upon under general anaesthesia, but without long-lasting curarization, to allow detection of the motor responses evoked by electrical stimulation of the nerve branches. This is the only means of identifying them with certainty.

Nerve branches are dissected under the operating microscope with a 200 mm lens and low magnification, and identified using bipolar electrostimulation at low intensity (to avoid much electrical diffusion).

All the branches corresponding to the muscles considered to be responsible for harmful spasticity are individually marked with differently colored tapes. Then variable proportions (half to four fifth) of the selected nerves or fascicles, are resected according to the preoperative program. Resection is about 5 millimeters long to prevent regrowth of fibers from the proximal stump. The proximal stump of each resected fascicle is coagulated using a very sharp bipolar forceps to prevent proliferative neuroma formation. The effect of each surgical lesion is evaluated by comparing muscular responses provoked by the successive stimulation (at a constant intensity, slightly above the threshold) of the distal and proximal segments of the nerve, on either sides of the resected portion. Should stimulation of the remaining fibers result in an intense muscular response, the nerve is subjected to further resection.

Post-operative care

After surgery on the lower limb, the leg is covered with an anti-varicose vein stocking and raised to facilitate its venous drainage. Anticoagulant therapy is administered for ten days, and the patient is encouraged to walk and resume physiotherapy as soon as the second post-operative day. For the upper limb, casts or splints are sometimes needed; the limb is raised to avoid oedema and mobilized as early as possible.

The surgical result is assessed just before discharge on the 10th day. Immediately thereafter, a program of physical therapy is undertaken either in a rehabilitation center or at home. All patients are re-examined at regular intervals as out-patients.

I. Neurotomies for spasticity in the lower limb

A) Selective neurotomy of the tribial nerve (STN) for the spastic foot

1) The so-called spastic foot is characterized by one or several of the following features depending on which muscles are involved by spasticity.

– Equinus and ankle clonus depend on the soleus muscle and/or the medial and lateral gastrocnemius. When equinus and/or ankle clonus are significantly decreased by flexing the knee, it may be assumed that gastrocnemius spasticity is predominantly responsible since the flexion reduces gastrocnemius tone. Conversely, if this manoeuvre is negative, spasticity may be considered predominant in the soleus muscle.
– Varus essentially depends on the tibialis posterior muscle. Occasionally, the tibialis anterior muscle, innervated by the peroneal nerve, can contribute, especially when varus affects the anterior part of the foot. A block of the tibial nerve allows one to differentiate between the respective involvement of these muscles.
– Tonic flexion of the toes depends mainly upon flexor hallucis longus and flexor digitorum longus muscles.

2) Surgical technique. The patient is operated on in the prone position, with the knee slightly flexed (10–15°) to relax the hamstring and gastrocnemius muscles and thereby facilitating popliteal access. The leg is draped to allow the surgeon to get a sufficient view of the foot to check its muscle responses.

The skin incision is made in the midline vertically for 7 cm down, from the transverse popliteal line. The incision may start 3 cm higher (with a bayonet shape) when identification of the gastrocnemius branches is

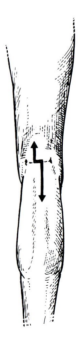

Fig. 1. Skin incision in the right popliteal fossa for STN

necessary. To get an easy access to the flexor fascicles inside the distal tibial trunk under the soleus arch, it may be necessary to extend the incision 3 cm downward (Fig. 1).

During the popliteal approach, care must be taken to avoid injury to the sensory sural nerve. It is situated in the subaponeurotic space between the two gastrocnemius muscles, just behind the satellite sural vein.

Tibial nerve dissection begins by locating the proximal segment of the nerve in the fat of the upper popliteal region. This area can be the site of fibro-

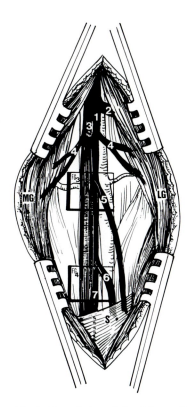

Fig. 2. Dorsal view of the right popliteal region.
– Tibial nerve (1), Peroneal nerve (2).
– The sensory sural nerve (3) lies superficially just beneath the subcutaneous aponeurosis between the two gastrocnemius muscles
– The medial and lateral gastrocnemius nerves (4) may arise either separately from the both sides of the tibial trunk or posteriorly from a common origin, sometimes including the sensory sural nerve. Each gastrocnemius nerve usually divides into two distal branches when approaching the muscle.
– The one or two soleus nerves (5) may arise from a common origin or quite separately from the tibial nerve.
– The posterior tibialis nerve (6), like the soleus nerve, originates from the ventro-lateral aspect of the tibial nerve, but more distally at the level of the soleus arch. Sometimes it may originate from a common trunk with the inferior branch of the soleus nerve.
– The distal trunk of the tibial nerve (7) contains 5 to 8 fascicles averaging 1 mm in diameter each; two thirds of them are motor fascicles, one third are sensory ones.
– Muscles: lateral and medial gastrocnemius (LG-MG), Soleus (S)

atrophic scar tissue, if the patient has been previously treated with alcohol injections. The tibial branches are dissected and identified proximally to distally using the operating microscope and the bipolar stimulation (Fig. 2). When correction of flexion of the toes is needed, the epineurium of the tibial trunk is opened at the level of the soleus arch to allow dissection of the responsible motor fascicles (Fig. 4).

Then the selected branches are partially resected according to the pre-operative program (Fig. 3).

3) Results in our personal series (Sindou et al. 1985, Sindou and Mertens 1988). At the present time, this series amounts at 150 cases. Only the results concerning 62 procedures (9 bilaterally and 44 unilaterally) in 53 patients with a follow-up of more than 3 years will be described below (average follow-up 4.8 years).

Spasticity resulted from lesions of the spinal cord in 12 cases and of the cerebral hemisphere in 41. Most of the patients were adults; there were only 6 children with cerebral palsy in the series.

Equinus was the most frequent component (54 times out of 62 cases). It was associated with varus in 45 and with flexion of the toes in 34.

STN eliminated equinus in 85%, varus in 89%, flexion of the toes in 74% and clonus in 67% of the cases.

Comparison of pre- and post-operative mobility was evaluated for ankle dorsiflexion using Lovett's motor scale (Fig. 6). Voluntary mobility, when present, was improved in 87% and remained unchanged in 13%. A similar comparative study was done for plantar flexion. The strength was worsened only in two cases, resulting in a talus foot in one.

From a functional point of view, all of the 41 patients with hemispheric deficit could walk, 32 with a stick. Seven of the 12 patients with spinal cord lesions were able to walk with one person helping, while the remaining 5 were in a wheelchair. An excellent result (i.e. complete suppression of excess of spasticity with a normal plantar positioning of the sole of the foot when standing and walking) was achieved in 82% of the cases. The pre- and post-operative degree of spasticity was quantified using the Ashworth scale (Fig. 5). The average score decreased from 3.84 to 1.53 after surgery. No significant recurrence had occurred at the 2 year follow-up.

The most serious complications were of the sensory and trophic types, due to excessive manipulations to the sural nerve (when occurring in the lateral aspect

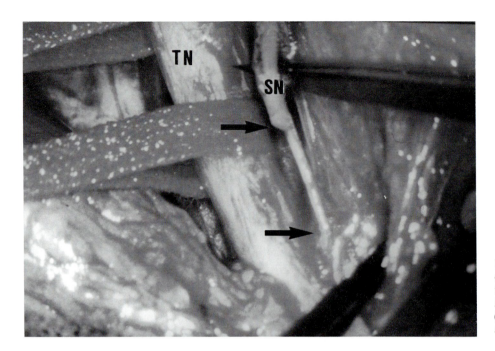

Fig. 3. Operative view of resection, over 7 millimeters length (between the two arrows) of the 2/3 of the *Soleus nerve* (S.N.). The *Tibial nerve* (T.N.) is medially under the loop of a tape

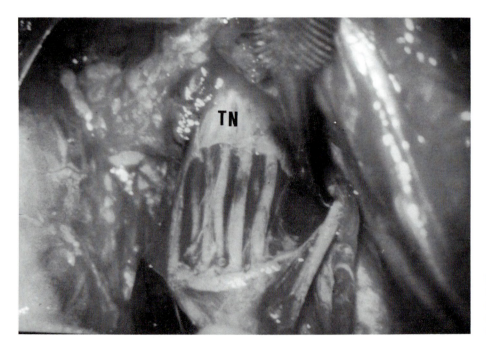

Fig. 4. Operative view of five dissected fascicles inside the distal part of the *Tibial nerve* (T.N.), at the level of the soleus arch, after opening of the epineural envelop

of the foot), and injury of the sensory fascicles inside the tibial trunk (when occurring in the plantar region). In 3 cases, pain characterized by electrical discharges with hyper-aesthesia, occurred on the lateral side of the foot. The painful phenomena responded to carbamazepine and fortunately disappeared within a few weeks. In 5 other cases who underwent a section

of the flexor fascicles of the toes, the neurotomy produced hypo-aesthesia with hyper-algesia in the sole of the foot. In 3 cases these disturbances were transient, but 2 were permanent.

4) Results in the literature series. Gros et al. (1977) have reported 52 cases of STN, mainly in children with

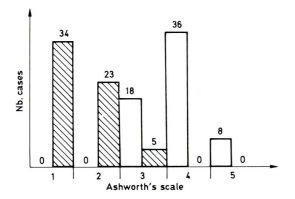

Fig. 5. *Results on spasticity*
–Pre (white) and post-operative (hatched) repartition of the spastic feet (62 cases), according to the Ashworth's scale.
–*Asworth's scale:*
1 no increase in tone
2 slight increase in tone, giving a catch when part is moved in flexion or extension
3 more marked increase in tone, but affected part easily flexed
4 considerable increase in tone, passive movement difficult
5 complete rigidity in flexion or extension

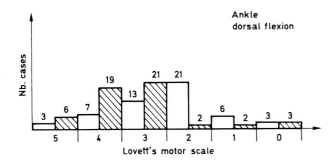

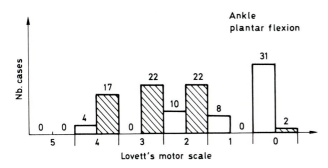

Fig. 6. *Results on voluntary motility*
–Pre (white) and post-operative (hatched) repartition of voluntary motility, calculated for 53 spastic feet according to the Lovett's motor scale.
–*Lovett's motor scale*
0 no muscular contraction
1 muscular contraction, no movement
2 possible movement without gravity
3 movement against gravity
4 movement against strength superior to gravity
5 normal motor strength

cerebral palsy. Spasticity decreased in all cases and functional improvement was seen in 68%. In 40% the splint was removed and in 28% walking, absent pre-operatively, occurred.

Siegfried and Lazorthes, in their monograph on neurosurgery for cerebral palsy (Siegfried and Lazorthes 1985), reported 14 patients treated by STN with long lasting complete suppression of spasticity in 8, and partial in 5 cases.

In Cahuzac's series of 89 procedures (Cahuzac 1980), consisting only in a complete section of nerves to the gastrocnemius in children with cerebral palsy and equinus, a reduction in equinus was observed in 71 cases (80%). In 18 cases recurrence was reported and 6 transient talus feet were noted.

In Peragut's 27 adults (Peragut et al. 1989), a decrease in spasticity was obtained in all cases, with improvement of walking: with normal shoes in 66,6% and with a splint or high shoe in 33,3%.

These data show that in the treatment of the spastic foot, STN is an effective procedure for suppressing excess of spasticity, correcting the abnormal posture and reducing pain. Residual voluntary mobility in the muscles innervated by the peroneal nerve often reappeared or improved, due to re-equilibration of the tonic balance between the palsied agonist muscles and the spastic antagonist muscles.

B) Obturator neurotomy for spastic hip adductors

1) The main components of the spastic hip are: adduction, flexion and internal rotation. They are harmful at rest during walking, and threaten the stability of the hip. These abnormal postures, especially adduction, can lead to coxa valga, subluxation and then dislocation of the hip. This is especially common in cerebral palsy.

The muscles responsible for adduction of the hip are the obturator externus, adductor brevis-longus-magnus, gracilis and pectineus. Some of them are also accessory flexors of the hip: i.e., the adductor brevis-longus and pectineus; and internal rotator: gracilis (Table 1). All these muscles are innervated by the obturator nerve, but some also have an innervation from the femoral nerve (adductor longus-pectineus), or by the sciatic nerve (adductor magnus). Consequently, even a complete obturator neurotomy will not achieve total denervation of the adductor muscles.

The problem is made even more complex by the necessity to preserve some of the useful function of

Table 1.

Muscles	Functions ( ) = useful function	Innervations Obturator n. anterior branch	Posterior branch	Femoral n.	Sciatic n.
Obturator externus	–adduction –(static of the head of the femur)	proximal to the division of the nerve			
Adductor brevis	–adduction –flexion –(external rotator)	*			
Adductor longus	–adduction –flexion	*		*	
Adductor magnus	–adduction		*		*
Gracilis	–adduction –internal rotation –(flexion of the knee)	*			
Pectineus	–adduction –(external rotation)		*	*	

these muscles; i.e., the obturator externus for stabilization of the hip, the adductor brevis and pectineus for their external rotation function (Table 1). In children, neurotomy of only the anterior branch of the obturator nerve is sufficient and avoid hypercorrection. But neurotomy of the posterior branch is necessary when there is a threat of subluxation of the hip.

As muscular contraction is often associated with spasticity in the adductors, a tenotomy of adductor longus, gracilis and adductor brevis may be added to obturator neurotomy at the same operation, using the same approach (Keats 1957).

2) Surgical technique. The patient is placed in the supine position, the thigh in adduction, with knee and hip slightly flexed. The approach is subpubic (3 cm below the pubis), allowing obturator externus branches to be preserved (Privat et al. 1981). The skin incision – 8 cm long – is made just below the subpubic canal in the upper-medial region of the thigh, at the level of the adductor longus tendon (Fig. 7).

The anterior branch of the obturator nerve is identified between the adductor longus laterally and the gracilis medially. The nerve lies behind these muscles, anterior to the adductor brevis (Fig. 8). To check all its muscular branches, it is necessary to dissect the proximal part of the nerve, as it leaves the subpubic canal. The branches to adductor longus and gracilis, which can be identified with bipolar stimulation, are partially or totally cut, according to the

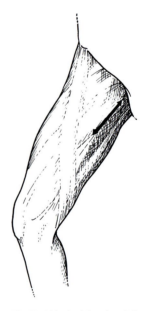

Fig. 7. Skin incision for right obturator neurotomy, on the relief of adductor longus muscle

preoperative plan. Branches to adductor brevis may or may not be preserved.

The posterior branch of the obturator nerve can be reached under the gracilis, anterior to the adductor magnus. If necessary, the branches to the adductor magnus are cut, taking into account that there may be residual innervation by branches from the sciatic nerve. The branches for pectineus must be preserved.

An additional tenotomy or myotomy of adductor longus and gracilis can be performed, through the

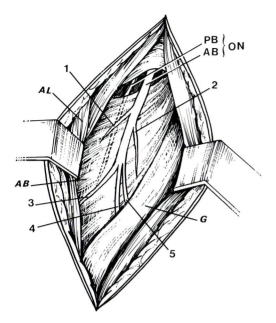

Fig. 8. Dissection of the anterior branch (AB) of the right obturator nerve (ON). The adductor longus (AL) is retracted laterally and the gracilis (G) medially. The nerve is anterior to the adductor brevis (*AB*). Adductor brevis nerve (1), (2), adductor longus nerve (3), gracilis nerve (4), (5). The posterior branch (PB) of the obturator nerve lies under the adductor brevis (*AB*)

same incision, close to their origin from the pubis. Its effectiveness can be checked by passive mobilization of the hip during sectioning.

3) Results. Due to the small number of children with cerebral palsy in our experience and because of preference for surgery in the dorsal root entry zone target in adult patients, our series of obturator neurotomies consists only of 14 procedures in 9 patients (4 uni- and 5 bilaterally). In our patients the sectioning was limited to the anterior branch and was accompanied by additional tenotomies when contractures were present. The result was good (i.e. passive abduction-adduction amplitude more than 60°), with a follow-up longer than two years in 12 cases.

We have reviewed the literature for obturator neurotomies used to treat children with cerebral palsy. Banks and Green (1960) reported on 135 cases of complete section of the anterior division to the obturator nerve associated with tenotomies with an average follow-up of 10 years. They saw a complete correction of abnormal postures in 60%, a partial result (i.e. less than 60° of passive abduction) in 21% and failure in 19% of the cases.

In a series of 111 cases treated by Cahuzac (1980)

without any associated tenotomy, the results were good in 86% of cases after a two year follow-up.

C) Neurotomy of the femoral nerve for spastic hip flexors

1) Flexion of the hip is dependant on the rectus femoris, psoas iliacus, sartorius and tensor fasciae latae. All of these muscles, except the last one, are innervated by the femoral nerve. Only the rectus femoris and sartorius receive branches arising from below the inguinal ligament.

Because of this pattern of innervation, femoral neurotomy, performed through an extra-pelvic approach, can only be effective when hip flexor spasticity predominates in the rectus femoris muscle. This may be determined by the test of Thomas. This test consists of comparing the amplitude of flexion-extension of the hip, while the knee being flexed and then extended with the patient supine. If there is no modification, the psoas iliacus is considered responsible. If hip flexion increases with flexion of the knee, this means that rectus femoris is involved, and, consequently, an extrapelvic selective neurotomy of the femoral nerve will be effective.

2) Surgical techniqe. The patient is placed in the supine position, the thigh with incomplete abduction. The skin incision, 5 cm in length, is made at the femoral triangle, just below the inguinal ligament, lateral to the femoral artery (Fig. 9). The femoral branch of the

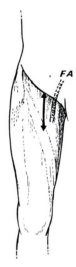

Fig. 9. Skin incision for right femoral neurotomy, below the inguinal ligament, laterally to the femoral artery (FA)

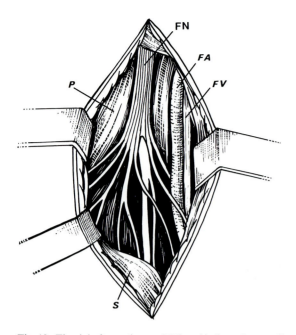

Fig. 10. The right femoral nerve (FN) and its branches are dissected, after opening the anterior fascia of the psoas muscle (P). The bipolar stimulation allows to identify the two or three branches to sartorius muscle (S) and three or four to rectus femoris muscle, which produce flexion of the hip. Femoral artery (FA), femoral vein (FV)

genito-femoral nerve lies superficially and must be preserved. After opening the deep fascia of the thigh, the femoral nerve is dissected lateral to the femoral artery, under the anterior fascia of the psoas muscle. The nerve terminates 4 cm below the inguinal ligament by dividing into its terminal branches (Fig. 10). The 2 or 3 branches to sartorius and the 3 or 4 to rectus femoris are identified, with bipolar stimulation.

A partial resection (1/2 to 4/5th) of each nerve is done according to the preoperative program.

3) Results. As far as we know, no detailed reports have been devoted to femoral neurotomy. However, it is sometimes mentioned in chapters on nerve sections for spasticity (Bardot 1979, Cahuzac 1980), that this procedure may be useful, but – if performed alone – that it frequently leads to hypocorrection since adductor muscles are accessory flexor muscles; when flexion-adduction of the hip is encountered obturator and femoral neurotomies may be combined. Femoral neurotomy can also be combined with orthopaedic procedures, like psoas tenotomy (if walking is definitively lost) or tendinous lengthening of the rectus femoris and/or psoas muscles.

D) Selective neurotomy of the hamstring branches of the sciatic nerve for spastic knee flexors

1) Spasticity of hamstring muscles (i.e. semi-tendinous, semi-membranous and biceps femoris) is responsible for spastic flexion of the knee. This syndrome must be differentiated from knee flexion secondary to flexion of the hip and/or equinus of the foot, which necessitate a compensatory flexion at the knee. Because hamstring muscles are biarticular muscles, their spasticity can also induce limitation of flexion of the hip.

These muscles are innervated by branches arising from the sciatic nerve in the upper part of the thigh. Even in the proximal part of the sciatic nerve, the fascicles destined to the tibial and the peroneal nerves as well as those destined for the hamstrings are organized into distinct bundles. The hamstring fascicles lie at the medial part of the sciatic trunk and they can be identified and isolated at this level of the sciatic trunk.

2) Surgical technique. The patient is placed in the prone position and the lower limb draped so as to make the muscular responses of the entire leg visible. The sciatic trunk is approached, at an equal distance between the greater trochanter laterally and the ischial tuberosity medially (Fig. 11). The sciatic trunk is reached after passing through the fibers of the gluteus maximus, at the lower border of the piriformis muscle, after lateral retraction of the gluteus medius (Fig. 12).

Under the operating microscope, the epineurium of the sciatic nerve is opened in its medial part and

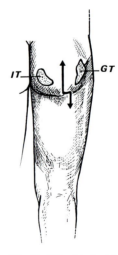

Fig. 11. The skin incision for hamstring neurotomies (on the right side) is located on the midline between the ischial tuberosity (IT) and the greater trochanter (GT)

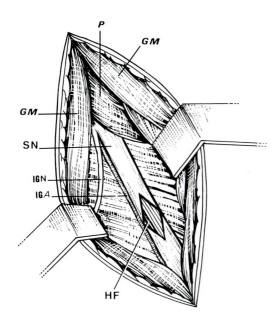

Fig. 12. Dissection of the right sciatic nerve (SN), under the piriformis muscle (P), after passing through the fibers of the gluteus maximus muscle (GM). The epineurium of the nerve is opened and fascicles for hamstring muscles (HF) are localized in the medial part of the nerve trunk. Inferior gluteal nerve (IGN), inferior gluteal artery (IGA)

an interfascicular dissection performed. After electrical identification of the fascicles responsible for flexion of the knee, 1/2 to 4/5 of these fascicles are resected, in accordance with the preoperative program. The epineurium is then closed with interrupted stiches.

3) Results. We have been able to find only a few cases in the literature. Cahuzac (1980) reported on 6 cases in children (4 of them operated upon bilaterally) with only 2 good results. Privat et al. (1981) reported on 5 procedures in adults, with a decrease in spastic flexion in all cases. Our personal experience amounts only to 2 paraplegic adult patients with a partial result in one, which required a complementary orthopaedic procedure to treat associated muscular contracture, and a complete release of the knee in the other.

E) Neurotomy of the deep peroneal nerve for spastic extension of the hallux

1) Permanent hyperextension of the hallux (which is an exacerbation of the Babinski sign) can be disabling for wearing shoes and/or during walking. Two muscles are involved: the extensor hallucis longus and the internal part of the extensor digitorum brevis. These two muscles are innervated by branches arising

from the deep peroneal nerve along the middle part of the leg and the dorsum of the foot. To be effective without a too extensive dissection, the neurotomy is performed by interfascicular dissection of the nerve trunk at the middle part of the leg.

2) Surgical procedure. A 5 cm linear skin incision is made, from the antefibularis depression to the midpoint between the malleoli, along the lateral aspect of the tibialis anterior muscle, beginning 5 cm below the apex of the patella. After opening the superficial aponeurosis, the intermuscular space between the tibialis anterior medially and the extensor digitorum longus laterally, is explored, until the deep peroneal nerve is found anterior to the interosseus membrane, along the anterior tibial artery. Under the microscope the epineurium of the nerve trunk is opened and its fascicles identified.

Stimulation of fascicles to extensor hallucis longus gives an extension of the hallux alone; stimulation of fascicles to extensor digitorum brevis: an extension of the toes, except the 5th, while with those to extensor digitorum longus: an extension of the toes, except hallux. Then the fascicle(s) to the extensor hallucis muscle are resected partially and those for the extensor digitorum brevis as well, but only if the main response to its stimulation is for the hallux.

3) Results. We have not been able to find any report on this procedure. We have performed it in a hemiplegic patient with a spastic foot and associating equino-varus, flexion of the 4 lateral toes, and also a hyperextension of the hallux very disabling for wearing shoes and walking. A selective tibial neurotomy was performed and was associated at the same time with a selective section of the fascicles to extensor hallucis longus as described. This procedure allowed complete reduction of the abnormal posture of the hallux as well as the equino-varus and flexion deformity of the other toes.

II. Neurotomies for spasticity in the upper limb

A) Neurotomy of the musculo-cutaneous nerve for the spastic elbow in flexion

1) Flexion of the elbow belongs to the common condition of the spastic upper limb. Elbow flexion of near 90° is necessary for the hand to be in a functional position. But excessive flexion, without sufficient reducibility, which impairs dressing and/or creates pain, justifies surgical correction.

The two main flexor muscles, i.e. biceps brachii and brachialis, are innervated by the musculo-cutaneous nerve. The third one: the brachio-radialis is innervated by the radial nerve and thus will not be involved by the procedure. Preservation of tone and strength in this last muscle will play a useful role in avoiding complete flexion paralysis.

2) Surgical technique. The patient is placed supine, the arm in abduction, draped in such a way as to be able to check muscular responses to electrical stimulation of the nerves. Extension of the elbow is tested under general anaesthesia. If the elbow cannot be extended beyond 75°, release of soft tissues is performed concomitantly with the neurotomy. A longitudinal incision is made along the medial aspect of the biceps brachii, lateral to the brachial artery, and extending from the inferior edge of the pectoralis major, down for 5 cm (Fig. 13).

The superficial fascia is opened, and the space between the bicepts (laterally) and the coraco brachialis (medially) is dissected. The musculo-cutaneous nerve lies in between, anterior to the brachialis muscle (Fig. 14). Branches to biceps and brachialis muscles are identified and partially resected.

Under magnification, the epineurium is opened and the fascicles dissected. Motor fascicles still present inside the nerve trunk, are isolated using bipolar

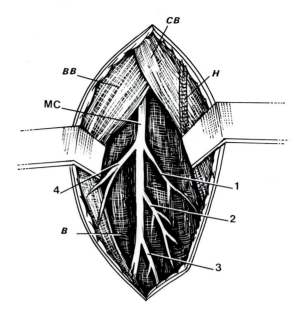

Fig. 14. Dissection of the right musculocutaneous nerve (MC) in the space between the biceps brachii (BB) laterally, the coraco brachialis (CB) medially and the brachialis (B) posteriorly. Branches to brachialis (1), (2) and to biceps brachii (3), (4) are recognized by stimulation giving elbow flexion. Humeral artery (H) with median nerve are situated medially and are not dissected

stimulation and resected according to the pre-operative program, while the sensory fibers are preserved to avoid loss of sensation to their cutaneous distribution.

3) Results. The most important series published was by Garland et al. (1981). It consists of 30 musculo-cutaneous neurotomies, performed completely without selectivity, in 29 adults with a non functional upper limb. A complementary release of soft tissue was performed when irreducible flexion was more than 75°. A cast was applied with the elbow in extension when flexion was fixed at more than 30°. In those with less than 30° of pre-operative flexion, a complete excursion of articular movement was obtained by surgery. In those with more than 30° of preoperative flexion, the average decrease in flexion was 40°. Over all, surgery improved the cosmetics of the patient and made passive mobilisation, nursing and dressing easier.

We have recently performed a musculo-cutaneous neurotomy in a hemiplegic patient, who kept a functional hand for prehension. Preoperatively the elbow was fixed at 110° of flexion, with only a few degrees of active flexion – extension. Two of the 3 motor fascicles of the nerve were cut. Surgery led to an active amplitude of flexion – extension of 100°

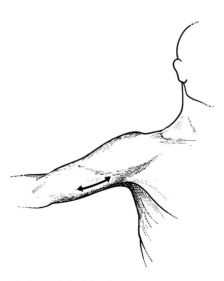

Fig. 13. Skin incision for right musculocutaneous neurotomy, along the medial aspect of the biceps brachii, under the inferior edge of the pectoralis major muscle

without spasticity and allowed the patient to place the hand in a functional position.

4) Discussion. Preoperative assessment should include motor examination of the brachio-radialis muscle which is not involved in the procedure. The purpose is to keep active elbow flexion; so without an active brachio-radialis, musculo-cutaneous neurotomy has to be done with care. Sometimes the procedure is performed only to improve nursing, with the aim of getting the arm into extension.

B) Neurotomies of the median and ulnar nerves for spastic wrist and fingers

1) The spastic abnormal postures of the upper extremity are generally characterized by several of the following components:

a) Pronation of the forearm. Pronator teres and pronator quadratus are the responsible muscles. They are innervated by the median nerve.

b) Flexion – adduction of the wrist. This is due to palmaris longus and flexor carpi radialis muscles both supplied by the median nerve, and to flexor carpi ulnaris tributary to the ulnar nerve.

c) Flexion of the fingers. Both the flexor digitorum superficialis, innervated by the median nerve, and the flexor digitorum profundus, innervated by both the median and ulnar nerves, are responsible for this.

d) Adduction of the thumb. This is under the action of adductor pollicis supplied by the deep terminal branch of the ulnar nerve. In the case of "thumb in palm" deformity, abductor pollicis brevis and opponents muscles, innervated by the median nerve, are involved too.

e) "Swan-neck" finger deformity. This deformity consists of hyperextension of the proximal interphalangeal articulation with flexion of the distal articulations. It can be explained either: by an excessive traction by the extensor muscles, or by spasticity in the lumbrical and interosseous muscles (innervated by the ulnar nerve, excepted the 1st and 2nd lumbrical which are supplied by the median nerve). In the first case the deformity is corrected by passive extension of the wrist. In the second, the deformity is not improved by this manoeuvre, but only by a block of the ulnar nerve.

Spasticity in the wrist and the hand is usually harmful, only a mild spasticity in flexion of the fingers is useful for prehension. With the aim to open the hand, so as to improve prehension, neurosurgery may be indicated:

– to correct excessive pronation of the forearm, so that the hand can be placed in functional position, i.e. in semi-pronation.

– to decrease spasticity in the flexor muscles, while sparing their voluntary control, and increase or reactivate voluntary command of the extensors by re-equilibrating the tonic balance between agonist and antagonist muscles.

– to reduce thumb and/or finger deformities such as the "thumb in palm" and the "swan-neck" fingers.

If the patient retains residual voluntary mobility in the extensor and supinator muscles and sensation, a significant functional improvement will be achieved. If these conditions are not present, there will be no gain in function. However, improvement in nursing care and comfort, as well as a better appearance of the hand, can be reasonably expected.

These aims can be achieved by selectively cutting the median and/or the ulnar nerve branches innervating the muscles supporting harmful spasticity. Selection of muscles to be denervated, requires a detailed preoperative clinical analysis of each spastic or deficient muscle. Local anaesthetic blocks of the median and/or ulnar nerves can be useful to determine the target(s) of surgery.

As the fascicular organization of the median and ulnar nerves at the level of their trunk do not allow one to differentiate motor from sensory fascicles [as pointed out by Sunderland (1968)], it is necessary to dissect the motor branches after they have left the nerve trunk. This makes it essential to perform an extensive exposure and careful dissection of the forearm muscles from the elbow to the wrist (Brunelli and Brunelli 1983).

2) Surgical technique. The cutaneous incision begins 4 cm above the flexion line of the elbow. It passes down along the medial aspect of the biceps brachii, and extends distally in the midline of the forearm, with a sinuous course to avoid skin retraction, ending 5 cm above the wrist (Fig. 15a).

The dissection is started proximally by the sectioning of bicipital aponeurosis. The median nerve which lies deeply between the 2 heads of the pronator teres, is found medial to the brachial artery. Median nerve branches to pronator teres are found deeply on its medial side. Then the pronator teres is retracted upward and laterally, the flexor carpi radialis down-

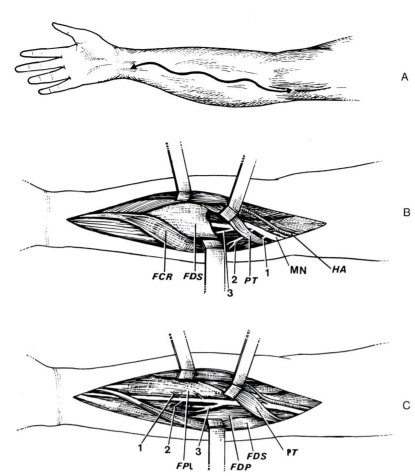

Fig. 15. Right median neurotomy in accordance with Brunelli's technique. **A** Skin incision on the right forearm, from the medial aspect of the biceps brachii at the level of the elbow, to the midline above the wrist. **B** First stage of the dissection, the pronator teres (PT) is retracted upward and laterally, the flexor carpi radialis (FCR) medially. Branches from the median nerve (MN), before it passes under the fibrous arch of the flexor digitorum superficialis (FDS), are dissected: to the pronator teres (1), and two nerve trunks to the flexor carpi radialis, palmaris longus and flexor digitorum superficialis (2), (3). **C** Second stage of the dissection, the fibrous arch of the FDS is sectioned to allow to dissect more distally the median nerve. The FDS is retracted medially and branches from the median nerve are identified: (1) to the flexor pollicis longus (FPL); (2) to the flexor digitorum profundus (FDP); (3) the interosseous nerve and its proper branches to these muscles

ward and medially (Fig. 15b). The branches from the medial aspect of the median nerve to the flexor carpi radialis–palmaris longus and flexor digitorum superficialis–can then be dissected. These branches originate from 1 or 2 trunks.

As the median nerve continues downward, it passed under a fibrous arch between the 2 heads of the flexor digitorum superficialis. This muscle is displaced medially, allowing one to find branches for the deep flexor muscles (Fig. 15c); i.e., flexor digitorum profundus and flexor pollicis longus. These branches arise from the trunk of the median nerve and from the anterior interosseous nerve. To make dissection easier, it may sometimes be useful to divide the fibrous arch of the flexor digitorium superficialis.

In the lower part of the forearm, the flexor digitorum superficialis is retracted medially, the branches from the anterior interosseous nerve to the pronator quadratus are dissected in front of the interosseous membrane.

In cases where it is necessary to denervate flexor carpi ulnaris, the skin incision is performed more medially than in the previous description, i.e., between the medial epicondyle of the humerus and the medial side of the biceps brachii. This approach allows one to dissect the ulnar nerve as it passes through the 2 heads of flexor carpi ulnaris, where it generally gives 2 branches to this muscle. Then, branches to the medial half of the flexor digitorum profundus are dissected more distally on the nerve.

These extensive exposures allow one to make selective neurotomies of the extrinsic spastic muscles innervated by the median and the ulnar nerves, as determined pre-operatively.

If denervation of the opponens muscle and abductor pollicis brevis are needed for correction of "thumb in palm" deformity, a complementary incision is performed in the midline of the palm, medially to the adduction line of the thumb. The flexor retinaculum is divided and the median nerve and terminal branches are exposed. The branch to the muscles of the thenar eminence is isolated. The fascicles responsible for opposition of the thumb with flexion of the metacarpo-phalangeal joint are identified.

In cases where contrature of tendons is associated with spasticity, a post-operative splint is useful for a few weeks to keep the hand and fingers in the functional position.

3) Results. Stoffel (1912) was the first to report on neurotomies of the median nerve, but with variable results. Fascicular sectioning of the nerve trunk led to disappointing results, with sensory disturbances and neuropathic pain. He then performed neurotomies of the muscular branches distally, but the results were inconstant with regard to the spasticity.

More recently, Cahuzac (1980), reported on 6 cases of children with cerebral palsy and spastic pronation of the forearm. They had undergone a complete section of the median nerve branches to pronator teres. In all cases, supination was improved, 5 times passively and once actively. As the pronator quadratus, innervated by branches from the anterior interosseous nerve, was not denervated, active pronation was maintained.

The extensive neurotomies of median and ulnar branches through an extensive forearm approach were described by Brunelli and Brunelli (1983, 1988). In their series of 53 patients, improvement was obtained in almost all of the cases, 40 cases required a second and 3 cases required a third operation to correct an excessive residual spasticity.

An unpublished series of neurotomies of the median nerve by Guegan et al. (1989) has been reported. These preliminary reviews had encouraged the authors to continue to perform this surgical treatment.

Personally we have performed 3 median neurotomies for a non-functional upper extremity to treat a spastic wrist and fingers in flexion with tendinous contracture. We used Brunelli's technique and the Page–Scaglietti procedure in combination through the same approach. Over a long term follow-up a complete correction of abnormal postures was obtained.

4) Discussion. Neurotomies can be directed to one or several of the components of spasticity of the upper extremity: – to branches of pronator teres and pronator quadratus for spastic pronation – to branches of the flexor carpii muscles and palmaris longus for spastic flexion of the wrist – to the flexor digitorum muscles for spastic fingers in flexion. For intrinsic spasticity of the hand, neurotomies can be directed to thenar branch of the median nerve for adduction of the thumb. For "thumb in palm" deformity, it may be difficult to perform a neurotomy of the ulnar branches to adductor pollicis in the palm of the hand, so an

alternative is a myomectomy of the adductor pollicis (Brunelli and Brunelli 1983, 1988), but with the risk of only a transient result.

When the hand is non-functional with spasticity due principally to intrinsic muscles, denervation can be much more extensive by sectioning of the deep branches of the ulnar nerve in the palm of the hand.

When tendinous contractures exist in association with spasticity, tendon lengthening or even tenotomies, such as the Page–Scaglietti procedure can be done during the same surgical session. Complementary orthopaedic procedures also may be indicated to correct residual deformities (as in "swan-neck fingers") or to supplement deficient muscular strength by non-spastic muscle transfers.

General discussion

1) Selective peripheral neurotomy (SPN) can be performed when spasticity is localized to muscles or muscular groups supplied by a single or a few peripheral nerves easily accessible. By suppressing excess spasticity, correcting the abnormal postures and reducing pain, SPN is able to achieve dramatic improvement in the functional status of these patients. If muscular strength has not been completely lost, surgery, by re-equilibrating the tonic balance between agonist and spastic antagonist muscles, results in improvement or reappearance of voluntary mobility.

2) Effectiveness of SPN is conditioned by an accurate preoperative determination of the various spastic components and a precise intraoperative identification of the nerve branches. The use of bipolar stimulation and microtechniques are of considerable help in this aim.

The extent of nerve resection is also critical: excessive lesioning will increase motor deficits, while insufficient lesioning leads to incomplete effectiveness.

Special care must be taken to avoid any damage to the sensory fibers. This inevitably leads to transient or permanent painful phenomena and sensory deficits, as well as trophic disturbances. So when the fascicular organization of the nerve trunk is not propicious for separating motor from sensory fascicles, SPN should be performed as distally as possible, at the level of the muscular branch; i.e., in the forearm for spasticity in the upper extremity.

3) The place of SPN in the surgical management of spasticity is precise. Chemical neurolysis with alcohol or phenol is the more classical alternative to surgical neurotomy. Performed percutaneously, it is a less invasive method and, if spasticity recurs, it may be easily repeated. In addition to recurrence, chemical neurolysis has the disadvantage of lesser selectivity with regard to both the choice of muscular targets and the sparing of sensory fibers. It is because of these limitations, that SPN may be prefered, even as the first procedure. The effectiveness of percutaneous selective radiofrequency neurotomies, an elegant procedure introduced by Kanpolat et al. (1987); may also be considered; but they have still to be evaluated with long term follow-up.

The ideal indications for SPN are focalized harmful hyperspastic disorders. By contrast, when spasticity severely affects the entire limb with multiple abnormal postures, surgery at the spinal root or a spinal cord level (DREZ-tomy) seems preferable.

SPN may be also considered in association with the previous procedures, especially microsurgical DREZ-tomy or rhizotomies, for treating very severe spasticity in the upper or lower limb. Such a combination reduces the extent and depth of the surgical lesion in the spinal cord.

Several types of neurotomies can be combined for the treatment of "multifocal" spasticity of the upper and lower limb(s) (as for example musculo-cutaneous and median neurotomies or obturator, sciatic and tibial neurotomies). This can be an alternative to spinal root or spinal cord procedures.

When orthopaedic factors participate in the irreducibility of abnormal spastic postures, their surgical correction may be indicated. But it seems to us logical to perform SPN as the first step when hypertonia is predominant. Then, if irreducible musculo-tendinous contractures and/or articular anky-loses persist, in spite of intensive postoperative physical therapy, complementary orthopaedic surgery is performed. The more the decrease in spasticity with neurological surgery, the more effective the ortho-paedic surgery will be. By contrast, when deformities predominate in, or are strictly the result of a deficiency in the agonist muscles, and excessive spasticity in the antagonist muscles is not present, orthopaedic oper-ations are the appropriate first procedure.

References

Banks HH, Green WT (1960) Adductor myotomy and obturator neurotomy for the correction of adductive contracture of the hip in cerebral palsy. J Bone Joint Surg [Am] 42: 111–126

Bardot A (1979) Neurotomies périphériques chez les spastiques. In: Pathologie des nerfs périphériques: le membre inférieur. 3ème cours sur la pathologie des nerfs périphériques, Marseille, pp 243–246

Brunelli G, Brunelli F (1983) Hyponeurotisation sélective microchirurgicale dans les paralysies spastiques. Ann Chir Main 2(3): 277–280

Brunelli G, Brunelli F (1988) Hyponeurotization in spastic palsies (selective partial denervation). In: Textbook of microsurgery. Masson, Paris, pp 861–865

Cahuzac M (1980) L'enfant infirme moteur d'origine cérébrale, 2ème ed. Masson, Paris

Garland DE, Thompson R, Waters RL (1981) Musculocutaneous neurotomy for spastic elbow in flexion in non-functional upper extremities in adults. J Bone Joint Surg [Am] 62: 108–112

Gros C, Frerebeau P, Benzech J, Privat JM (1977) Neurotomie radiculaire sélective. In: Simon L (ed) Actualités en rééducation fonctionnelle. Masson, Paris, pp 230–235

Guegan Y, Brassier G, DE Labarthe J, Dufour T (1989) Neurotomie fasciculaire du nerf médian: approache chirurgicale de la spasticité distale du membre supérieur. Communication à la Société de Neurochirurgie de Langue Francaise

Kanpolat Y, Caglar C, Akis E, Erturk A, Ulug H (1987) Percutaneous selective R.F. neurotomy in spasticity. Acta Neurochir (Wien) [Suppl 39]: 96–98

Keats S (1957) Combined adductor—gracilis tenotomy and selective obturator nerve resection for the correction of adduction deformity of the hips in children with cerebral palsy. J Bone Joint Surg 39: 1087–1090

Lorenz F (1887) Über chirurgische Behandlung der angeborenen spastischen Gliedstarre. Wien Klin Rdsch 21: 25–27

Mertens P (1987) Les neurotomies périphériques dans le traitement des troubles spastiques des membres. Thèse Médecine n° 471, Lyon

Peragut JC, Allovon E, Fabrizi A, Bardot A (1989) Chirurgie fonctionnelle nerveuse du membre inférieur. In: Bardo A, Pelissier J (eds) Neuro-orthopédie des membres inférieurs chez l'adulte. Masson, Paris, pp 81–86

Privat JM, Privat C, Frerebeau P, Benezech J, Gros C (1981) Renouveau de la neurotomie obturatrice. In: Simon L (ed) Actualités en rééducation fonctionnelle et réadaptation, 6ème série. Masson, Paris, pp 70–76

Privat JM, Privat CH, Benezech J, Gros C (1981) Spasticité et chirurgie fonctionnelle du nerf sciatique. In: Simon L (ed) La sciatique et le nerf sciatique. Masson, Paris, pp 300–306

Siegfried J, Lazorthes Y (1985) Radicotomies et neurotomies sélectives. In: La neurochirurgie fonctionnelle de l'Infirme moteur d'origine cérébrale. Neurochirurgie 31 [Suppl 1]: 44–54

Silfverskiold N (1923) Réduction of the uncrossed two muscles of the leg to one joint muscle in spastic condition. Acta Chir Scand 56: 315–322

Sindou M, Mertens P (1988) Selective neurotomy of the tibial nerve for treatment of the spastic foot. Neurosurgery 23: 738–744

Sindou M, Abdennebi B, Boisson D, Eyssette M, Goutelle A (1985) Traitement du pied spastique par la neurotomie sélective du nerf tibial. Neurochirurgie 31: 189–197

Stoffel A (1912) The treatment of spastic contractures. Am J Orthop Surg 10: 611–644

Sunderland S (1968) Nerves and nerve injuries. E and S Livingstone

Correspondence: Dr. P. Mertens, Service Neuro-Chirurgie, Hopital Neurologique P. Wertheimer, 59 Boulevard Pinel, 69003 Lyon, France

The different (open surgical, percutaneous thermal, and intrathecal chemical) rhizotomies for the treatment of spasticity

F. Segnarbieux and **Ph. Frerebeau**

Department of Neurosurgery, C.H.R. Saint Eloi–Gui de Chauliac, University of Montpellier, France

Part I. Open surgical rhizotomies

Using the animal model of mesencephalic transection, Sherrington (1940) demonstrated in 1898 that decerebrate rigidity was abolished by posterior rhizotomy. The first posterior rhizotomies were attempted independently by Bennet (1889) and Abbe (1911), the procedure having been suggested to the latter by Dana. On the background of Sherrington's work, Foerster in 1908 (Foerster 1908) applied the posterior rhizotomy procedure from L1 to S2 for the treatment of spasticity in four patients. His results in 159 patients operated on for pain or spasticity were published in 1913 (Foerster 1913).

A renewed interest in posterior rhizotomy using more selective procedures appeared in the sixties and seventies with the reports of Gros et al. (1967) and several other European authors (Sindou et al. 1974, Fasano et al. 1976, Privat et al. 1976, Fraioli and Guidetti 1977, Gros 1979, Siegfried and Lazorthes 1985).

Each dorsal root divides into several rootlets (4 to 8 in general), and the morphology of these have been carefully studied by Hovelacque (1927), Sindou et al. (1976), Sindou and Goutelle (1983), D'Avella and Mingrino (1979). Each of these rootlets can be considered as the elementary target for surgery. The electro-physiological work by Kuhn (1953) demonstrated that in almost all rootlets, muscular proprioceptive and cutaneous exteroceptive afferent fibers are present. According to anatomical studies in animals by Ranson and Billingsley (1916), Earle (1952), Szentagothai (1964) and in man by Sindou et al. (1974), each anterior and posterior rootlet is working as a "rootlet reflex arch".

A) Posterior rhizotomies at the lumbo-sacral level

1. Excision of posterior spinal nerve roots

In his article "on the indications and results of the excision of posterior spinal nerve roots in men" in which 36 personal cases operated on for spasticity in the lower limbs were analyzed, Foerster (1913) gave the following recommendations: "For severe spastic paraplegia, I recommend resecting at least five roots. It is necessary to leave the fourth lumbar root, since this root generally guarantees the extensor reflex of the knee so very necessary for standing and walking. Thus the general rule is resection of the second, third and fifth lumbar, and first and second sacral roots. Unfortunately, there exist individual differences; in some cases, the fourth lumbar does not affect knee extension but knee flexion, as the fifth lumbar and first sacral do; the knee extension is affected only by the second and third lumbar roots. In order to know by which lumbar roots the extension reflex of the knee is effected, we must have recourse to the electrical current during the operation."

Concerning the results Foerster stated in the same article that: "We must bear in mind that the resection of the posterior roots relieves only the spastic symptoms, but not the paralysis, if such exists besides the spastic state". And he concluded: "The disappearance of the spasticity after the root resection is the best proof of the sensory origin of the spastic contracture. But a certain degree of spasm sometimes returns, owing to the fact that the spinal gray matter is gradually recharged by the remaining posterior roots".

In 1936, Lehman (1936) reported on 210 patients

operated on by Foerster. Among 23 patients who had been followed for sufficiently long periods, the result was good in 15 cases. In some cases, the immediate result was satisfactory, but later spasticity recurred, and such recurrences were seen up to 3 years after the treatment.

2. Posterior selective rhizotomy

In order to reduce the sensory side-effects of the original Foerster method, Gros et al. (1967) introduced in 1967 a technical modification consisting of sparing one rootlet only of the five of each root, from L1 (located at the L1-L2 laminotomy level) to S1 root (spotted by intra-operative assessment of the ankle jerk). This preservation of 1/5th of the rootlets allows one at the same time to respect the radicular arteries and the peripheral sensation. With this method, a long term (3 years and 8 months on average) release of spasticity was obtained in 76% of the 25 assessed patients. The spared afferents were enough to preserve normal sensation of the lower limbs in 70% of cases. A global effect on spasticity, including distal effects on upper limbs, speech, writing and self-feeding, were noticed in 18 of the 25 cases.

On similar principles Ouaknine, a pupil of Gros, developed a microsurgical technique consisting of resecting from 1/3 to 2/3 of each group of rootlets of all the posterior roots, from L1 to S1. The importance of the resection depends upon the intensity of spasticity in the corresponding muscular groups. Analysis of the results obtained in his 75 patients (36 with cerebral palsy, 18 with trauma, 15 with multiple sclerosis and 6 with a degenerative disease) followed over a period of at least one year shows a 70% success rate, without trophic or motor complication, and with minimal sensory deficits (Ouaknine 1980).

3. Sectorial posterior rhizotomy

In an attempt to reduce the side-effects on the postural tone in walking patients, Gros and his pupil Privat (Gros 1977, 1979, Privat et al. 1976) proposed in 1976 a topographic selection of the rootlets. The procedure, called sectorial posterior rhizotomy, is based upon a pre-operative assessment differentiating useful spasticity, as related to postural tone (abdominal, quadriceps, gluteus medius muscles), from harmful spasticity in the hip flexors, adductors, hamstrings and triceps surae.

At surgery a mapping of the evoked motor activity of the exposed rootlets, from L1 to S2, by direct electro-stimulation of each posterior group of rootlets is performed. Sectioning is decided upon according to the pre-operative program.

Assessing the data from 22 cases using this technique, the authors found a mean (grouping) of evoked motor activity in accordance with classical radicular distribution but a wide range of responses into adjacent root territories. Nevertheless, stimulation of the rootlets to be divided, evoked motor responses in one of the three following sectors: superior (hip adductors), mid (hamstrings), and inferior (triceps surae).

Results of this method are given in other sections of this book (see chapters by Privat and Privat, and by Frerebeau)

4. Partial posterior rhizotomy

In 1977, Fraioli and Guidetti (1977) reported on a procedure consisting of dividing the dorsal half of each rootlet of the selected posterior roots, a few millimeters before their entrance into the postero-lateral sulcus.

In their series of 44 cases, affected mostly by cerebral palsy and followed over 7 years (Fraioli et al. 1984), there was a considerable improvement with complete disappearance of abnormal postures in 30 patients, a slight improvement in 12, and no improvement in 2. The 30 improved cases showed further improvement later on, with 4 becoming independent walkers, and 9 able to walk with support. The absence of significant sensory deficit was probably explained by the fact that partial section left intact a significant number of fibers of all types.

5. Functional posterior rhizotomy

The neurophysiological search for special organized circuits responsible for spasticity led Fasano et al. (1976) to propose in 1976 the so-called functional posterior rhizotomy. The method is based on bipolar intra-operative stimulation of the posterior rootlets and analysis of the type of muscle responses by EMG recordings. Responses characterized by a permanent tonic contraction (disinhibition), with an after-discharge pattern and a large spatial diffusion to distant muscle groups, are considered to belong to spinal circuits responsible for spasticity (Fasano et al. 1974, 1988).

In the reports by Fasano et al. on his cerebral palsy patients (62 cases) (Fasano et al. 1978), abnormally responsive rootlets were divided, with a quantitative section of 25–50% in 75% of cases, less than 25% in 23% of cases, and more than 50% in only 2% of the patients. Results were poor in 12%, fair in 27%, good in 52% and excellent in 19%. Voluntary motibility was unchanged in 14%, moderately or markedly increased in 32% and 49%, respectively, and returned to normal in 5%. Distant favourable motor effects were noticed at the rostral level in most cases; improvement was slight in 18%, moderate in 41%, marked in 28% and excellent in 13%. Facilitation in speech and reduction in swallowing were considered as slight in 52%, moderate in 24%, marked in 16% and excellent in 8%. Such effects could be obtained without significant reduction of the sensory functions and sphincter control.

The procedure was also used by other authors, especially for children with cerebral palsy (Arens et al. 1989, Peacock et al. 1982, 1987, Cahan et al. 1987, Abbott et al. 1989, or myelomeningocele (Storrs 1987). Methods, indications and results in children will be described in another section of this book by Abbott et al.

In 1983 Laitinen (1983) reported 9 adult patients operated upon by Fasano's technique; 6 of them had severe multiple sclerosis necessitating a wheelchair. 80% of selected rootlets were divided. Spasticity was abolished in the operated limbs in 4 cases, diminished in 5. A recovery of walking with support was obtained in 2 out of 6 wheelchair patients. The follow-up period ranged from 8 to 26 months.

6. Selective posterior rhizotomy in the dorsal root entry zone

This method, introduced by Sindou in 1972 (Sindou 1972) for somatogenic and neurogenic pain, and then developed for harmful spasticity in the limbs (Sindou et al. 1974, 1982, Sindou and Jeanmonod 1989), is detailed in a special chapter of this book.

B) Posterior rhizotomies at the cervical level

Only very few surgical attempts have been devoted to the correction of spastic disorders affecting the upper limb(s).

In his article entitled "On the indications and results of the excision of posterior spinal nerve roots in men"

Foerster (1913) mentioned 23 cases of spastic paralysis of the arm treated by resection of the posterior cervical roots from C4 to T2 except C6, or from three-fifth to four-fifths of the fascicles composing each root including C6. In contrast to paraplegia, he concluded that for spastic hemiplegia of the arm "in the majority the result was not good, a satisfactory improvement being obtained in only a few cases", and he did not recommend posterior rhizotomy as a valuable procedure for spasticity in the upper limb.

Many years later, Kottke (1970) and Heimburger et al. (1973) reported successful decreases of spasticity in the upper limbs after bilateral posterior cervical rhizotomy of C1 through C3 (or the upper rootlets of C4). Their series consisted of 6 and 15 patients, respectively, who were suffering from cerebral palsy. In both, lessening of spasticity was observed not only in the neck, but in the arms and the spine and legs. This was attributed to the abolition of the tonic reflexes of the neck. Similar favourable distant effects were noticed by Ouaknine (1980), Gros et al. (1967), and Gros (1977, 1979) in their series of Little's disease treated with lumbosacral posterior rhizotomies. Improvement in spine, arms, and even speech were considered by the authors as "related to a quantitative reduction in the stimulations transmitted by the intersegmentary connections through the spinal cord interneurons".

In the recent past, attempts to improve selectivity of posterior rhizotomies have been made in patients with good residual functions in the upper limb: among them, the sectorial posterior rhizotomy procedure sectioning 4/5th of the rootlets in the selected sectors (Gros 1979, Privat et al. 1976) and the so-called selective posterior rhizotomy in the dorsal root entry zone (Sindou 1972, Sindou et al. 1986). The latter – in maintaining intact a part of the afferent fibers – allows an effective preservation of neurological functions in the upper limb. This technique and its results will be developed in a following section of the book.

C) Anterior rhizotomies and combined (anterior and posterior) rhizotomies

Extensive anterior rhizotomy (from the lower thoracic to the first sacral segment inclusive) was recommended by Munro (1945) in paraplegic patients, when severe irreducible spasms endangered life. The method was found to be effective in nearly all cases of the series reported by Munro (1945): 42 patients, Freeman and Heimburger (1947): 28 cases, Kerr (1966): 30 cases. Of course this modality is only indicated when there is no residual voluntary movement in the legs.

Pollock and Davis (1930) found in a spastic cat model created by vertebral and carotid ligation that spasticity was not modified by posterior rhizotomy but yielded to anterior rhizotomy. Similar effectiveness of anterior rhizotomy – after failure of posterior rhizotomy – was reported by Tarlov (1967) in a case of hypertonia due to damage to spinal interneurones.

These data are in favour of a mechanism related to spontaneous hyperactivity of the motor neurons deprived from their inhibitory control and not to exaggerated segmental (stretch) reflexes.

An association of sectioning of some motor rootlets with posterior rhizotomy has been proposed by the Montpellier school (Gros et al. 1981) especially at the L2 level for severe adduction in the hip, and at C7-C8 and T1 level for hyperflexion of the wrist and fingers. 5 cases of such combined rhizotomies were mentioned by Gros et al. (1981), but details of results were not given.

Part II. Percutaneous thermo-rhizotomies

Percutaneous radiofrequency rhizotomy was initially performed for the treatment of pain (Uematsu et al. 1974, Lazorthes et al. 1976). Young and Mulcahy (1980) have subsequently proposed percutaneous sacral rhizotomy for neurogenic detrusor hyper-reflexia. Later, Kenmore (1983), Hertz et al. (1983), and Kasdon and Lathi (1984) reported on series of patients with intractable spasticity treated by the same procedure. We have used this simple and safe technique in 12 patients with severe spasticity of the knee.

Reports differ on which peripheral nerve fibers are affected by radiofrequency lesions. Letcher and Goldring (1968) demonstrated in vitro, early selective conduction block of smaller A delta and C fibers before those of the A alpha–beta group. That principle was applied to the management of peripheral neuralgia and spasticity. In contrast Uematsu et al. (1974) reported the first histological study about RF – thermocoagulation effects on the sciatic nerve of the cat and demonstrated an indiscriminate neuropathological effect in all sizes and all types of fibers. Smith et al. (1981) found unselective and delayed pathological damage in dogs. To date, there has not been

a clinical human study correlating electrophysiological and histological changes with pain and spasticity relief and the sparing of motor and touch function. In egg experimentation, Bogduk et al. (1987) described the cardinal finding that the radiofrequency lesion did not extent distal to the tip of the electrode but radially in the shape of an oblate spheroid and had a maximal diameter of only 2 mm. Because of the radial extent of this lesion, the electrode must be introduced parallel and not perpendicularly to the target nerve.

Letcher and Goldring (1968) supported the idea that the wattage necessary to abolish the action potentials was just below that necessary to begin coagulation of egg albumin (47°). With graded lesions using electrode tip temperatures from 45° to 75°, the breakdown of nerve fibers is similar to that occurring with the tip temperature at 85° (Smith et al. 1981). The maximal size of the lesion is attained once a thermal equilibrium is reached. There is no discernible increase of the lesion as this temperature is maintained but, with the same temperature, larger lesions occured when larger electrodes were used (Hertz et al. 1983).

The procedure requires general anaesthesia. The patients are placed with padding protection on the fluoroscopic table. The procedure in the lumbar spine is performed in the lateral recumbent position, the affected side up. Of course prone position would be very uncomfortable in the case of fixed tendons and joint with resulting abnormalties of posture. The entry point on the skin is about 5 to 7 cm from the midline just below the level of the intervertebral space and the 12 gauge needle is advanced obliquely upwards towards the appropriate foramen under fluoroscopic control so as to reach the target root tangentially (Kenmore 1983). Then the radiofrequency probe is placed through the spinal stylet and a ground electrode inserted into the buttock. Stimulation current is applied with an increasing voltage until a motor response is obtained in the appropriate muscle group. It is sometimes necessary to re-adjust the probe so as to obtain the best motor response with a threshold of less than 0.5 volts. The radio-frequency lesion can be made at 90°C for two minutes. Then a repeated stimulation is applied; an increase in threshold of at least 0.2 volts is desired to be certain of a significant relief of spasticity (Hertz et al. 1983). Otherwise the procedure must be repeated by repositioning the electrode, rather than repeating the coagulation. The same process can be performed at each selected level from L1 to L5 for different targeted muscle. It must be mentioned that there is considerable confusion and disagreement as to what constitutes "normal" neuro-anatomy for motor and sensory distribution of the nerve roots, especially at the lumbosacral level, because of bony segmental anomalies (Uematsu et al. 1974).

Kenmore (1983) described the placement of the electrode for radiofrequency lesion at S1: the needle is inserted percutaneously in the midline between the spinous processes of L5 and S1 and directed laterally towards the elbow of the S1 nerve root without penetration of the dura. Young and Mulcahy (1980) performed foraminal radiofrequency sacral rhizotomy from S1 to S4 with cystometric monitoring for neurogenic detrusor hyper-reflexia.

In the cervical spine, Uematsu et al. (1974) used a 17 gauge guide needle with the patient in the supine position on a Rosomoff head-holder. The tip of the needle was placed in the posterior compartment of the vertebral foramen to avoid damage to the vertebral artery.

The best results in the literature (Hertz et al. 1983, Kasdon and Lathi 1984, Kenmore 1983) as well in the authors' series, were obtained in patients with spasticity in the lower limb(s) and when multiple lumbar RF-rhizotomies were performed (from L1 or L2 to L5). In patients with a long follow-up, a high rate of recurrent spasticity was observed (6 to 9 months on average), but the pre-operative level of spasticity was not reached.

This method has the advantage of being less invasive than the open procedures in very debilitated patients. It seems more appropriate for spastic disturbances limited to a few muscular groups, corresponding to a small number of spinal roots. Frequently the effects are transient and this constitutes its main disadvantage. This is counterbalanced by the possibility of repeating the procedure.

Part III. Intrathecal chemical rhizotomies

Intrathecal injection of alcohol was introduced by Dogliotti (1931) for relief of cancer pain, and later on by Guttman (1953) for the treatment of hypertonia in patients with severe spastic paraplegia. After injection through lumbar puncture, the foot of patient's bed had to be kept elevated for 24 hours, because alcohol is lighter than the CSF.

In 1955, Maher (1955) replaced alcohol with phenol – a hyperbaric solution – as the neurolytic agent for pain relief, with the famous remark that: it is easier to lay a carpet than to paper a ceiling". Use of phenol for treatment of spasticity was then developed simultaneously in 1959 by Nathan (1959) and Kelly and Gautier-Smith (1959), because of a better selectivity than alcohol.

The most often used solution is 5% phenol in glycerine. It is obtained by dissolving 15 grams of crystalized phenol in 300 cc of anhydrous glycerine, followed by heating to 60°C and filtration. The preparation is contained inside small 5 cc ampules sterilized at 140°C for 4 hours. The ampules must be absolutely dry, as presence of water would render the preparation very neurotoxic. Such a solution can be safely stored for only a few days. In case of insufficient effect, the concentration of phenol can be increased to 10% or even 20%. When solutions in iophendylate (an oil contrast medium) are used, concentration of phenol must be higher (in the order of 20%), because of a slower release. Such a preparation, which has the advantage of allowing fluoroscopic control, cannot be stored.

The best candidates for intrathecal phenol injections are paraplegic patients suffering from severe spasms, without useful residual motor or sensory functions below the level of the lesion. When rhizotomy must be done bilaterally, it is prudent to perform the treatment in two separate sessions (i.e. one side at a time) and with an interval of one to two weeks.

The patient lies on the spastic side, the head raised 30°. In patients who retain useful automatic bladder function and sphincteric control, the pelvis must be elevated as well, to prevent phenol from coming into contact with the terminal roots of the cauda equina. Injection is done through lumbar puncture performed at the intervertebral space corresponding to the upper level of the radicular sleeves to be injected. Patients must be carefully immobilized to allow precise layering of the neurolytic material. Low lumbar injections can seriously endanger vesical, anal and sexual functions, while injections between L2-L3 or L3-L4 involve slighter risks of this occurrence.

In Greitz and Lindblom's (1966) refined technique, small doses of water – soluble absorbable contrast medium are used and the patient's position is adjusted until the medium fills the correct nerve root sleeves. The amount of medium also determines the necessary volume of phenol in glycerine (in the order of 1 ml), which will layer under the water-soluble medium.

When using oil contrast medium, it must be recalled that phenol-glycerine solution layers above the contrast. The patients are maintained in the lateral flexed lying position for 30 minutes after the injection and then flat in bed for 24 hours.

According to Dahm (1985), in patients with residual sacral nerve functions, the excitability of the H-reflex in the soleus muscle can be monitored during the procedure. If the amplitude of the response diminishes after the injection of 0.1 ml of phenol, the patient is repositioned until full recovery of the H-wave occurs. The total amount is then injected.

Extensive information about techniques and results of intrathecal phenol in the treatment of spasticity (and pain) are given in the review-articles by Papo and Visca (1976) and Wood (1978). As most patients operated on for spasticity were patients with very severe, pre-existent neurological deficits, exact evaluation of the risks of the procedure is very difficult. According to Wood's conclusions based on the data in the literature concerning patients with only pain problems, there is a risk of transient ill – effects including headache, weakness, numbness and sphincter problems of 1–33%, and of permanent complication from 1–13%; the higher the concentration, the higher the risk.

The human histo-pathological reports show that lesions may vary from minimal posterior root damage to additional anterior root damage, arachnoiditis, vascular thrombosis and even spinal cord infarction (Wood 1978, Sindou and Jeanmonod 1989).

In a recent series published by Dahm (1985), which includes 101 rhizotomies performed in 30 patients from June 1976 to October 1982, results were judged after a 6–8 weeks follow-up. Satisfactory effects were obtained in 8 out of 24 injections using 2% to 7.5% phenol and 23 out of 36 with a 10% solution. Patients with unsatisfactory results responded well to a stronger concentration later. 32 out of 41 injections using a 20% concentration had satisfactory effects. There were no severe complications in the series. Complications were limited to 8 cases of transient headache lasting up to 4 days and transitory retention of urine.

According to Papo and Visca (1976), two basic limitations must be borne in mind: the risk of urinary complications if the patient has bladder function and the transient duration of benefical effects (from several months to two years). Therefore most authors advocate limiting the indications of phenol rhizo-tomies to completely paraplegic patients with painful spasms, in whom bladder control has already been lost and life expectancy is short, or in patients who are too ill to withstand major surgery.

References

Abbe R (1911) Resection of the posterior roots of spinal nerves to relieve pain, pain reflex, athetosis and spastic paralysis. Dana's operation. Med Rec 79: 377–381

Abbott R, Forem SL, Johan M (1989) Selective posterior rhizotomy for the treatment of spasticity. Childs Nerv Syst 5: 337–346

Arens LJ, Peacock WJ, Peter J (1989) Selective posterior rhizotomy: a long term follow-up study. Childs Nerv Syst 5: 148–152

Bennet WH (1889) Subdivision of posterior roots of spinal nerve. Lancet 72: 329–348

Bogduk W, Macintosh J, Marsland A (1987) Technical limitations to the efficacy of radiofrequency neurotomy for spinal pain. Neurosurgery 20: 529–535

Cahan LD, Kundi MS, Mc Pherson D, Starr A, Peacock WJ (1987) Electrophysiologic studies in selective dorsal rhizotomy for spasticity in children with cerebral palsy. Appl Neurophysiol 50: 459–682

D'Avella D, Mingrino S (1979) Microsurgical anatomy of lumbo-sacral spinal roots. J Neurosurg 51: 819–823

Dahm LS (1985) Chemical modification of spasticity. In: Sir Eccles J, Dimitrijevic MR (eds) Recent achievements in restorative neurology. Upper motor neuron function and dysfunctions. Karger, Basel, pp 27–30

Dogliotti A (1931) Traitement des syndromes douloureux de la périphérie par l'alcoolisation sous-arachnoïdienne des racines postérieures à leur émergence de la moelle épinière. Presse Méd 39: 1249–1252

Earle K (1952) The tract of Lissauer and its possible relation to the pain pathway. J Comp Neurol 96: 93–111

Fasano VA, Barolat-Romana G, Ivaldi A, Squazzi A (1976) La radicotomie postérieure fonctionnelle dans le traitement de la spasticité cérébrale. Neurochirurgie 22: 23–34

Fasano VA, Broggi G, Barolat-Romano G, Squazzi A (1978) Surgical treatment of spasticity in cerebral palsy. Childs Brain 4: 289–305

Fasano VA, Barolat-Romano G, Squazzi A (1979) Electrophysiological assessment of spinal circuits in spasticity by direct dorsal root stimulation. Neurosurgery 4: 146–152

Fasano VA, Broggi G, Zemes S (1988) Intraoperative electrical stimulation for functional posterior rhizotomy. Scand J Rehab Med [Suppl 17]: 149–154

Foerster O (1908) Über eine neue operative Methode der Behandlung spastischer Lähmungen mittels Resektion hinter Rückenmarkswurzeln. Z Orthop Chir 22: 203

Foerster O (1913) On the indications and results of the excision of posterior spinal nerve roots in men. Surg Gynecol Obstet 16: 463–474

Fraioli B, Guidetti B (1977) Posterior partial rootlet section in the treatment of spasticity. J Neurosurg 46: 618–626

Fraioli B, Zamponi C, Baldassare L, Rosa G (1984) Selective posterior rootlet section in the treatment of spastic disorders of infantile cerebral palsy: immediate and late results. Acta Neurochir 33: 539–541

Freeman LW, Heimburger RF (1947) The surgical relief of spasticity in paraplegic patients; anterior rhizotomy. J Neurosurg 4: 435–443

Greitz T, Lindblom U (1966) Selective nerve root blocking with phenol under myelographic control. Invest Radiol 1: 257–261

Gros C (1977) Table ronde de la Société Française de Neurochirurgie sur le chirurgie de la spasticité. Neurochirurgie 23: 316–388

Gros C (1979) Spasticity–clinical classification and surgical treatment. In: Krayenbulhl (ed) Advances and technical standards in neurosurgery, vol 6. Springer, Wien New York, pp 55–97

Gros C, Ouaknine G, Vlahovitch B, Frerebeau PH (1967) La radicotomie selective posterieure dans le traitement neurochirurgical de l'hypertonie pyramidale. Neurochirurgie 13: 505–518

Gros C, Privat JM, Frerebeau PH, Benezech J (1981) Les radicotomies antérieures: leur place dans le traitement de la spasticité. In: Simon L (ed) Actualités en rééducation fonctionnelle et réadaptation, Gémé série. Masson, Paris, pp 63–70

Guttman L (1953) The treatment and rehabilitation of patients with injuries of the spinal cord. In: Cope 2 (ed) History of the Second World War; Her Majesty's Stationery Office. Vol Surgery pp 422–516

Hertz DA, Parsons KC, Pearl L (1983) Percutaneous radiofrequency foraminal rhizotomies. Spine 8: 729–732

Heimburger RF, Slominski A, Griswold P (1973) Cervical posterior rhizotomy for reducing spasticity in cerebral palsy. J Neurosurg 39: 30–34

Hovelacque A (1927) Anatomie des nerfs craniens et rachidiens et du système grand sympathique chez l'Homme. Doin, Paris

Kasdon DL, Lathi ES (1984) A prospective study of radiofrequency rhizotomy in the treatment of post-traumatic spasticity. Neurosurgery 15: 526–529

Kelly RE, Gautier-Smith PC (1959) Intrathecal phenol in the treatment of reflex spasms and spasticity. Lancet ii: 1102–1105

Kenmore D (1983) Radiofrequency neurotomy for peripheral pain and spasticity syndromes. Contemp Neurosurg 5: 1–6

Kerr AS (1966) Anterior rhizotomy for the relief of spasticity. Paraplegia 4: 154–160

Kottke J (1970) Modification of athetosis by denervation of the tonic neck reflexes. Dev Med Child Neurol 12: 236–237

Kuhn R (1953) Organization of tactile dermatomes in cat and monkey. J Neurophysiol 16: 109

Laitinen LV, Nilsson S, Fugl-Meyer AR (1983) Selective posterior rhizotomy for treatment of spasticity. J Neurosurg 58: 895–899

Lazorthes Y, Verdie JC, Lagarrigue J (1976) Thermocoagulation percutanée des nerfs rachidiens à visée antalgique. Neurochirurgie 22: 445–453

Lehmann W (1936) Chirurgische Therapie bei Erkrankungen und Verletzungen des Nervensystems. In: Bumke O, Foerster O (Hrsg) Handbuch der Neurologie, Bd 8. Springer, Berlin, pp 90–265

Letcher FS, Goldring S (1968) The effect of radiofrequency current and heat on peripheral nerve action potential in the cat. J Neurosurg 29: 42–47

Maher R (1955) Relief of pain in incurable cancer. Lancet i: 18–20

Munro D (1945) The rehabilitation of patients totally paralysed below waist: anterior rhizotomy for spastic paraplegia. Engl J Med 233: 456–461

Nathan PW (1959) Intrathecal phenol to relieve spasticity in paraplegia. Lancet ii: 1099–1102

Ouaknine GE (1980) Le traitement chirurgical de la spasticité. Union Méd 109 (10): 1–10

Papo I, Visca A (1976) Intrathecal phenol in the treatment of pain and spasticity. Prog Neurol Surg 7: 56–130

Peacock WJ, Arens LJ (1982) Selective posterior rhizotomy for the relief of spasticity in cerebral palsy. S Afr Med J 62: 119–124

Peacock WJ, Arens LJ, Berman B (1987) Cerebral palsy spasticity. Selective posterior rhizotomy. Pediatr Neurosci 13: 61–66

Pollock LS, Davis LE (1930) Reflex activities of decerebrate animal. J Comp Neurol 50: 377–411

Privat JM, Benezech J, Frerebeau Ph, Gros C (1976) Sectorial posterior rhizotomy: a new technique of surgical treatment for spasticity. Acta Neurochir 35: 181–195

Ranson S, Billingsley P (1916) The conduction of painful afferent impulses in the spinal nerves. Am J Physiol 40: 571–584

Sherrington C (1940) On the distribution of the sensory nerve roots. In: Denny Brown (ed) Selected writings of Sir Charles Sherrington Chapter II. Hoeber, New York, pp 532

Siegfried J, Lazorthes Y (1985) La neurochirurgie fonctionnelle de l'infirmité motrice d'origine cerebrale. Neurochirurgie 31 [Suppl 1]: 44–54

Sindou M (1972) Etude de la jonction radiculo-médullaire postérieure. La radicellotomie sélective postérieure dans la chirurgie de la douleur. Thèse Médecine, Lyon, p 182

Sindou M, Quoex C, Baleydier C (1974) Fiber organization at the posterior spinal cord-rootlet junction in man. J Comp Neurol 153: 14–26

Sindou M, Fischer G, Goutelle R, Schott B, Mansuy L (1974) La radicellotomie postérieure sélective dans le traitement des spasticités. Rev Neurol 30: 201–215

Sindou M, Fischer G, Mansuy L (1976) Posterior spinal rhizotomy and selective posterior rhizidiotomy. In: Krayenbuhl H, Maspes PE, Sweet WH (eds) Progress in neurological surgery, vol 7. Karger, Basel, pp 201–250

Sindou M, Millet MF, Mortamais J, Eyssette M (1982) Results of selective posterior rhizotomy in the treatment of painful and spastic paraplegia secondary to multiple sclerosis. Appl Neurophysiol 45: 335–340

Sindou M, Goutelle A (1983) Surgical posterior rhizotomies for the treatment of pain. In: Krayenbuhl H (ed) Advances and technical standards in neurosurgery, vol 10. Springer, Wien New York, pp 147–185

Sindou M, Mifsud JJ, Boisson D, Goutelle A (1986) Selective posterior rhizotomy in the dorsal root entry zone for treatment of hyperspasticity and pain in the hemiplegic upper limb. Neurosurgery 18: 587–595

Sindou M, Jeanmonod D (1989) Microsurgical Drez-otomy for the treatment of spasticity and pain in the lower limbs. Neurosurgery 24: 655–670

Sindou M, Jeanmonod D (1990) Structural approach to management of pain. In: Dimitrijevic M, Wall PD, Lindblom U (eds) Recent achievements in restorative neurology; altered sensation and pain. Karger, Basel, pp 64–78

Smith HP, Mc Whorter JM, Challa VR (1981) Radiofrequency neurolysis in a clinical model. Neuropathological correlation. J Neurosurg 55: 246–253

Storrs B (1987) Selective posterior rhizotomy for treatment of progressive spasticity in patients with myelomeningocele. Pediatr Neurosci 13: 135–137

Szentagothai J (1964) Neuronal and synaptic arrangement in the subtantia gelatinosa. J Comp Neurol 122: 219–239

Tarlov IM (1967) Rigidity in man due to spinal interneuron loss. Arch Neurol 16: 436–443

Uematsu S, Udvarhelyi GB, Benson D, Siebens A (1974) Percutaneous radiofrequency rhizotomy. Surg Neurol 2: 319–325

Wood KM (1978) The use of phenol as a neurolytic agent: a review. Pain 5: 205–229

Young B, Mulcahi JJ (1980) Percutaneous sacral rhizotomy for neurogenic detrusor hypereflexia. J Neurosurg 53: 85–87

Correspondence: Dr. Ph. Frerebeau, Department of Neurosurgery, CHR Saint Eloi–Gui de Chauliac, University of Montpellier, F-34059 Montpellier, France

Sectorial posterior rhizotomy for the treatment of spasticity in adults

J.M. Privat and **Ch. Privat**

Service de Neurochirurgie, Centre Gui de Chauliac, CHRU, Montpellier, France

Sectorial posterior rhizotomy (S.P.R.) aims to limit sectioning to the dorsal rootlets causing the "handicapping" spasticity (Gros 1979, Privat et al. 1976).

Rationale

Two notions are of paramount importance to the fundamental principles for the technique:

1. Handicapping versus useful spasticity. Handicapping spasticity is that which disturbs voluntary movement and creates tonic imbalance between muscular groups. Useful spasticity is that which allows sustained function such as standing and walking, when voluntary movement is insufficient.

Therefore functional and analytic testing (Fig. 1) is mandatory before deciding on surgery:

- functional, to define which kind of handicapping situation is affecting the patient, and decide on the goal of rhizotomy, as well as predict its postoperative limits;
- analytic, to establish the surgical program for each joint and the radicular sectors to be cut.

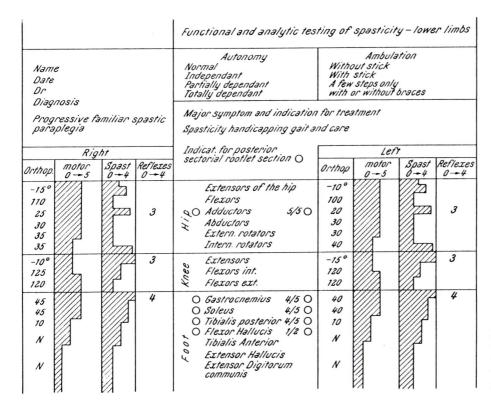

Fig. 1. Functional and analytic testing of spasticity (lower limbs). "Mapping chart" used to evaluate the indications and results of sectorial posterior rhizotomy

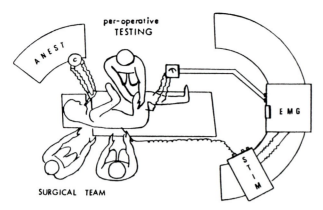

Fig. 2. Operative technique: the surgeon is behind the patient, who lies in a lateral position; the physiatrist, on the opposite side, performs the intra-operative testing, by assessing the responses to stimulation of rootlets

2. Agonist–antagonist crossed innervation as stated by Sherrington. This principle explains that surgical treatment limited to a sector may act on spasticity in adjacent territories.

Taking into account these two notions, a mapping chart – serving as a pre-operative program – is established, in order to guide the surgeon in selecting the rootlets to be cut, and those to be preserved (see Fig. 3).

Operative technique

The patient is operated upon in the lateral position, under general anesthesia without curare (Fig. 2). Through a T12-L1 laminectomy, rootlets are dissected and gathered in groups by colored threads so as to form functional sectors (Fig. 3).

While the surgeon stimulates each posterior rootlet (monopolar, square waves, 50–70 Hz, 0,1–4 volts, 1 msec), the physiotherapist records the clinical and EMG responses. This enables the team to establish a "mapping" of rootlet groups (i.e. "Functional sectors"). Every functional muscular group is usually dependant on 3 to 5 rootlets.

After several checks demonstrating a good correlation between responses obtained by intra-operative stimulation and the pre-operative muscle testing (Fig. 4), the surgeon is allowed to divide 4/5 th of the rootlets supporting those muscles with handicapping spasticity.

Intra-operative mapping can be made more accurate when the following measures are undertaken:

1. When beginning, it is useful to grossly localize the root levels. The best way for that is to stimulate the anterior rootlets before the posterior ones;

2. Even if the right threshold has been chosen, there may be a diffusion of responses into several muscular groups. So it is necessary to stimulate each group of rootlets, as if it was a "piano keyboard". After the first sections have been made, results must be confirmed by a second mapping, prior to sectioning of the remaining "handicapping rootlets", if necessary.

3. Stimulation of a single group of rootlets may evoke responses in several different muscles. For example, responses in the quadriceps femoris (supporting useful spasticity) and in the adductors (supporting handicapping spasticity) may occur after stimulation of the same rootlet group. In this case, it is necessary to perform further dissection of each rootlet and even to dissociate rootlets into thin bundles of fibers, in

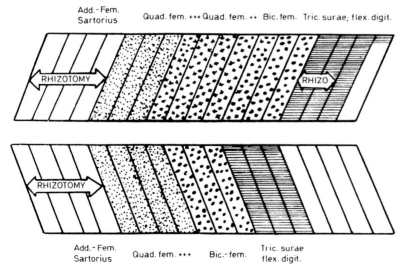

Fig. 3. Operative technique. Typical intra-operative mapping of rootlets, according to intra-operative stimulation and testing. Arrows indicate the extent of posterior sectorial rhizotomy

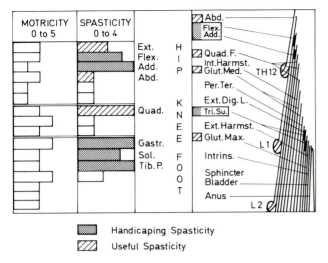

	Handicaping Spasticity
	Useful Spasticity

Fig. 4. Comparison of pre-operative (left) and intra-operative (right) testing of spasticity. Choice of the rootlets (supporting handicapping spasticity) to be divided by posterior sectorial rhizotomy

order to select those supporting handicapping spasticity.

Personal experience: results

Among our last 100 spastic patients who underwent functional surgery, we have performed SPR in 21. All were adults. The etiology was spinal cord injury in 12, multiple sclerosis in 2, Strumpell-Lorrain syndrome in 2, miscellaneous in 5.

The therapeutic goal (facilitation of nursing and physiotherapy, and/or improvement in function) was reached in 72% and surpassed (with better functional improvement than expected) in 16%. The failure rate was 12%.

Conclusion

SPR is based on operative identification of the posterior rootlets subserving harmful spasticity, with electrophysiological stimulation, muscle testing and EMG studies. The procedure is able to decrease the "handicapping", and preserve the "useful" spasticity.

References

Gros C (1979) Spasticity: clinical classification and surgical treatment. In: Krayenbuhl H (ed) Advances and technical standards in neurosurgery, vol 6. Springer, Wien New York, pp 55–97

Privat JM, Benezech J, Frerebeau Ph, Gros C (1976) Sectorial posterior rhizotomy: a new technique of surgical treatment of spasticity. Acta Neurochir 34: 181–195

Correspondence: Dr. J.M. Privat, Service de Neurochirurgie, Centre Gui de Chauliac, CHRU, F-34059 Montpellier, France

Sectorial posterior rhizotomy for the treatment of spasticity in children with cerebral palsy

Ph. Frerebeau

Department of Neurosurgery, C.H.R. Saint Eloi – Gui de Chauliac, University of Montpellier, France

From 1967 to 1982, 60 children or young adults have been operated on in the neurosurgical clinic of Montpellier, using the successive evolutive technical modalities of posterior rhizotomy. Quantitative Posterior Rhizotomy (Gros et al. 1967, Ouaknine 1980) and Sectorial Posterior Rhizotomy (Privat et al. 1975, Gros 1979) [see previous chapter by J.M. Privat and Ch. Privat for technical description]. The present study analyzes the long term results obtained in this cerebral palsy series.

Patients and methods

– The patients' ages ranged from 5 to 26 years (11 on average). The suspected aetiology was prematurity in 13 cases, neonatal hypoxia in 17, other perinatal insults in 8, and was unknown in 22. The handicap was: spastic hemiplegia in 5 cases, spastic diplegia in 18, pure spastic quadriplegia in 9, mixed spastic and athetoid quadriplegia in 28.

– The I.Q. level was classified as of a superior level (above 75) in 22 cases (most of them had hemiplegia or pure diplegia), moderate retardation (from 40 to 75) in 19, profound retardation (below 40) in 19.

Developing motor skill was analyzed using a three level scale: level 2 (stand up and walk) in 29 cases; level 1 (acquired axial tone and sitting position) in 9; level C (absence of previous items) in 22.

Functional status was assessed according to three criteria. 1. Ambulatory function (walking) was classified using 5 levels: independant walking (5 cases), walking with help (19 cases), wheelchair with occasional walking (10 cases), permanent wheelchair (10 cases), bed-ridden (16 cases). 2. Activities of daily living were assessed for dressing, washing, sphincter continence, feeding, writing. Independence in three items was considered positive (29 cases). 3. Social integration was classified as follows: working, independant, partly dependant, fully dependant, bed-ridden.

Assessment of joint imbalance (due to weakness and spasticity) was analyzed in 4 main muscle groups: hip flexor-extensor; hip adductor-abductor; knee flexor-extensor; ankle flexor-extensor. Great attention was paid to differentiating the harmful spasticity and possible associated lesion (muscle shortening, athetosis) versus useful spasticity and negative symptoms (disturbances of postural tone, decrease in voluntary muscle strength).

– Surgery was indicated for improving: walking in 29 cases, bracing adaptation in 19, sitting in the wheelchair in 12, nursing and prevention of orthopaedic complications in 10.

The final overall result was assessed for these criteria with a mean follow-up time of 5 years. All the patients underwent a pre-operative, six month full-time physiotherapy course in order to increase the postural tone. In the post-operative period, 39 children were sent to a rehabilitation center, 15 were treated at home, (6 had unknown data). 34 underwent associated orthopaedic surgical procedures, before rhizotomy in 21 patients, and after in 20.

– Patients operated on to improve nursing and/or prevent orthopaedic complications had a Quantitative Posterior Rhizotomy (Q.P.R.), from L1 to S1, cutting 66% to 80% of the rootlets.

Patients who underwent Sectorial Posterior Rhizotomy (S.P.R.) for improving walking or bracing had 27% to 65% (average 40%) of the rootlets divided, especially those for the hamstrings and/or triceps surae.

An Anterior Rhizotomy (20% to 54% of the anterior rootlets) was combined to posterior rhizotomy (30% to 80% of the posterior rootlets) in bedridden patients, especially those with severe spasticity in the hip adductors, in whom the anterior rhizotomy was targeted on the adductor rootlets.

Operative results

Results could be evaluated in only 40 of the 60 cases. Data are summarized in Table 1.

The pre-operative spasticity was dominant in hip adductors and ankle flexors. Figure 1 shows the mean value of pre and post-operative spasticity.

The selectivity of the procedures has been analyzed by comparing the effect on spasticity related to divided versus saved rootlets. A 51% mean decrease of spasticity was obtained in muscles related to divided rootlets, versus 22% in muscles related to saved rootlets, with 2 discordant results.

Figure 2 which displays the pre and post-operative

Table 1. Posterior rhizotomy in cerebral palsy

Rehabilitation goal	nb cases	Results
Nursing		6/7 facilitated
	8	Associated goals } 4/6 obtained
Orthop. prevent.		3/4 avoided
Sitting	13	13/13 improved or acquired
Walking		Improved 7 } 13
	19	Acquired 6
Bracing		Reduced 8 } 11
		Suppressed 3

analysis of muscle strength, shows that surgery does not significantly decrease voluntary mobility.

A positive result in the functional status (walking, activities of daily living and social integration) was obtained in 70% of cases.

Discussion

"In patients suffering from cerebral palsy, the muscle imbalance by impairing voluntary control of motor function and abnormal stretch reflex is the deforming force that limits or precludes ambulation" (Drenamm). Treating the rootlet reflex arch using rhizotomy seems to be a adaptable procedure.

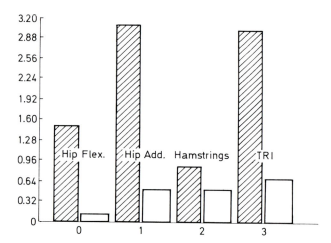

Fig. 1. Mean value of pre (hatched) and post-operative (black) spasticity (HELD score) in four main muscle groups; *0* hip-flexor; *1* hip-adductor; *2* hamstrings; *3* triceps surae

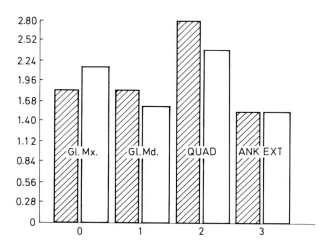

Fig. 2. Mean value of pre (hatched) and post-operative (black) muscle strength (HELD score) in four main groups (*0* gluteus maximus; *1* gluteus medius; *2* quadriceps femoris; *3* ankle extensor), related to saved rootlets

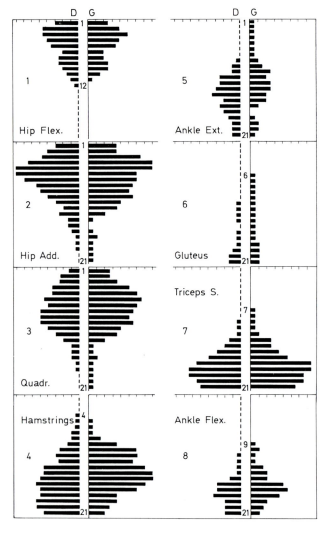

Fig. 3. Histogram of positive responses to stimulation of the posterior rootlets from L_1 to S_2, in each main muscle group *1* hip-flexor; *2* hip-adductor; *3* quadriceps femoris; *4* hamstrings; *5* ankle extensors; *6* gluteus; *7* triceps surae; *8* ankle flexor. D: right, G: left

Sectorial Posterior Rhizotomy – based on intra-operative rootlet detection by electrostimulation – aims at saving the useful spasticity of antigravity muscles related to postural tone. In SPR, the average number of divided rootlets was less important (in the order of 40%) than in Q.P.R (66% to 80%). In their publications, Fraioli and Guidetti (1977), Fraioli et al. (1984) mentioned a range of 33% to 66%, and Fasano et al. (1979) of 10% to 75%. Our experience leads us to advocate a mean cutting of 50 to 60% of rootlets to achieve a satisfactory result.

A good level of strength in the quadriceps femoris is a pre-operative criteria for selection. Unrecognized athetosis remains the main factor for bad results. As demonstrated by Stein and Carpentier (1965) in an experimental work, athetosis may be increased by the decrease in tone and remains intact after reduction of proprioceptive afferents. Patients with extensive forms of brain lesions, quadriplegia, athetosis and low I.Q. remain the most difficult to treat.

References

Fasano VA, Barolat-Romano G, Squazzi A (1979) Electrophysiological assessment of spinal circuits in spasticity by direct dorsal root stimulation. Neurosurgery 4: 146–152

Fraioli B, Guidetti B (1977) Posterior partial rootlet selection in the treatment of spasticity. J Neurosurg 46: 618–626

Fraioli B, Zamponi C, Baldassare L, Rosa G (1984) Selective posterior rootlet section in the treatment of spastic disorders of infantile cerebral palsy: immediate and late results. Acta Neurochir 33: 539–541

Gros C (1979) Spasticity. Clinical classification and surgical treatment. In: Krayenbuhl (ed) Advances and technical standards in neurosurgery, vol 6. Springer, Wien NewYork, 55–97

Gros C, Ouaknine G, Vlahovitch B, Frerebeau Ph (1967) La radicotomie selective postérieure dans le traitement neurochirurgical de l'hypertonie pyramidale. Neurochirurgie 13: 505–518

Gros C, Privat JM, Frerebeau Ph, Benezech J (1981) Les radicotomies anterieures: leur place dans le traitement de la spasticité. In: Simon L (ed) Actualités en rééducation fonctionnelle et réadaptation, 6ème serie. Masson, Paris, pp 63–70

Ouaknine G (1980) Le traitement chirurgical de la spasticité. Union Méd 109: 1–10

Privat JM, Benezech J, Frerebeau Ph, Gros C (1976) Sectorial posterior rhizotomy – a new technique of surgical treatment for spasticity. Acta Neurochir 35: 181–195

Stein BM, Carpentier MB (1965) Effects of dorsal rhizotomy upon subthalamic dyskinesia in the monkeys. Arch Neurol 13: 567–583

Correspondence: Prof. Ph. Frerebeau, Department of Neurosurgery, C.H.R. Saint Eloi–Gui de Chauliac, University of Montpellier, F-34059 Montpellier, France

Selective functional rhizotomy for the treatment of spasticity in children

R. Abbott and **M. Johann-Murphy**, with the collaboration of **J.T. Gold**

Division of Pediatric Neurosurgery, New York University Medical Center, New York, U.S.A.

Introduction

During the past three years interest in the use of selective functional rhizotomy to treat spasticity has increased, particularly in the United States. This is due largely to the positive experiences of surgeons employing various techniques of sensory rhizotomies during the 1960's, 1970's and early 1980's in Europe and South Africa (Fasano et al. 1980, Fraioli and Guidetti 1977, Gros et al. 1973, Laitinen et al. 1983, Peacock et al. 1987, Privat et al. 1976, Sindou et al. 1974, 1987). To understand the rationale of this procedure, a summary of the current theories of the pathophysiology is helpful.

Physiology of the procedure

At the segmental level, Ia sensory fibers synapse not only with the alpha motor neurons (Stretch Reflex), but also with interneurons (Baldissera et al. 1981, Rymer 1984, Scheibel 1984). The interneuronal pool also receives innervation from flexor reflex afferents (FRA) and high threshold afferents (secondary muscle afferents, joint receptors afferents and cutaneous receptors afferents) (Baldissera et al. 1981, Lundberg 1969). It is the interneuron pool's function to modulate the pattern and degree of responsiveness of the spinal cord reflex circuitry (Dimitrijevic 1985, Lundberg 1969, Rymer 1984). The interneuronal pool is in turn modulated by descending fiber tracts from the brain, segmental spinal afferents, renshaw fibers and spinal propriospinal fibers (Jankowski et al. 1973, 1974, Lloyd 1942, Lundberg 1964, 1969, Nathan and Smith 1959, Stelzner 1982).

In a spastic individual there is a loss of modulation of the interneuronal pool in the spinal cord and, thus, there is a loss in the ability to handle the incoming afferent signals in an appropriate manner (Dimitrijevic and Nathan 1967). With the loss of descending fibers from the brain there is an imbalance in the facilitory and inhibitory tone at the segment in question and, consequently, in the ability of that segment to appropriately handle afferent signals from Ia fibers, propriospinal fibers, high threshold afferent fibers, and FRA (Ashby et al. 1974, Dimitrijevic and Nathan 1967). Additionally, a reordering of the pattern of synaptic connections may occur in the developing nervous system when it sustains an injury. A mechanism termed sprouting whereby vacated synapse sites are filled by sprouting axons surviving neurons may also occur (Liu and Chambers 1958). This reordering allows the possibility of reversing the polarity of axonal influence on the interneuron in question.

Regardless of the exact mechanism, the alterations in the segment's circuitry results in a spreading activation of muscle contraction in response to afferent stimuli arriving at the spinal cord. This activation is further enhanced by the stretching of antagonistic muscles. The gamma loop reflex circuits of these antagonistic muscles may have loss modulating influence of the descending fiber tracts because of the brain injury. Further spreading of muscle contraction results in response to the afferent gamma loop action potentials. The end result is a hypertonic limb with the pattern and degree of its hypertonicity being a function of the location and extent of the CNS lesion. The expression of a lesion due to a static encephalopathy (cerebral palsy or cp) will differ from that due to a post-infectious encephalopathy arising after birth, and these will differ from the patterns seen with a post-traumatic or post-CVA encephalopathy. This is related to the variation in the pattern of injury to the CNS and to the timing of the injury with regards the degree of development in the nervous system. These variables no doubt account for the variation in efficacy seen with the different treatments available for spasticity.

Surgical technique

The surgery is most commonly performed in the lumbar canal (as advocated by Peacock) and utilizes the selection criteria devised by Fasano (Fasano et al. 1979, Peacock and Arens 1982). Anesthesia presents difficulties since a muscle relaxant must be used for induction given the predisposition of these patients for reactive airways and gastric reflux. The relaxant, however, must be cleared by the time rootlet stimulation starts so the examination of the pattern of response in the muscles may proceed. The L1 through S1 lamina are removed either by routine rongeuring or by using a power saw (which allows replacement of the lamina at the end of the procedure) (Raimondi et al. 1976). The laminotomy/laminectomy need not be wide so care should be taken to stay well medial of the facets thus avoiding subsequent difficulties with spinal lordosis. Stimulation of the sensory roots or rootlets is bipolar using modified micro ball-tipped dissectors or Samii micro dissectors* (Fig. 1). The stimulator source is a constant current generator attached to the EMG equipment with the train lasting for one second and having 50 square wave pulses per second (Abbott et al. 1989). A multi-channel EMG recorder is preferred to allow electrical monitoring outside of the myotome of the root being stimulated. One must be well versed in the idiosyncrasies of these pieces of equipment to avoid misinterpretation of operative responses. Additionally, it is of the utmost importance to have an individual palpating the leg muscles for evidence of contraction as there will be instances of false-positive EMG activity due to volume conduction of electrical activity to electrical leads at a distance from the muscle contracting (Fig. 2) (Abbott et al. 1989). To help reduce movement artifact a low

---

* Aesculap Instruments Corp.

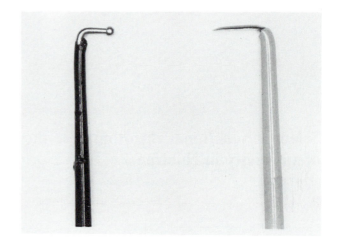

Fig. 1. Stimulating electrodes used in dissecting and stimulating the roots and rootlets. Note that the instruments are modified microdissectors with a nonconductive coating except for the bared ends used for stimulating. Not shown are the other ends of these instruments which have been modified to receive the "banana" jack of the stimulating circuit line

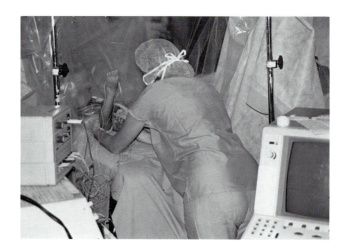

Fig. 2. Examination configuration used in surgery. Shown is the patient being monitored by both a trained examiner skilled in muscle examination and a multichannel EMG machine

frequency filter is set to 50 Hz and the high frequency filter is set to 5 Kz (Abbott et al. 1989). Most centers test the L2 through S2 dorsal roots bilaterally. *Roots which when stimulated cause either muscle activity outside of its myotome or activity lasting after cessation of the stimulus current are deemed abnormal* and they are separated into their component rootlets (Fasano et al. 1979) (Fig. 3). The rootlets are in turn stimulated and the same criteria are used to judge their normality. Abnormally responsive rootlets are candidates to be cut.

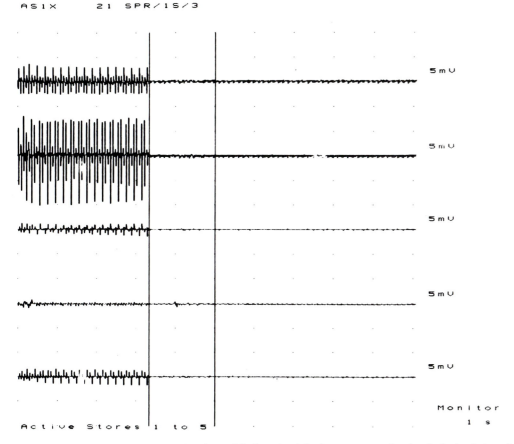

Fig. 3. Multichannel EMG tracing showing a diffusion of activity in response to the electrical stimulation of the right S1 root. The channel protray, from top to bottom, activity in the right quadriceps, right hamstrings, right gastrocnemius, left quadriceps and left gastrocnemius. The duration of stimulation was for one second and total duration of monitoring for activity was for three seconds

It is not infrequent that a majority of the roots and rootlets respond abnormally. The question then arises, how many can be safely cut. Foerster found, when doing complete rhizotomies, that he could deafferent two adjacent levels of the spinal cord without causing a sensory deficit. In fact, he reported lesioning 4 adjacent levels with only a small area of anesthesia resulting (Foerster 1913). As a rule we (at NYUMC) will only do a partial rhizotomy (<50%) at a level adjacent to two levels which have been completely lesioned (Abbott et al. 1990). Using this guideline we have only experienced a 2% incidence of sensory loss which has been confined to a small, subdermatomal area. This loss has been of no functional importance (Abbott et al. 1990).

There are several variations of the above protocol being employed today. Park has advocated stimulating the ventral roots, as a preliminary step, to obtain the individual's myotomal map. This is because he has found that the myotome can be pre- or post-fixed in some of his patients (Park and Phillips 1988). It is his feeling that he can better appreciate when diffusion of activity is occurring. This phenomena has not been observed by others however. At NYUMC we routinely test for each root's threshold of reactivity and then repetitively stimulate the roots three times in order to optimally appreciate each root's responsiveness and to identify which roots are consistently responding normally (Abbott et al. 1990). It is only at this point that lesioning commences for it has been our experience that there can be a great degree of variation in response pattern seen in "abnormal" roots with repetitive stimulation (Abbott et al. 1990). We have found, with repeated stimulation of a group of roots, that some of the roots will have a persistently normal pattern of response regardless of whether they are stimulated with the same intensity of current or with a progressively greater intensity of current. Conversely, there is a group of roots which will vary in their pattern of response, sometimes responding normally and at other times responding abnormally. Their response pattern does not seem to be dependent upon the intensity of the stimulation current. Lastly, there seems to be a group of roots which respond abnormally on every estimation. At the present time we use a protocol which emphasizes repetitive stimulation of the roots to insure that all roots which have the potential to trigger abnormal reflexive responses are identified.

We have as yet been unable to demonstrate a correlation between postoperative tone and the patterns of response seen in the leg muscles with stimulation of the remaining rootlets of the cauda equina following the completion of lesioning (Abbott et al. 1989). This is inspite of our being able to demonstrate a relationship between preoperative tone and the patterns of muscle response to root stimulation seen in surgery (Fig. 4). Consequently, there is as yet no known marker for adequate lesioning in the cauda equina and a question still exists as to whether or not sensory root stimulation with monitoring of the evoked muscle response truly reflects the pathophysiology of spasticity.

Storrs and McLone (1989) have reported on a different technique for the determination of lesioning targets and that will be reported on in a subsequent chapter. Of note is the fact that they are testing the excitability of the segment's reflex circuitry while standard selective posterior rhizotomy is monitoring for diffusion of muscle activity. When available, it will be most interesting to compare patients treated with the two methods since there are several points about the technique which make it attractive (need for only a single, migrating EMG electrode; less chance of false positivity due to volume conduction; and less

movement artifact because the stimulation is at a subthreshold intensity).

Post-operative management

The post-operative therapy of the selective posterior rhizotomy patient is critical for, in reality, the surgery is not curative of the individuals functional disabilities; it just diminishes the spasticity (Abbott et al. 1989, Elk 1980, Irwin-Carruthers et al. 1985). The patterns of limb use remain post-operatively as does the individual's underlying weakness. Three issues must be dealt with in the post-operative therapy plan: muscle stretching to gain the range which has been lost in the muscle (due to the long standing spasticity), muscle strengthening to increase endurance, and reeducation to impart a better pattern of muscle use and control (Elk 1980, Irwin-Carruthers et al. 1985). Also of importance is reassessment of any orthotic and adaptive equipment (e.g., eating utensils, wheelchairs, etc.) needed to improve the patient's functional status. Our experience in treating these individuals has lead us to feel that post-operative therapy must be consistent and of a intense, long-term nature (Abbott et al. 1989). To shorten the time needed to achieve the goals set for the pattern of limb use, we initially limit the individual's active movements outside of the therapeutic setting. This is to discourage his/her reinforcing the old patterns of limb movement which will remain as the preferred pattern of use in the immediate post operative period (Abbott et al. 1989).

It is of the utmost importance that the therapist working with the individual be observant for indications of development of new motor skills and to foster this development (Elk 1980). There is no set therapy which the individual must be taken through. We have found that a heterogeneous therapy program incorporating principles of motor control, neuro-developmental treatment, proprioceptive neuromuscular facilitation, sensory integration and the Rood approach to therapy allows us the versatility in treating these individuals (Bobath 1980, Carr et al. 1987, Knott and Voss 1969, Stockmeyer 1967).

Patients with moderate to severe muscle tightness will require vigorous, daily stretching by the therapist to attempt to reacquire the lost range in the muscle (Abbott et al. 1989). With an aggressive stretching program, functional range should be accomplished by 3–6 months. This is usually possible in children under 6 years of age. The therapist may experience difficulty

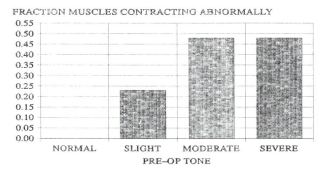

RELATIONSHIP BETWEEN PRE-OP TONE
AND INTRA-OP PRE-LESIONING RESPONSES

Fig. 4. Abnormal muscle activity seen in response to dorsal root stimulation. Shown is the fraction of muscles within each tone grouping (normal, slightly, moderately or severely spastic preoperatively) which responded abnormally

in stretching muscles in older individuals because of extensive contracture within the muscle being stretched. If the desired range has not been achieved within 8–12 months, tenotomies can be considered. Once the desired range has been achieved, the stretching program must be continued or a progressive loss in range will occur, particularly as the individual grows. Five minutes a day for 3–5 days per week is usually adequate to maintain the range unless active growth is occurring. During active growth daily stretching is frequently required. The stretching can be reenforced by using appropriate orthotics for at least 6 hours per day (Tardieu et al. 1988).

Muscle strengthening is usually required postoperatively to supplant the lost spasticity because most spastic ambulators use their spasticity to assist in bearing weight while standing and walking (Elk 1980, Irwin-Carruthers 1985). While isolated muscle strengthening may be useful to increase strength and improve the child's body awareness, it is imperative to integrate this muscle back into functional movements. The muscle must work with its synergists to produce the correct pattern of movement (Abbott et al. 1989, Elk 1980, Irwin-Carruthers 1985). Also, the strengthening exercises should be tailored to foster graded movements which require alternate contraction of muscles in a concentric and eccentric manner. Emphasis on strengthening the end ranges of movement must be incorporated in the program as spastic children tend to move in mid range only (Bobath and Bobath 1982). This is especially apparent during ambulation as exemplified by lack of terminal knee extension at the terminal swing phase of gait as well as a loss of hip extension during the terminal phases of stance. Endurance is another important goal of strengthening therapy, and at NYUMC we use activities such as tricycle/bicycle riding to accomplish this (Abbott et al. 1989).

Increasing a muscle's range of movement and its strength is preparatory to the reeducation of the pattern of limb use. While in reality all three types of therapy are being delivered at the same time, there must be adequate strength and range in a muscle in order for an individual to learn to control the muscle appropriately. Key to the minimization in time devoted to this reeducation process is allowing only normal patterns of limb use after surgery (Elk 1980, Irwin-Carruthers 1985). To aid in this we frequently place the individual in a wheelchair or on a tricycle to give them mobility when not in a therapy session.

These modes of movement maintain the child's motor independence while discouraging abnormal patterns of limb use (Abbott et al. 1989). We have also found that these individuals will show improvement in balancing skills prior to improvement in muscle control, especially when the individual was ambulatory preoperative (Dzialga 1988). Until the individual gains adequate control over the muscles of the legs, it is helpful to slow down the rate at which they walk by using assistive devices such as canes, crutches or walkers (Abbott et al. 1989). The degree of assistance is gradually lessened as the individual gains in their ability to control the limbs.

These patients will require orthotic devices postoperatively due to poor control of ankle joint musculature and characteristic pronation foot deformity (Abbott et al. 1989). The poor control of musculature at the ankle join is a reflection of the disuse of the anterior tibial group due to a spastic antagonist. Also, the voluntary control of the gastroc-soleus is poorly developed because of persistent spasticity in the muscles. The result, post-rhizotomy, is a lack of control at the ankle joint with a resultant foot slap at initial contact and a pronated foot throughout the stance phase of the gait cycle. Added to a poorly controlled foot and ankle joint immediately post-rhizotomy is the weakness of hip and knee musculature. At NYUMC we have found success in dealing with the above problems by prescribing a hinged or jointed ankle-foot orthosis with a dorsi-flexion check strap and a plantar flexion stop (Fig. 5). This strap

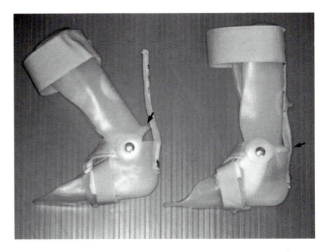

Fig. 5. A pair of hinged or jointed ankle-foot orthosis showing the check strap to prevent dorsiflexion to a varying degree as well as the plantar flexion stop (arrow)

allows simulation of a solid ankle foot orthosis. With improvement of muscle strength around the hip and knee joints, the check strap can be loosened and the plantar flexion stop can be shaved back to slowly encourage more active movement around the ankle joint. The foot plate of the brace maintains the subtalar joint in better biomechanical alignment, thereby allowing the active movement to come from the ankle joint.

Results

1. There are currently *three centers* who have reviewed the outcome in their patients who have undergone selective, functional dorsal rhizotomy.

The first center in *Torino* (Italy) is headed by Fasano and published an article in 1980 outlining the outcome at 2–7 years in 80 of their spastic, cerebral palsy patients (Fasano et al. 1980). All patients with hypertonicity and no contracture experienced complete normalization of the muscle tone post-operatively and this improvement persisted through follow-up examination. In those patients with hypertonicity and muscle contracture, there was a 91% normalization or near-normalization in the muscle tone and, again, this persisted through follow-up. If, however, there was dystonia present in addition to the hypertonicity, the improvement seen was not as great as in the other groups.

The second center in *Cape Town* (South Africa) was headed by Peacock and in 1987 they published a report of the 1–5 year follow-up examinations in 60 of their patients (Peacock et al. 1987). These were children with cerebral palsy upon whom selective, functional dorsal rhizotomy had been performed. Two third of his patients were spastic diplegics preoperatively and, post-operatively, 22 had normalization of their tone while 18 became hypotonic. 16 of the 60 patients were spastic quadriplegics and, post-operatively, 9 had normalization of their tone while 5 had some persisting hypertonicity. There is no mention of the outcome of the 4 individuals who had hypertonicity and choreoathetoid movement disorder, but in a personal communication the author has discouraged operating on individuals with this type of mixed picture.

Laitinen's group in *Umea* (Sweden) reported on the outcome in 9 patients who underwent functional dorsal rhizotomy (Laitinen et al. 1983). These patients had spasticity of differing etiology (multiple sclerosis, nonspecific myelopathy, spinal injury and cerebral

hemorrhage) with the onset of the spasticity occurring in adulthood. Four of the nine experienced a normalization in their tone while 5/9 saw their hypertonicity "much diminished" at follow-up examinations occurring 6–26 months after the surgery.

Assessment of an individual's functional abilities is difficult since there is no accepted, standardized grading system to quantify changes seen. *Improvement of the functions* of sitting and standing are the goal of this procedure. Thirty one of sixty five of Fasano's patients had a greater than 30% improvement in their sitting posture with 8 of these patients gaining a normal posture while sitting (Fasano et al. 1980). Peacock reported that 39/40 diplegic patients experienced an improvement in stability while in the side sitting position, while 15/16 of the quadriplegics who received this operation experience improvement in their ability to side sit (Peacock et al. 1987). 15/65 of Fasano's patients had a greater than 30% improvement in their walking ability while another 7 patients had a greater than 70% improvement in walking (Fasano et al. 1980). Of the fourteen independent ambulators operated upon by Peacock (individuals not requiring an assistive device to walk), 12 had a documented increase in their stride length because of an increase in their ability to extend at the knee (Peacock et al. 1987). Of the eight dependent ambulators (those requiring a cane, crutch or walker), five became independent of their assistive devices while walking but one experienced a decline in function as he had been dependent on his spasticity to assist in standing (Peacock et al. 1987). Post-operatively, this individual required long leg bracing in order to stand. Thirteen of the sixteen quadriplegics reciprocated when held preoperatively. Nine of these individuals showed improvement in their ability to ambulate after the surgery (Peacock et al. 1987).

2. *At NYUMC* we have now performed this procedure on 140 individuals. We have been able to examine 56 of these patients with the same protocol pre-operatively and at 6 months post-operatively. 29 of these patients have also undergone evaluation one year after their surgery. We have found that there has been a statistically significant change (p < .001) in the tone in the leg muscles with a resolution of functionally debilitating spasticity. When we compared our goniometric data obtained pre-operatively to that obtained at six and twelve months, the improvement in the range of hip abduction, and knee extension (with the hips flexed) were significant to p < 0.05. We have

found that this improvement in range is especially dramatic in children less than 8 years in age.

To analyze functional changes we have divided our patients into three groups based upon the loco-motive abilities pre-operatively. Thus, there is a group whose primary mode of locomotion was walking preoperatively, a group whose primary mode of locomotion was crawling pre-operatively and a nonambulatory group who required wheelchairs to move about. We examined each individual's ability to get into a position (the transitional score), the amount of assistance required to maintain the position (the assistance score) and the individual's appearance in the position (the alignment score). We summed the scores obtained for the long, short and side sit positions to obtain an overall score for sitting and, similarly, we summed scores for the 1/2 kneeling and standing positions to obtain an overall score for standing. This was done for the transitional, assistance and alignment scores. We have noted a trend of improvement in the transitional scores and assistance scores, especially in the crawling group. There is a statistical significant change (p < 0.05) in the alignment score in standing in all groups.

This is a patient population who is at high risk for *operative complications* (Abbott et al. 1989). We have seen in five of the 140 patients upon whom we have operated bronchospasm of such severity as to ter-minate the surgery prematurely. Because of this we now administer intravenous aminophylline the night before surgery and during surgery to any child with a history of bronchodilator use. Also, all crawlers and nonambulators receive this treatment since these are groups who have sustained more significant brain injuries and usually had a more stormy perinatal period frequently punctuated by hyaline membrane disease. Any child with a recent upper respiratory tract infection does not undergo surgery for a 4–6 week period. We have also had five of our patients develop aspiration pneumonia post-operatively owing to a tendency toward gastric reflux. As a consequence, all severely involved individuals (physical and cognitive impairment) are placed at NPO for at least 18 hours and, if an enlarged gastric bubble is seen on x-ray, the child has a nasogastric tube inserted prior to going to surgery.

Post-operatively, we have been most impressed with the *transient side-effects*. Approximately 30% of our patients experience dysesthesias of the feet for a period from one to three weeks. Nearly all children undergoing this procedure can be expected to experience severe pain aggravated by back spasm typically lasting 48 hours. We have seen a transient bladder dysfunction with urinary retention in 10 patients of a degree to necessitate intermittent catheterization. Fasano reports one of his 80 patients had this difficulty and Laitinen saw this in 1 of his 9 patients (Fasano et al. 1980, Laitinen et al. 1983).

We have seen *hypesthesia* in three of our 140 patients with two experiencing a focal loss in proprioception in a single digit of a foot and one loss of pain sensation in the right S1 dermatome (Abbott et al. 1989). Fasano reports a 5% incidence of sensory "disorder" with half being of a transient sort and half a focal area of hypesthesia (Fasano et al. 1980). Laitinen found that 2/9 of his patients had a diminution of pin-prick sensation (Laitinen et al. 1983). Cahan performed somatosensory evoked potential testing in 20 of his patients finding abnormal patterns in 3 of the 11 patients who had normal patterns pre-operatively (Cahan et al. 1987). Interestingly, none of these individuals experienced any subjective changes in sensation.

Given the length of spinal canal exposure there is a theoretical concern about *spinal stability*. Peacock mentions in his paper that one young lady experienced a progression of a spondylolisthesis (Peacock et al. 1987). On retrospect a lumbar pars interarticularis defect was noted on her preoperative x-rays. There have been no other reports of iatrogenic spinal pathology in individuals undergoing this type of procedure. The location of the surgery is probably the key to this for Yasuoka, reporting on a series of children undergoing spinal surgery with lamin-ectomies, found that secondary scoliosis was a function of the level of the surgery with the incidence being nearly 100% for the cervical region while none of the three children undergoing lumbar laminectomy experienced curvature (Yasuoka et al. 1981).

Conclusion

The early reports of the outcome of children with spastic cerebral palsy undergoing functional dorsal rhizotomy are encouraging and support proceeding with this procedure in investigational centers. It is important to understand, however, that little can be stated in an objective manner about the functional outcome in patients undergoing this procedure at the present time. Given the heterogeneity of the patient population we must await the time when several centers have accumulated a large patient population who have undergone an adequate length of post-operative therapy and have been subject to pre- and post-operative protocol evaluation using verified examination tools.

References

Abbe R (1896) Intradural section of the spinal nerves for neuralgia. Boston Med Surg J 135: 329–335

Abbott R, Forem S, Johann M (1989) Selective posterior rhizotomy for the treatment of spasticity, a review. Childs Nerv Syst 5: 337–346

Abbott R, Johann M, Spielholz N, Espstein F (1989) Selective posterior rhizotomy and spasticity; relationship between intraoperative abnormal muscle contractions and the tone examination. In: Park TS, Phillips LH, Peacock WJ (eds) Management of spasticity in cerebral palsy and spinal cord injury. Hanley & Belfus, Philadelphia, pp 471–476

Abbott R, Deletes V, Spielholz N, Wisoff JH, Epstein FJ (1990) Selective posterior rhizotomy, pitfalls in monitoring. In: Marlin A (ed) Concepts pediatric neurosurgery. Karger, Basel, pp 187–195

Ashby P, Verrier M, Lightfoot E (1974) Segmental reflex pathways in spinal shock and spinal spasticity in main. J Neurol Neurosurg Psychiatry 37: 1352–1360

Baldissera PW, Hultborn H, Illert M (1981) Integration in spinal neuronal systems. In: Brooks VB (ed) Handbook physiology, sec 1. The nervous system, vol 2. Motor control. American Physiology Society, Bethesda, pp 509–595

Barolat-Romana G, Davis R (1980) Neurophysiological mechanisms in abnormal reflex activities in cerebral palsy and spinal spasticity. J Neurol Neurosurg Psychiatry 43: 333–342

Bennett WH (1889) Acute spasmotic pain in the left lower extremity was completely relieved by subdural division of the posterior roots of certain spinal nerves, all other treatment having proved useless. Medico Chir Trans 79: 329–348

Bobath K (1980) A neurophysiological basis for the treatment of cerebral palsy. Clin Dev Med 75: 1–88

Bobath B, Bobath K (1982) Motor development in the different types of cerebral palsy. W Heinemann, London, pp 1–100

Cahan LD, Kundi SM, McPherson D, et al (1987) Electrophysiologic studies in selective posterior rhizotomy for spasticity in children with cerebral palsy. Appl Neurophysiol 50: 459–460

Carr JH, Shepherd RB, Gordon J, et al (1987) Movement science: foundations for physical therapy in rehabilitation. Aspen Systems, London, pp 27–143

Dimitrijevic MR, Nathan PW (1967) Studies in spasticity in man. Brain 90: 1–31

Dimitrijevic MR (1985) Spasticity. In: Swash M, Kennard C (eds) Scientific basis of clinical neurology. Churchill Livingstone, Edinburgh, pp 108–115

Dzialga MJ (1988) Early ambulation patterns in cerebral palsy children who have undergone selective posterior rhizotomies. Thesis, New York University, pp 22–32

Elk B (1980) Preoperative assessment and postoperative surgical occupational therapy for children who have undergone a selective posterior rhizotomy. South African J Occ Ther 14: 49–50

Fasano VA, Barolat-Romana G, Zeme S, et al (1979) Electro-physiological assessment of spinal circuits in spasticity by direct dorsal root stimulation. Neurosurgery 4: 146–151

Fasano VA, Broggi G, Zeme S, et al (1980) Long-term results of posterior rhizotomy. Acta Neurochir [Suppl] 30: 435–439

Foerster O (1913) On the indications and results of the excision of posterior spinal nerve roots in men. Surg Gynecol Obstet 16: 463–475

Fraioli B, Guidetti B (1977) Posterior partial rootlet section in the treatment of spasticity. J Neurosurg 46: 618–625

Gros C, Frerebeau PH, Kuhner A, et al (1973) Technical modification in the Foerster operation. Selective posterior lumbar root section. The results of 18 years of practice. Presented at the International Congress of Neurosurgery, Tokyo 1973

Irwin-Carruthers SH, Davids LM, VanRensburg CK, et al (1985) Early physiotherapy in selective posterior rhizotomy. Fisioterapie 41: 44–49

Jankowski E, Lundberg A, Stuart D (1973) Propriospinal control of last order interneurons of spinal reflex pathways in the cat. Brain Res 53: 227–231

Jankowski E, Lundberg A, Roberts WJ, et al (1974) A long propriospinal system with direct effects on motoneurons and on interneurons in the cat lumbosacral cord. Exp Brain Res 21: 169–194

Knott M, Voss DE (1969) Proprioceptive neuromuscular facilitation. Patterns and techniques. Hoeber Medical Div, Harper and Row, New York, pp 83–185

Laitinen LV, Nilsson S, Fugl-Meyer AR (1983) Selective posterior rhizotomy for treatment of spasticity. J Neurosurg 48: 895–899

Liu CN, Chambers NW (1958) Intraspinal sprouting of dorsal root axons. Arch Neurol Phychol 79: 46–61

Lloyd DP (1942) Mediation of descending long spinal reflex activity. J Neurophysiol 5: 435–458

Lundberg A (1964) Supraspinal control of transmission in reflex paths to motoneurons and primary afferents. In: Eccles JC, Schade JP (eds) Physiology of spinal neurons. Elsevier, Amsterdam, pp 197–221

Lundberg A (1969) Convergence of excitatory and inhibitory action on interneurons in the spinal cord. In: Brazier MAB (ed) The interneuron. Univ Calif Press, Los Angeles, pp 231–265

Nathan PW, Smith MC (1959) Fasciculi proprii of the spinal cord in man: review of present knowledge. Brain 82: 610–688

Ouaknine G-E (1980) Le traitement chirurgical de la spasticité. Union Med Can 109: 1424–1443

Park TS, Phillips LH (1988) Electrophysiological studies of selective posterior rhizotomy patients. Presented at Pathophysiology and management of spasticity in spinal cord injury and cerebral palsy symposium. Charlottesville, VA, May 25–27, 1988

Peacock WJ, Arens LJ (1982) Selective posterior rhizotomy for the treatment of spasticity in cerebral palsy. SA Med J 62: 119–124

Peacock WJ, Arens LJ, Berman B (1987) Cerebral palsy spasticity. Selective posterior rhizotomy. Ped Neurosci 13: 61–66

Pederson E (1969) Spasticity: mechanisms, measurement, management. Charles C Thomas, Springfield, pp 91–98

Privat JM, Benezech J, Frerebeau P, et al (1976) Sectorial posterior rhizotomy, a new technique of surgical treatment for spasticity. Acta Neurochir 35: 181–195

Raimondi AJ, Gutierrez FA, DiRocco C (1976) Laminotomy and total reconstruction of the posterior arch for spinal canal surgery in childhood. J Neurosurg 45: 555–560

Raymer WZ (1984) Spinal mechanisms for control of muscle length and tension. In: Davidoff RA (ed) Handbook of the spinal cord, vols 2 and 3. Marcel Dekker, New York Basel, pp 609–646

Scheibel AB (1984) Organization of the spinal cord. In: Davidoff RA (ed) Handbook of the spinal cord, vol 2. Marcel Dekker, New York Basel, pp 47–77

Sherrington CS (1898) Decerebrate rigidity and reflex coordination of movements. J Physiol (Lond) 22: 319–337

Sindou M, Fischer G, Goutelle A, et al. (1974) La radicellotomie postérieure sélective dans le traitement des spasticités. Rev Neurol 30: 201–215

Sindou M, Mifsud JJ, Rosati C, et al (1987) Microsurgical selective posterior rhizotomy in the dorsal root entry zone for treatment of limb spasticity. Acta Neurochir [Suppl] 39: 99–102

Stelzner DJ (1982) The role of the descending systems in maintaining intrinsic spinal function: a developmental approach. In: Sjolund B, Bjorklund A (eds) Brainstem control of spinal mechanisms. Elsevier Biomedical Press, Amsterdam, pp 297–321

Stockmeyer SA (1967) An interpretation of the approach of rood in the treatment of neuromuscular dysfunction. Am J Phys Med 46: 900–926

Storrs BB, McLone DG (1989) Selective posterior rhizotomy in the treatment of spasticity associated with myelomeningocele. In: Marlin A (ed) Concepts Pediatr Neurosurg, vol 9. Karger, Basel, pp 173–177

Tardieu C, Lespargot A, Tabary C, Bret MD (1988) For how long must the soleus muscle be stretched each day to prevent contracture? Dev Med Child Neurol 30: 3–10

Yasuoka S, Peterson HA, Laws ER, et al (1981) Pathogenesis and prophylaxis of postlaminectomy deformity of the spine after multiple level laminectomy: difference between children and adults. Neurosurgery 9: 145–152

Correspondence: Prof. R. Abbott, Division of Pediatric Neurosurgery, New York University Medical Center, 550 First Ave, New York, NY 10016, U.S.A.

Electrophysiological monitoring in selective posterior rhizotomy for spasticity: principles, techniques and interpretation of responses

T. Nishida and **B.B. Storrs**

Northwestern University Medical School and Children's Memorial Hospital, Chicago, Illinois, U.S.A.

Since the introduction of intraoperative electro-stimulation technique by Fasano et al. (1978, 1979, 1988), selective posterior rhizotomy (SPR) has gained renewed interest as an effective treatment of spasticity associated with cerebral palsy. A monitoring technique which identifies those posterior rootlets that are to be sectioned requires the ability to yield quick and reliable data. Over the past two years at the Children's Memorial Hospital (CMH) in Chicago, more than 100 SPRs have been performed and this article details our monitoring technique (Storrs et al. 1988) and compares it to that of Fasano et al. (1978) (Table 1).

Principles

H reflex

Stimulation of the posterior tibial nerve at the popliteal fossa elicits a short latency high amplitude M (motor) response and a delayed H (Hoffman) response of low amplitude in the soleus muscle. It is generally understood that the neural pathway of the H response is similar to that of the muscle stretch reflex hence the H reflex. That is, the nerve impulse is conveyed by way of Ia fibers to the alpha motoneuron

Table 1

	Fasano (1978)	CMH (1987)
1. Amplifier		
sensitivity mv/cm		0.2–0.5
bandpass Hz		8–8 K
sweep velocity msec/cm		200
2. Recording electrode		surface
3. Stimulator		
rate Hz	1, 50	1, 2, 5, 10, 20, 50
duration msec	0.5	1
intensity v	0.1–0.5	5–50
train duration sec	1	less than 2
4. Stimulating electrode		
interpolar distance mm	10	10
5. Anesthesia	Ketamine	Halothane Nitrous Oxide Fentanyl
6. Normal	inhibition (50 Hz)	decrement > 50%
7. Abnormal	high threshold tonic contraction diffusion interferential pattern afterdischarge	tonic or clonic contraction diffusion increment or decrement < 50%

to contract a muscle, although the H reflex bypasses annulospiral endings. In normal adults, the H reflex is restricted to only soleus and flexor carpi radialis muscles.

H max/M max ratio, expressed as a percentage, reflects the excitability of the motor neuron pool. The ratio is increased in the spastic subjects (Angel and Hoffmann 1963). After SPR, significant decrease or absence of H max/M max ratio has been reported in 7/8 patients by Cahan et al. (1987) confirming decrease in tone.

The current monitoring technique differs from the classical H reflex in two ways. First, the stimulus is delivered to the dorsal root proximal to the ganglion, not to a mixed nerve at the knee. Second, the recording electrode is placed over the appropriate muscle group innervated by its corresponding root.

H reflex recovery curve

When a pair of stimuli with a varying interstimulus interval (ISI) is applied to the posterior tibial nerve at the knee and the amplitude ratio of initial and subsequent H responses (H2/H1) is plotted against the ISI, the H reflex recovery curve follows a characteristic pattern in normal subjects and those with upper motor neuron lesion. Normal subjects exhibit four different phases:

1. early facilitation ISI up to 15 msec
2. early inhibition ISI 20–100 msec
3. late facilitation ISI 100–200 msec
4. late inhibition ISI 200–1000 msec

The early facilitation has been attributed to the increased EPSPs in the alpha motoneurons (Taborikova and Sax 1969). The early inhibition is considered to be due to the combination of Renshaw cell inhibition on alpha motorneuron, Golgi tendon inhibition and reduction of excitatory neurotransmitter at the interneuronal level, although the contribution of Golgi tendon inhibition is questionable.

Those with upper motor neuron lesion exhibit more rapid and complete recovery with less late inhibition than normal (Fig. 1). Magladery et al. (1952) was the first to describe a difference in the recovery curve of normal and patients with upper motor neuron lesions. In spastic patients, increased excitability of the motor neuron and reduced presynaptic inhibition modify the recovery curve. Futagi and Abe (1985) and Futagi et al. (1988) demonstrated significant differences in the H

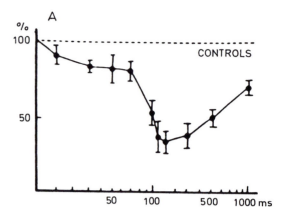

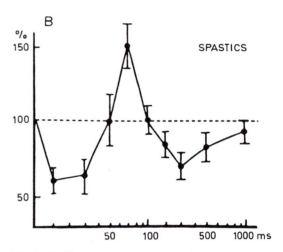

Fig. 1. H reflex recovery curves comparing control and spastic limbs Delwaide PJ (1980) In: Spasticity: disordered motor control. Feldman RG, Youn RR, Koella WP (eds) Year Book Medical Publishers, Chicago

reflex recovery curve between normal children and patients with cerebral palsy. Recovery and facilitation of the amplitude were significantly increased among spastic children especially at ISI of 100–900 msec. There was also a strong correlation between the degree of recovery and the severity of spasticity. Ioku et al. (1969), by applying ten consecutive stimuli at a rate varying from one to 60 Hz, plotted the averaged value of the amplitudes against the rate of stimulation. This "frequency depression curve" showed a similar distinction between normal adults and patients with internal capsule lesions.

Techniques

Recording parameters

At the CMH, a standard EMG equipment (TE-4, TECA Corp) is used with a storage oscilloscope

(511A1, Tektronix). An amplifier (AA6-MK11) with a frequency filter setting of 8 Hz to 8K Hz identical to the routine motor nerve conduction study is utilized. A sensitivity of 200–500 uV/cm is employed depending on the amplitude of the response elicited. Sweep velocity is set at 200 msec/cm (sweep duration 2 sec) to accommodate responses recorded at various rates of stimulation.

A disposable, pre-gelled, silver/silver chloride electrode with hypoallergic rectangular transparent tape (Ver Med) is placed over the belly of each muscle group with a reference to its tendon. An active recording electrode for the L2 rootlet stimulation is placed over the adductors, L3 quads, L4 either quads or anterior tibialis, L5 either medial hamstrings or peroneous longus, S1 lateral gastrocnemius, and S2 intrinsic toe flexors. The placement of the electrode over the posterior aspect of the leg is more convenient since the patient is in the prone position on a surgical bolster. Active, reference and ground electrodes are connected via snap-on short lead wires to a pre-amplifier located near the recording site to reduce electrical interference.

Stimulus parameters

Each rootlet is stimulated by a hook shaped fixed interval bipolar stimulator (Radionics, Inc.) with the interpolar distance at 5–10 mm and the cathode situated proximally. Submaximal stimulation (usually 5–50 V) is delivered through a constant voltage stimulator (NS6) at a rate of 1 Hz with a duration of 1 msec to elicit minimal twitch response and to be at least 200–500 uV in amplitude which should be stable without amplitude fluctuation. Then the stimulation is repeated with the same intensity at the rate of 2, 5, 10, 20, 50 Hz. Stimulus train duration varies depending on stimulus frequency (usually less than 2 sec). The identical procedure is performed for all sensory rootlets sequentially from S1 (at times S2) through L2 bilaterally.

Anesthesia

Halothane is utilized as an induction and maintenance anesthesia with Nitrous Oxide and Fentanyl as an adjunct. A non-depolarizing short-intermediate acting neuromuscular blockage (Atracurium or Vecuronium) is added for the initial part of the procedure which is totally reversed by Neostigmine prior to the electrostimulation.

Technical hints

In our experience recording from the surface electrode is superior to the needle electrode since the latter produces unstable responses in the event of a strong muscle contraction. Neuromuscular blockade should be reversed completely before the electro-stimulation because we found, a decremental response at a low rate of stimulation may give spurious results. Stimulus intensity should be adjusted to a level that produces minimal twitch but a stable response. Maximal or supramaximal stimulus can overflow to the adjacent rootlets and cause brisk muscle contraction in a widespread distribution. The interpolar distance of stimulating electrodes should be kept close to prevent current spread. It is also important that the stimulating electrodes are free from blood or CSF to ensure the stable response. Usually motor and sensory roots can be easily identified visually, however on rare occasions when it is difficult, the motor root can be confirmed electrically by its lower threshold. Multi-channel recording will detect a spread of evoked response to adjacent root levels or other limbs, however in our experience these can be easily identified clinically. The main sources of electrical interference in the operating room are the electrocautery unit and/or pulse oxymeter.

Interpretation of responses

At the CMH, the total number of rootlet tested ranged from 17–61 per patient and the number of rootlet sectioned ranged from 6–41 per patient (18–80%).

Each rootlet was stimulated at the rate of 1, 2, 5, 10, 20, 50 Hz and the ratio of subsequent H over H1 was determined at each rate of stimulation. Figures 2, 3, 4, 5, and 6 illustrate some of the responses. Those rootlets considered normal have a ratio of less than 50% at any frequency, and those rootlets considered abnormal have a ratio of more than 50% or at times over 100% at all frequencies tested.

This value is derived from the previously published data by several investigators particularly Mayer and Mosser (1969) who demonstrated that the reduction in amplitude from H1 to H2 in normal children (3–7 years) averaged 82.3% (70–91%) at 100 msec ISI. For average adults (20–50 years) the reduction in amplitude was 56.2% (30–70%) which was similar to that of 6–12 months old infants. *Their study indicates*

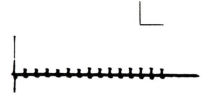

Fig. 2. Decremental response (or inhibition) at 10 Hz stimulation. Calibration: horizontal bar = 200 msec, vertical bar = 0.5 mv

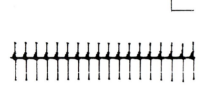

Fig. 3. Sustained response (or interferential pattern) at 10 Hz stimulation. Calibration: horizontal bar = 200 msec, vertical bar = 0.5 mv

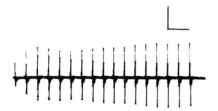

Fig. 4. Incremental response (or facilitation) at 10 Hz stimulation. Calibration: horizontal bar = 200 msec, vertical bar = 0.5 mv

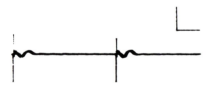

Fig. 5. Polysynaptic response following monosynaptic response at 1 Hz stimulation. Calibration: horizontal bar = 200 msec, vertical bar = 0.5 mv

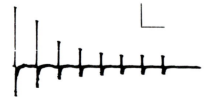

Fig. 6. Decremental response due to the effect of neuromuscular blockade at 5 Hz stimulation. Calibration: horizontal bar = 200 msec, vertical bar = 0.5 mv

that children between the age 3–7 years exhibit the greatest distinction between "normal" and "abnormal" rootlets, therefore this is a favorable age group to undergo SPR.

Other criteria of abnormality are clinically observed, sustained tonic or clonic contraction that persists following the cessation of stimulus and the spread ("diffusion") of contraction to other muscle groups in the same limb or to the opposite limb. A long duration wave of lower amplitude following each response is also noted especially at a slower rate of stimulation and in proximal muscle groups. This may represent a polysynaptic response activated by multisegmental circuitry, however it is not certain whether this is a pathological phenomenon.

Our findings are somewhat different from those of Fasano et al. (1978) (Table 1).

The stimulus threshold in the normal dorsal root was reported by Fasano et al. to be between 0.1 and 0.5 v with 0.5 msec square wave and the threshold higher than 2 v was considered abnormal. We have never been able to elicit a response at such a low intensity except for the ventral root.

When the stimulus rate was increased to 50 Hz, "normal" rootlet responded only to the first stimuli. In our experience this is not usually the case. Regardless of stimulus frequency, a response can be obtained for each stimulus although the amplitude may be lower.

"Interferential pattern" or sustained response at 50 Hz without the reduction of amplitude was considered to be an "abnormal" rootlet by Fasano et al. (1978)." "Afterdischarge phenomenon", i.e., prolonged electrical response after the cessation of stimulus, has not been observed by us, nor were tonic muscle contractions associated with this phenomenon.

Triple flexion contraction of the homolateral limb was also considered to be abnormal by Fasano.

"Cyclic fluctuation", the decrescendo–crescendo response and "excess inhibition", the irregular response at a low rate of stimulation appear to be more technical in origin, most likely due to the motion of the bipolar stimulator or uneven stimulus strength.

Fasano's technique was based on a study by DeCandia et al. (1967) which showed that repeated stimulation of the afferent fibers of a monosynaptic reflex induces frequency dependent amplitude reduction of the reflex response, presumably due to neurotransmitter depletion or presynaptic inhibition.

As mentioned earlier, the distinction between normal and abnormal rootlets is set somewhat arbitrarily at 50% reduction of the amplitude at any stimulus frequency (1 to 50 Hz). However at higher stimulus frequencies (over 10 Hz), the difference between normal and abnormal recovery curves are not as marked as that of lower frequencies. Therefore the decision to resect a rootlet should be made based on the findings of slow rate stimulation. As demonstrated by Futagi and Abe (1985, 1986) the facililation of the response at slow rate of stimulation may be the most important feature of the recovery curve in spastic subjects.

Conclusions

Our technique has provided excellent results for more than 100 patients without significant sensory compromise. The reduction in spasticity was noted in 95.5% of the cases at one year post-operatively and no patients were made worse. Two patients had plantar dysesthesia that persisted for 6–8 weeks.

Needless to say, it is imperative to develop a reliable, non-time consuming monitoring technique that provides quantitative and reproducible measures to distinguish normal from abnormal rootlets. Consensus on the standardization of this intraoperative technique and criteria for sectioning is urgently needed.

Acknowledgement

We thank Mrs. Jeanne Toguri, RN for secretarial assistance.

References

Angel RW, Hoffman WW (1963) The H reflex in normal, spastic and rigid subjects. Arch Neurol 8: 591–596

Cahan LD, Kundi MS, McPherson D, Starr A, Peacock W (1987) Electrophysiologic studies in selective dorsal rhizotomy for spasticity in children with cerebral palsy. Appl Neurophysiol 50: 459–682

DeCandia M, Provini L, Taborikova H (1967) Mechanisms of the reflex discharge depression in the spinal motoneuron during repetitive orthodromic stimulation. Brain Res 4: 284–291

Fasano VA, Broggi G, Barolat-Romana G, Squazzi A (1978) Surgical treatment of spasticity in cerebral palsy. Childs Brain 4: 289–305

Fasano VA, Barolat-Romana G, Zemes S, Squazzi A (1979) Electrophysiological assessment of spinal circuits in spasticity by direct dorsal root stimulation. Neurosurgery 4: 146–151

Fasano VA, Broggi G, Zemes S (1988) Intraoperative electrical stimulation for functional posterior rhizotomy. Scand J Rehab Med [Suppl] 17: 149–154

Futagi Y, Abe J (1985) H-reflex study in normal children and patients with cerebral palsy. Brain Dev 7: 414–420

Futagi Y, Abe J, Tanaka J, Okamoto N, Ikoma H (1988) Recovery curve of the H-reflex in normal infants, central coordination disturbance cases and cerebral palsy patients within the first year of life. Brain Dev 10: 8–12

Ioku M, Nakatani S, Oku Y, Jinnai D (1969) The H reflex study with high frequency stimulation. Electromyography 9: 219–227

Magladery JW, Teasdall RD, Park M, Languth HW (1952) Electrophysiological studies of reflex activity in patients with lesions of the nervous system. I. A comparison of spinal motoneurone excitability following afferent nerve volleys in normal persons and patients with upper motor neurone lesions. Bull Johns Hopkins Hosp 91: 219–244

Mayer RF, Mosser RS (1969) Excitability of motoneurons in infants. Neurology 19: 932–945

Storrs BB, Nishida T (1988) Use of the H reflex recovery curve in selective posterior rhizotomy. Pediatr Neurosci 14: 120–123

Taborikova H, Sax DS (1969) Conditioning of H-reflexes by a preceding subthreshold H-reflex stimulus. Brain 92: 203–212

Correspondence: Dr. T. Nishida, Northwestern University Medical School, 303 E. Chicago Ave, Chicago, Illinois 60611, U.S.A.

Surgery in the dorsal root entry-zone: microsurgical DREZ-tomy (MDT) for the treatment of spasticity

M. Sindou and **D. Jeanmonod**, with the collaboration of **P. Mertens**

Department of Neurosurgery, Hopital Neurologique, Lyon, France

Introduction

Microsurgical-DREZ-tomy (MDT) was first introduced for the treatment of pain. In the 1960s' a large amount of anatomical and physiological work drew clinicians' attention to the dorsal horn (Melzach and Wall 1965) as the first level of modulation for pain sensation. This research convinced the senior author to consider the dorsal root entry zone (DREZ) as a possible target for pain surgery. Therefore in 1972 anatomical studies and preliminary surgical trials were undertaken in man, in order to determine whether a destructive procedure at this level was feasible (Sindou 1972, Sindou et al. 1974c).

This method – initially named: "selective rhizotomy in the posterior root-spinal cord junction" – was applied as early as 1972 to somatogenic and then neurogenic pain (Sindou 1972, Sindou et al. 1974a, 1982, Sindou and Lapras 1982, Sindou and Daher 1988). Post-operative assessment revealed, in addition to pain relief, a decrease in muscular tone and abolition of the stretch reflexes in the territories corresponding to the spinal cord segments operated on. The following year, it was decided to extend indications of MDT to severe spasticity (Sindou et al. 1974b, 1984, 1985).

The substance of this chapter corresponds to a sixteen-year experience of dealing with spasticity mainly in adults. During this period, the MDT procedure was applied to 31 patients at the cervical and 78 at the lumbo-sacral level.

Rationale

MDT was developed on the bases of *human anatomical studies* (Sindou 1972, Sindou et al. 1974c, 1976, 1983) revealing the existence in the DREZ of a spatial segregation of afferent fibers according to their size, and thus presumably destination and function. The procedure consists of microsurgical lesions performed in the ventro-lateral part of DREZ at a depth of 2 mm and orientated at 45° angle ventrally and medially. The lesions interrupt 1) the fine myelinated and unmyelinated (mainly nociceptive) fibers as they head directly for the dorsal horn (DH) or travel to other segments in the medial part (demonstrated as excitatory by Denny-Brown et al. 1973) of the tract of Lissauer, and 2) the large A alpha (myotatic) fibers. These fibers are located respectively laterally and centrally in the DREZ (Figs. 1 and 2). This procedure spares most of the large (lemniscal) fibers which are grouped medially, as well as the lateral (inhibitory) portion of the tract of Lissauer. MDT is thus expected: 1) to interrupt selectively the afferent components of the (myotatic) mono- and (nociceptive) polysynaptic reflexes, which have been cut off from their suprasegmental inhibitory control by pathological conditions (Dimitrijevic and Nathan 1967a, b, 1968), and 2) to deprive the somatosensory relays of the DH of most of their excitatory inputs, while preserving their inhibitory segmental (i.e. lemniscal), intersegmental (i.e. lateral part of Lissauer tract), and also suprasegmental influences.

Owing to its special location: *at the junction between the peripheral and central parts of the somatosensory system*, MDT can exert on the DREZ and the dorsal horn – which have been shown to play an important role in spinal cord modulation –, a specific inhibitory action on pain and muscle tone. This is achieved while producing both marked hypoalgesia and marked

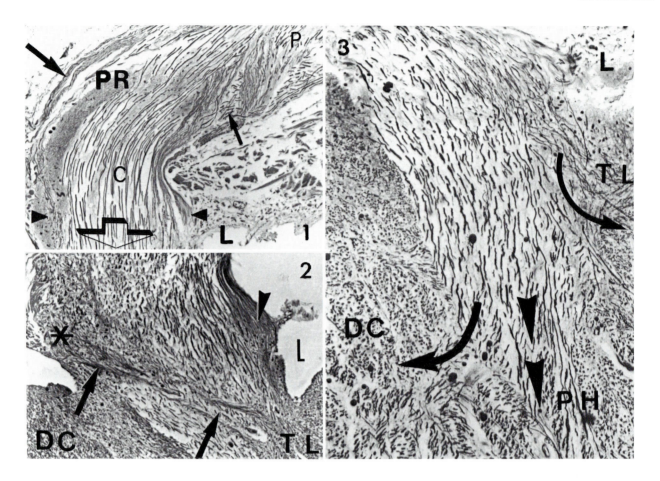

Fig. 1. *Course of nerve fibers at the Dorsal Root Entry Zone (DREZ) in man* (Sindou 1972). Rootlet diameter: 1 mm (axons stained by Bodian) **(1)** Longitudinal section of a C6 rootlet before entry into the spinal cord. At the peripheral segment (P), the large and small fibers have no particular organization. Just before the pial ring (PR), the small fibers reach the rootlet surface (arrows), mostly in the lateral region (L). In the central segment (C), the small fibers are arranged in two bundles (triangles) located on either side of the large fibers. **(2)** Longitudinal section of a C7 rootlet at its entry into the spinal cord. The large fibers constitute the center of the rootlet and run towards the dorsal column (DC). The small fibers form two bundles. One is lateral (triangle), the other medial (asterisk). The medial portion runs obliquely across the rootlet (arrows) to reach the tract of Lissauer (TL) Thus, most of the small fibers are regrouped at the lateral region (L) of the DREZ. **(3)** Longitudinal section of a cervical rootlet with its afferent endings in the spinal cord. The large lemniscal fibers (thick curved arrows) are grouped medially to enter the dorsal column (DC). The large myotatic fibers (double arrow) penetrate deeper into the posterior horn (PH) to reach the anterior horn. The small nociceptive fibers (thin curved arrow) are regrouped laterally to enter the tract of Lissauer (TL)

thermic hypoaesthesia, with a less important decrease in proprioception and cutaneous discrimination senses (see Sindou et al. 1986, Sindou and Jeanmonod 1989, for details).

These clinical data correlate well with the electrophysiological findings that we have obtained by *intra-operative recordings of the evoked electrospinogram (EESG) from the surface of the spinal cord*, after stimulation of the median and the tibial nerve, for the cervical and the lumbo-sacral spinal cord segments, respectively. These recordings showed: 1) an only moderate effect of MDT on the cervical (N11) or lumbo-sacral (N21) presynaptic compound action potentials, which probably correspond to the entrance of the lemniscal fibers into the dorsal column, 2) a more marked effect on the post-synaptic dorsal horn waves related to the larger primary afferent fibers (N 13 for cervical and N24 for lumbo-sacral) and 3) a complete disappearance of the dorsal horn waves related to the finer afferents (N2 and N3) (Fig. 3) (see Jeanmonod et al. 1989 for details). Of course intra-operative EESG recordings are useful to the surgeon to guide him to the accurate location and adequate control in depth of the surgical lesion.

The contralateral parietal N20 potential was recorded by a scalp electrode. When acutely decreased

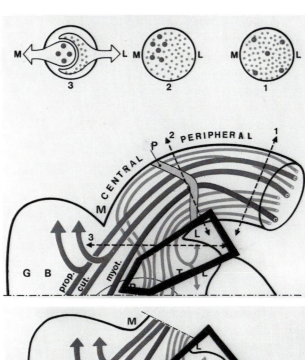

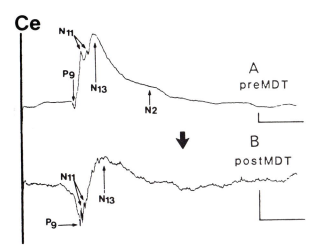

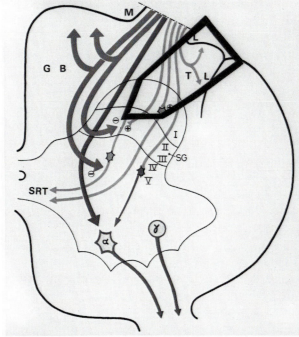

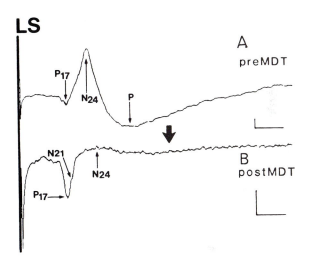

Fig. 3. *Effects of MDT on the EESG.* Recordings from the surface of the dorsal column, medially to the DREZ at the C7 cervical (Ce) and the L5 lumbo-sacral (LS) segments, ipsi-lateral to the stimulation of the median and the tibial nerve, respectively, before (**A**: pre MDT) and after (**B**: post-MDT).

– The initial positive event P9 (for cervical) [P17 (for lumbo-sacral)] corresponds to the farfield compound potential originating in the proximal part of the brachial (lumbo-sacral) plexus. The small and sharp negative peaks N11 (N21) correspond to nearfield pre-synaptic successive axonal events, probably generated in the proximal portion of the dorsal root, the dorsal funiculus and the large-diameter afferent collaterals to the dorsal horn. After MDT all these pre-synaptic potentials remain unchanged.

– The large slow negative wave N13 (N24) correspond to the post-synaptic activation of the dorsal horn by group I and II peripheral afferent fibers of the median (tibial) nerves. They are diminished after MDT (in the order of 2/3 rds).

– The later negative slow wave N2 (just visible in the cervical recording) corresponds to a post-synaptic dorsal horn activity consecutive to the activation of group II and III afferent fibers. N2 is suppressed after MDT

Fig. 2. *Upper part: Organization of fibers in the DREZ in man* (Sindou et al. 1974c). Each rootlet consist of a peripheral and a central segment; the junction of the two portions – called pial ring (P) – is on average 1 mm from the penetration of the rootlet into the dorso-lateral sulcus. Peripherally, the fibers have no organization. In the neighbourhood of the pial ring, the small fibers are situated under the rootlet surface, predominantly on its lateral side. In the central segment, they regroup laterally to enter the tract of Lissauer (TL). The large fibers are located centrally for the myotatic fibers and medially for the lemniscal ones which enter the tracts of Goll and Burdach (GB). The black triangle indicates the proposed extent of the surgical lesion, i.e., the lateral and central bundles formed by the nociceptive and myotatic fibers, as well as the (excitatory) medial part of the TL and the apex of the dorsal horn. *Lower part: Posterior rootlet projections to the spinal cord.* The small fibers terminate on the spino-reticulo-thalamic (SRT)

cells, which they activate, through interneuronal pathways on the moto-neurons of the anterior horn. The short recurrent collaterals of the large fibers (of cutaneous or proprioceptive origin) terminate on the SRT cells, which they inhibit

by the operation, it recovered totally leading to a normal pattern a few days after surgery. This attests the preservation of the ascending lemniscal system.

All these data provide evidence for an acceptably *selective action of MDT*: 1) a block of the activation of the segmental spinal cord mechanisms for tone and/or pain and 2) a relative preservation of the discriminative and proprioceptive dorsal column system, as well as the inhibitory circuitry of the dorsal horn – thus retuning the spinal cord regulation towards inhibition.

Selection and assessment of patients. Quantification of data

Up to the present time, *selection* for MDT was restricted to patients who had deficits accompanied by harmful spasticity. Therefore, at present, we can only recommend MDT for severe disabling hyperspastic states, like those encountered in:

–upper limb hemiplegias with abnormal postures in flexion of the elbow, wrist and fingers;
–paraplegias with spontaneous flexion or irreducible extension, making washing and dressing difficult, placement in a wheelchair uncomfortable, and kinestherapy ineffective.

Of course, MDT – like all the other ablative methods – can only be indicated when spasticity has resisted all forms of physiotherapy and drug treatments, especially diazepam, baclofen, and dantrolene.

–*Assessment* of the patient must be performed by a multidisciplinary team. In our department this team includes the neurosurgeon, an anaesthetist, a neurologist, a psychiatrist, an orthopaedic surgeon, a specialist in urodynamics, and a physiotherapist.

Once the spastic state has been demonstrated as being harmful, one has to determine the respective involvement in the abnormal postures of spasticity – to be treated with MDT –, and of bony, articular, muscular, tendinous, and/or ligamentous limitations – to be relieved by orthopaedic procedures. If doubt persists after detailed clinical and radiological examination, a testing of passive articular mobility is performed using brief general anaesthesia with curare derivatives. When spasticity plays the larger part in the articular limitations, abnormal postures are significantly diminished during this test. If not,

orthopaedic surgery may be the answer, as the initial or only treatment.

If after MDT, the articular gains are not deemed sufficient, despite intensive physiotherapy, orthopaedic surgery should be performed without delay, before passive mobilization triggers the reappearance of abnormal motor postures.

–For *quantification of data*, we have used the scales and scoring systems based on clinical examination and those detailed in the chapter seven.

Most of our patients were so severely affected that their spasticity could not be quantified by measurement of the strength of the stretch reflex, i.e., the Held's test. Muscular hypertonia was graded by using a grading system modified from the Ashworth scale (Table 3A) and spasms (especially occurring in patients with spinal cord lesions) according to their frequency and/or the disability they produced (Table 3B).

The score to quantify spontaneous abnormal postures, was obtained by calculating the angle between the posture and the reference position of each joint involved.

Articular limitations were estimated by performing angular measurements of both extreme positions during passive forced movement. The grading was the same as for spontaneous abnormal postures.

Voluntary motor activity was evaluated using the classical five grade of Lovett's scale or, if the patient had severe deficits, by sub-classifying motor function as: absent, nonfunctional or functional.

Pain, when present, was designated using the as severe, marked, moderate, mild and absent, and somatosensory function as normal; mildly, markedly, and severely impaired; and abolished.

The global functional disability in relation to spasticity, was scored using a grading system which differed for hemiplegic (Table 4) and paraplegic (Table 6) patients. These functional evaluations were easily performed by any member of the team.

Surgical technique

Surgery is performed under general anaesthesia, but with only an initial short-lasting curarization to allow intra-operative observation of motor responses to electrical stimulation of the nerve roots. Roots are identified by electrical stimulation using bipolar neurostimulation with an increasing voltage from 1 to 6 volts. Stimulated ventral roots have a

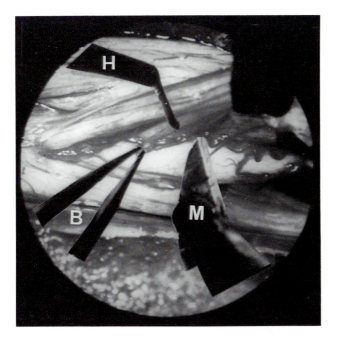

Fig. 4. *Technical principles of MDT*. Exposure of the dorso-lateral aspect of the conus medullaris on the left side. The rootlets of the selected dorsal roots are retracted postero-medially with a micro-sucker or a small hook (H) to gain access to the ventro-lateral part of the dorsal root entry zone. After dissection of the arteries running along the dorso-lateral sulcus and coagulation of the small pial vessels using a sharp bipolar microforceps (B), the incision is performed using a microknife made with a small piece of razor-blade (M). The cut is at a 45 degree angle and to a depth of 2 mm. The surgical lesion is completed by doing microcoagulations, under vision, at a low intensity, inside the incision down to the apex of the dorsal horn

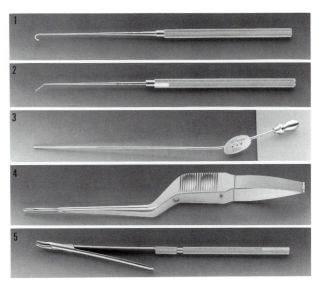

Fig. 5. *Necessary instruments for performing MDT*. From top to bottom: **1** Curved and buttoned micro-hook for manipulating and holding the spinal roots. **2** Malleable micro-probe (of the Jacobson type) for gentle dissection and sustained retraction of the rootlets. **3** Buttoned micro-sucker (of an original design) which can be used not only as a sucker, but also as a probe and/or a retactor. **4** Curved sharp micro-scissors to divide the fine arachnoidal filaments, the pia-mater and the tiny pial vessels. **5** Curved razor-blade holder; its jaws are strated to allow a better stability of the piece of razor blade. (Set of instruments for Microsurgical DREZ-tomy made by FL Fischer. Fischer *MET* GmbH, Bötzinger Strasse 6, D-7800 Freiburg, West Germany)

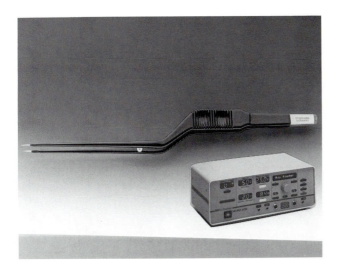

Fig. 6. *Special bipolar forceps for performing MDT*. This bipolar forceps is bayonet-shaped, insulated except at the tip over 5 mm, sharp and graduated every millimeter over its 5 mm extremity

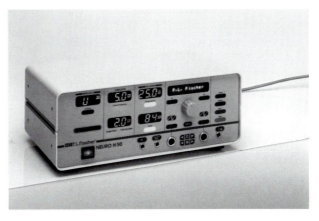

Fig. 7. Neurosurgical stimulator, lesion generator and impedance monitor (Type: neuro N50, also developed by FL Fischer). This lesion generator can be connected with the bipolar forceps (see Fig. 6)

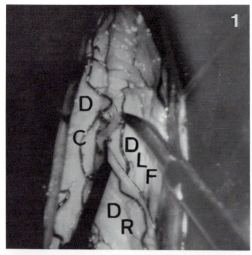

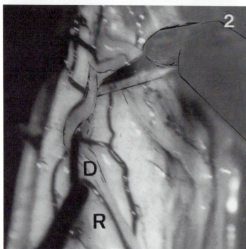

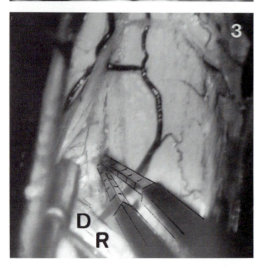

motor threshold at least 3 times lower than the dorsal roots.

Standard microsurgical techniques are used with magnification in the order of $10 \times$ to $25 \times$. Special micro-instruments have been designed for MDT by the senior author (MS), and made by F.L. Fischer (Fischer MET GmbH, Bötzinger Strasse 41, D-7800 Freiburg, West Germany). They are shown in Figs. 4–7.

1. Operative procedure at the cervical level (Fig. 8)

The sitting position – with the neck in flexion – has the advantage of offering the surgeon a comfortable approach, and of lessening oozing because of a lower venous pressure in the cervico-cephalic region. But the prone position – the head and neck flexed, in the "Concorde" position has the advantage of avoiding collapse due to CSF depletion, especially in patients with brain atrophy. Because of a lower incidence of drowsiness, mental confusion and headaches after operation, the prone position is used in most patients. The sitting position is still preferred in individuals with a short and fat neck. Whatever the position, the head is always fixed with a three pin head-holder.

The level of laminectomy is determined after identification of the prominent spinous process of C-2 by palpation. A hemilaminectomy, generally from C4 to C7, with preservation of the spinous processes, allows sufficient exposure to the posterolateral aspect of the cervical spinal cord segments corresponding to the upper limb innervation, i.e., the rootlets of C5 to T1 (T2).

After opening the dura and the arachnoid longitudinally, the exposed roots and rootlets are dissected free by separation of the tiny arachnoid filaments that bind them to each other, to the arachnoid sheath and to the spinal cord pia mater. The main radicular vessels are preserved.

Each ventral (and dorsal root) from C4 to T1 is electrically stimulated at the level of their corresponding foramen to identify precisely their dominant muscular innervation: the diaphragm for C4 (the response is palpable below the lower ribs), shoulder

Fig. 8. *MDT technique at the cervical level.* Exposure of the right dorso-lateral aspect of the cervical cord at C6. **1** The rootlets of the selected dorsal root (DR) are displaced dorsally and medially with a hook or a micro-sucker, to obtain access to the ventro-lateral aspect of the DREZ in the dorso-lateral sulcus. Using microscissors, the arachnoid adhesions are cut between cord and dorsal rootlets.

DC = dorsal cord, DLF = dorso-lateral funiculus. **2** After having coagulated exclusively the tiny pial vessels, an incision—2 mm in depth, at 45 degrees ventrally and medially—is made with a microscalpel in the lateral border of the dorso-lateral sulcus. **3** Then, microcoagulations are performed down to the apex of the dorsal horn, using a thin, sharp, graduated, bipolar microforceps

abductors for C5, elbow flexors for C6, elbow and wrist extensors for C7, intrinsic muscles of the hand for C8 and T1.

Microsurgical lesions are then performed at the selected levels, i.e., those which correspond to the harmful spastic muscles. The attachment of the rootlets to the spinal cord is sufficiently solid to allow them to be retracted posteriorly and medially to give access to the ventro-lateral region of the DREZ. The small pial vessels at this level are separated and moved, whenever possible, or coagulated by means of a sharp bipolar forceps, thus allowing the incision to be made without bleeding. The incision is made with a microknife (made of a small piece of razor blade maintained in a blade-holder) at the very entry zone of the rootlets in the dorsolateral sulcus. The incision is 2 mm deep into Lissauer's tract and obliquely oriented at 45° down to the apex of the dorsal horn, recognizable under the microscope by its gray-brown colour. Then the surgical lesion in the target is completed by microcoagulation of short duration and low intensity inside the incision.

If the laxity of the root is sufficient, the incision is performed continuously in the dorsolateral sulcus ventrolaterally along all of the rootlets of the targeted root thus accomplishing a sulcotomy. If not, a partial ventrolateral section is made successively under on each rootlet of the root, after the surgeon has isolated each one by separating the tiny arachnoid membranes which hold them together.

Recording of surface spinal cord evoked potentials by stimulation of the tibial and the median nerve (EESG) can be helpful in checking the integrity of the dorsal column and the extent of MDT, respectively (Jeanmonod et al. 1989).

2. Operative procedure at the lumbo-sacral level (Fig. 9)

The patient is positioned prone on thoracic and iliac supports, the head placed 20 cm lower than the level of the surgical wound, to minimize the intra-operative loss of CSF. The desired vertebral level is identified by palpation of the spinous processes, or, if this is doubtful, by obtaining a lateral X-ray including S1 vertebra. A given interspinous level, identified by a needle, can then be marked with methylene blue.

A bilateral (or unilateral) laminectomy from T11 to L2 is performed. The dura and arachnoid are opened longitudinally. The filum terminale is identified.

Identification or roots is then performed by electrical stimulation. Stimulation of the S1 dorsal root produces a motor response of the gastrocnemius-soleus group (this can be confirmed later, by repeatedly checking the ankle reflex before, during, and after MDT at this level). The roots L1 and L2 are easily identified at the penetration into their respective dural sheaths. Stimulation of L2 produces a response of the iliopsoas and adductor muscles. Stimulation of the S2-S4 dorsal roots can be assessed by the recording of the motor vesical or anal response using cysto- or rectomanometry or an electromyogram of the anal sphincter. These procedures are difficult in the operating theatre. We have found that measurements of the conus medullaris is sufficient, especially for patients already having severe preoperative impairment of their vesico-anal functions. These measurements, based on human postmortem studies, have shown that the division between the S1 and S2 segments is situated around 30 mm above the exit from the conus of the tiny coccygeal root. The identification of the remaining roots – L3 to L5 – is difficult for many reasons: 1) The exit through their respective dural sheaths is caudal to the operative site. 2) The dorsal rootlets enter the DREZ along an uninterrupted line. 3) The ventral roots are hidden in front of the dentate ligament. 4) The motor responses in the leg to stimulation of the roots are difficult to observe intraoperatively, because of the patient's prone position, and because of the severe paralysis and orthopaedic articular limitations impeding the leg movement. 5) Our experience (in 43 patients) has been that isolated stimulation of the dorsal roots is often non conclusive in spastic patients because of diffusion of activity into a large number of leg muscles.

After stimulation of the roots has been completed, recordings of spinal cord surface evoked potentials can be obtained in order to complement root stimulation for identification of spinal cord segments and in order to study the effects of MDT on DREZ physiology (Jeanmonod et al. 1989).

All the dorsal roots of the cauda equina on one side are then displaced dorsally and medially to obtain proper access to the lateral aspect of the DREZ, in the postero-lateral sulcus. A careful dissection has to be carried out to cut all arachnoid adhesions, thus freeing all rootlets and related vessels. In a few patients, an arachnoiditis can make this dissection difficult. The postero-lateral spinal artery courses along the postero-lateral sulcus. Its diameter is between 0.1 and 0.5 mm. It is fed by the posterior radicular arteries and joins caudally with the descending anterior branch of the artery of Adamkiewicz through the anastomotic loop of Lazorthes of the conus medullaris. This artery has to be preserved by being freed from the sulcus. The tiny pial vessels situated on the lateral aspect of the DREZ are coagulated with a pointed and graduated microforceps and cut with a curved, sharp microscissors. A continous incision (i.e. a postero-lateral sulcotomy) is then performed with a microscalpel. The cut must be 2 mm deep, with an angle of 45 degrees

ventrally and medially – similar to the cervical MDT. The borders of the incision are spread slightly apart with the forceps, so that the grey-brown colour of the most dorsal part of the DH can be seen. The lesion is then completed by microcoagulation inside the cut with the graduated bipolar microforceps. We use a blunt microaspirator to keep the rootlets gently out of the way and to control CSF flow and bleeding.

For patients with severe paraplegia (80%) – especially those with flexor spasms – we perform uninterrupted MDT from L2 down to S2 (and sometimes to S5). For patients with limited harmful spasticity, we try to spare some of the roots which innervate non

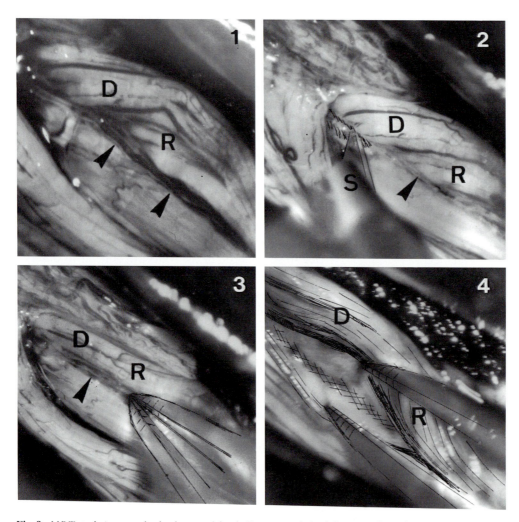

Fig. 9. *MDT technique at the lumbo-sacral level.* Exposure of the left posterolateral aspect of the conus medullaris. **1** The rootlets of the selected lumbosacral dorsal roots (DR) are displaced dorsally and medially to obtain proper access to the ventrolateral aspect of the DREZ in the posterolateral sulcus. Only the tiny pial vessels (arrows) will be coagulated with a thin, pointed, graduated, bipolar microforceps. **2** A microscalpel (S) made with a small, elongated fragment of a razor blade mounted on a holder is ready to start the incision, which will be at an angle of 45° ventromedially and 2 mm deep (arrow, posterolateral sulcus). **3** Microcoagulations are performed inside the incision, 2 mm in depth, down to the upper layers of the dorsal horn. The line of incision is opened (between the two tips of the bipolar forceps and reveals its depth and the apex of the dorsal horn)

Table 1. MDT for treatment of the hemiplegic upper limb (summary of our 16 case series)

					Preoperative status							Postoperative Status						
Case	Sex	Age (yr)	Cause	Duration (yr)	Voluntary mobility (n= +++ +)	Sensation (n= ++)	Pain	Functional status	MDT Level	Side	Follow up (yr)	Spasticity	Voluntary mobility (n= +++ +)	Sensation (n= ++)	Pain	Functional status	Complications	Patient appreciation
1	F	52	V	2	+	++	Intense N–S	0	C-5–T-1	R	12	MR	+	↗+	0	PM	No	VU
2	M	45	T	2	+	++	Intense S	0	C-5–T-2	L	12	A	++	++	0	AM+	No	VU
3	M	22	T	2	0	++	Intense S	0	C-5–T-1	L	10	A	0	++	0	PM	Yes[b]	VU
4	M	57	T	2	+	++	0	PM	C-6–C-8	R	8	A	+	↗+	0	PM	No	F
5	M	23	T	2	+	++	Intense N–S	0	C-5–T-1	L	5	A	↗++	++	M	AM+	No	VU
6	M	32	V	2	0	++	Moderate N–S	0	C-5–T-1	L	4	MR	↗+	+	0	PM	No	VU
7	M	29	T	6	+	++	Intense S	0	C-5–T-1	R	3	MR	++	++	M	AM+	No	VU
8	M	65	T	5	0	++	0	0	C-5–T-8	L	3	MR	0	++	0	PM	No	VU
9	M	24	T	1	++	++	Intense N–S	AM+	C-5–T-1	L	3	MR	↗+++	↗+	0	AM++	No	VU
10	M	43	V	2	++	++	Moderate S	AM+	C-6–T-1	L	2	SD	↗+++	++	0	AM++	No	Rec[c]
11	M	48	V	3	+	++	0	0	C-7–C-8	R	2	MR	↘0	↗+	0	PM	No	VU
12	M	49	T	7	0	++	0	0	C-5–T-1	R	2	A	0	↗+	0	PM	No	F[d]
13	M	25	T	1	++	+	Intense N–S	AM+	C-5–C-8	L	2	MR	↗+++	+	0	AM++	No	Vu
14	M	62	V	4	++	+	Intense[e] N	AM+	C-5–T-1	R[f]	2	MR	+++	+	0	AM++	No	Vu
15	M	40	T	3	+	++	Moderate S	0	C-5–T-1	L	1	MR	↗+	↗+	0	AM+	No	MU
16	M	42	T	2	++	++	Intense N–S	0	C-5–T-1	L	1	SD	++	↗+	M	AM+	No	MU

[a] Abbreviations: Cause – V vascular; T traumatic. Voluntary Mobility – 0 none; + poor proximal; ++ good proximal but poor distal; +++ good both proximal and distal; ↗ more than preoperatively; ↘ less than preoperatively. Sensation – ++ preserved or nearly normal; + diminished; Pain – N neurogenic; S somatogenic; N-S combination of the previous two; 0 no pain. Functional status – 0 no function; PM easy passive mobilization only; AM + slightly but useful voluntary movements; AM + + slightly but useful voluntary movements with prehension in the hand. Spasticity – A abolished; MR markedly reduced; SD slightly diminished. Patient Appreciation – F failure; MU moderately useful; VU very useful.

[b] Loss of mobility in the right leg.

[c] Spasticity recurred in 5 months; reoperation: anterior rootlet section of C8–T-1.

[d] Patient hoped to recover voluntary motility.

[e] Capsulothalamic syndrome.

[f] Combined MDT and Dorsal Column Stimulation

hyperspastic muscles, although it is difficult to differentiate these roots, because of the limitations of root stimulation described above.

When there is a localized arachnoiditis or undissectable, important vessels embedded inside the posterolateral sulcus along one or a few cord segments, the appropriate target, i.e. the lateral aspect of the DREZ, cannot be easily and safely reached. Section of the corresponding rootlets is then performed more peripherally, so that there is no risk of misplacing the incision and of compromising cord vascularization.

Post-operative care and rehabilitation program

Considering the precarious pre-operative state of a large majority of spastic patients and the severity of their basic disease, hospitalization in the intensive care unit for a few days is strongly recommended. Intensive physiotherapeutic measures for respiration and positioning in bed are used to prevent pulmonary complications and pressure sores. As soon as the patient is stabilized and the wound healed, he is transferred to the department of rehabilitation for intensive physiotherapy. If the articular limitations are not overcome with therapy at the end of the first month, orthopaedic surgery is performed without delay.

Pressure sores, if severe and without a natural tendency to heal, are surgically repaired. This is easier to do after reduction of the abnormal postures. The urinary function is checked by urodynamic evaluation and an medical and/or surgical treatment is undertaken if needed.

After discharge from the rehabilitation center, an ambulatory physiotherapy program is initiated to allow the patient to stay home. Thereafter he is followed regularly as an outpatient by the multidisciplinary team.

Results

This section, which describes the long-term effects of MDT, has been taken from the data of patients in whom the results could be carefully studied with a minimum follow-up of 2 years (5 years on average). These patients belong to two different series, already published in detail (Sindou et al. 1986, Sindou and Jeanmonod 1989).

One of the series (Sindou et al. 1986) concerns 16 patients – 15 males and 1 female, 23 to 65 years old (average 41 yrs) suffering from hyperspastic *hemiplegia*

Table 2. Causes of spasticity in the lower limb(s) (personal series: 53 cases)

– *Spinal cord lesions*	
Post-traumatic paraplegia (T_4:2, T_{10}:1, T_{12}:2)	5
Non-traumatic paraplegia (Mills syndrome: 1, Strumpell–Lorrain: 1, AVM with arachnoiditis: 1, chondroma at T_9:1, meningo-myelitis at T_6:1)	5
Post-traumatic tetraplegia (C_6:2, C_7:1)	3
Non-traumatic tetraplegia (Arnold–Chiari)	1
Post-traumatic Brown-sequard syndrome (C_4)	1
Total = 15	
– *Cerebral lesions*	
Encephalopathies (cerebral palsy: 2, degenerative disease: 1)	3
Stroke	2
Brain stem trauma	5
Total = 10	
– *Spinal cord and cerebral lesions*	
Multiple sclerosis	28
Total (all lesions) = 53	

Table 3. Scoring system for spasticity and spasms in paraplegic patients

A *Spasticity*	Score	Description
Absent	0	
Mild	1	No spontaneous abnormal posture, normal passive mobility; no disability
Moderate	2	Passive mobilization completely reduces the abnormal posture; moderate disability
Marked	3	Passive mobilization incompletely reduces the abnormal posture; marked disability
Severe	4	Passive mobilization reduces the abnormal posture minimally or not at all; severe disability

B *Spasms*	Score	Description
Absent	0	
Mild	1	Rare and mild spasms, only during mobilization; no disability
Moderate	2	Frequent, spontaneous, but moderate spasms; moderate disability
Marked	3	Very frequent, spontaneous and marked spasms; marked disability, some problems for sitting or lying
Severe	4	Almost constant and severe spasms; severe disability, major problems for sitting or lying

in the upper limb. These patients had irreducible, abnormal postures in flexion, making even passive mobilization, washing, and dressing difficult (Table 1). The cause of the spasticity was vascular in 5 cases and traumatic in 11; the duration of disability ranged from 1 to 7 years (average 2 years and 10 months). Pain was associated with spasticity in 12 cases. Although recognition of the mechanisms of the pain was often difficult, it was considered purely neurogenic in 1 case, somatogenic in 5, and mixed in the 6 others. Voluntary motor activity was totally abolished in 4 cases and severely affected in the other 12. Only 5 in the latter group retained some voluntary movement in the affected hand, but this was without any use for prehension, as extension of wrist and fingers remained very difficult. Cutaneous and deep sensations remained normal or nearly so in 14 cases while markedly diminished in only 2.

The other series (Sindou and Jeanmonod 1989) consists of 53 patients – 30 females and 23 males, aged from 11 to 67 years (mean age: 41). They were all selected on the basis of the presence of a severe disabling *spasticity which affected one* (6 patients) *or both* (47 patients) *lower limbs*. Multiple sclerosis (MS) was the most frequent (28 patients) cause of the spasticity (Table 2). Duration of the causal diseases was between 4,5 months and 30 years (mean 16.3 months). Spasticity was associated with unvoluntary flexion in 38 patients, and caused abnormal postures, more or less reducible, in all pattients but one (flexion in 49 and extension in 3). These abnormal postures made any lying position in bed very uncomfortable, and sitting, washing and dressing, difficult or even impossible. Moreover pain, present in 37 patients (69.8%) multiple pressure sores, in 22 patients (43.1%), and urinary problems, in 48 (90.6%), increased the discomfort and aggreviated the spasticity. Only 3 patients had voluntary motor activity scored as functional, and only 8 had strictly normal somato-sensory function.

MDT was performed at the cervical level for spasticity in the upper limb (in most patients from C5 to T1), and *in the conus medullaris* for spasticity in the lower limbs (in 80% cases all segments between and including L1 and S2).

Repeated clinical follow-up has shown that the post-operative progress of patients was complete at between 1 month and 1 year according to the different items studied. All later examinations, up to a maximum of 15 years (5 years on average), showed no

further, significant changes thus demonstrating very little long term loss of effectiveness of MDT.

1. Relief of spasticity

Immediately after operation, the muscular tone is usually less than normal, but returns to a more or less normal level within several weeks. The final result can only be judged after a three month follow-up.

A total or marked effect on spasticity – i.e. a "useful" result, allowing withdrawal of antispasmodic medications – was obtained in 87% of our patients with a spastic *upper limb* (see Table 1).

A similarly useful effect on spasticity was obtained in 75% of the patients with spasticity in the *lower limbs*. When spasms were present in paraplegic patients, they were suppressed or markedly decreased in 88% of the cases (see Table 3 and Fig. 10). The analysis of the results in relation to the localization of the lesions showed that the best outcome was seen in spasticity (and spasms) due to pure spinal cord lesions (in the order of 80% useful results), followed by multiple sclerosis (75%). The least improvement was observed in patients with spasticity due to cerebral lesions (60%) (Fig. 11).

2. Effects on abnormal postures and articular limitations

Reduction in spasticity usually leads to a significant improvement of abnormal postures and articular limitations. This was achieved, in about 90% of our cases.

For the hemiplegic *upper limb* (16 cases) the increase in articular amplitude was most remarkable for the elbow and the shoulder (when not "frozen"), and much more limited for the wrist and fingers, especially if there was retraction of the flexor muscles and no residual voluntary motor activity in the extensors. In the later situation complementary orthopaedic surgery can be most useful in gaining a better position of the hand. Our three patients who underwent such a secondary correction, experienced benefit in comfort and even function from the orthopaedic operation.

For the *lower limbs* with abnormal postures in flexion (49 cases), the increase in articular amplitude was very dependant upon the degree of severity of the pre-operative retractions. The fact that in a number of cases the increase in amplitude was better after MDT than during the test under general anaesthesia,

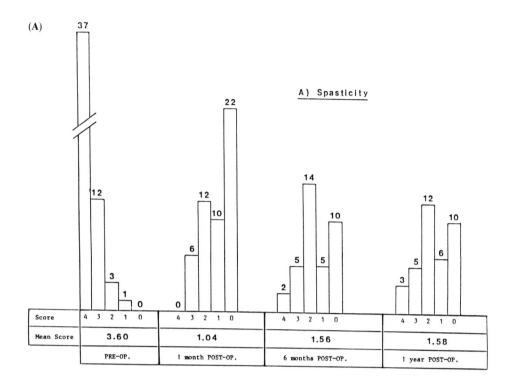

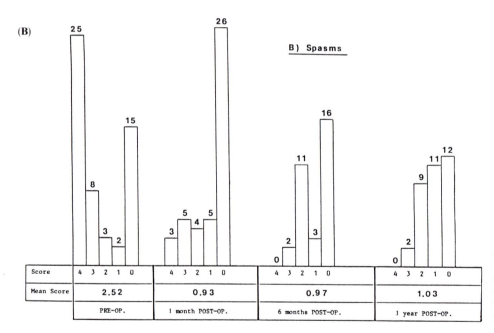

Fig. 10. *Postoperative evolution of spasticity* (A) *and spasms* (B), with distribution of patients scores (see Table 3) in relation to different postoperative follow-up times. Ordinates represented patient numbers

was probably due to the positive effect of the early, intensive post-operative physiotherapy. When the post-MDT gains were deemed insufficient because of persistant joint limitations, complementary ortho-paedic surgery was indicated, not only to increase the articular mobility, but also to prevent reactivation of flexion reflexes through nociceptive stimulations provoked during intensive mobilization.

With regard to the 3 patients who had paraplegia and irreducible hyperextension, all were completely relieved.

3. Effects on voluntary motor activity

In the patients with some voluntary movements hidden behind their spasticity, reduction in the

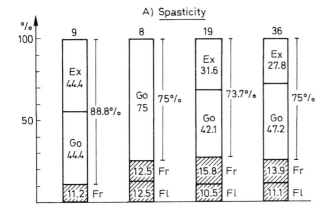

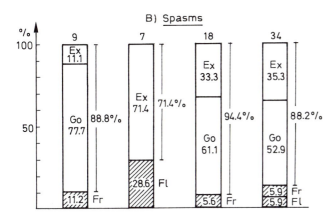

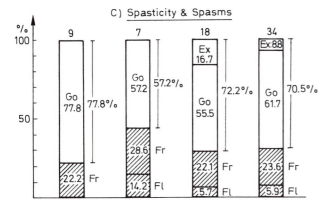

Fig. 11. *Results on spasticity and spasm in relation to the localization of the responsible lesions (Fl* failure; *Fr* fair; *Go* good; *Ex* excellent; *hatched* fair results plus failures; *SC* spinal cord lesions; *CER* cerebral lesions; *MS* multiple sclerosis; *CUM* cumulated data). All numbers are percentages, except those at the top of each column, which indicate the total number of patients

hypertonia results in an improvement in voluntary motor activity. Its functional quality depends upon the pre-operative level of the motor function.

Motor improvement occurred in 50% of the patients operated on for spasticity in the *upper limb*, allowing

better voluntary motor activity of their shoulder and arm during dressing and washing. But only half of those who had some pre-operative distal motor function, obtained additional hand prehension.

In the series of patients with spasticity in the *lower limbs* only 10% had a significant motor improvement after surgery. Among the others, 80% remained unchanged (most of them were non functional preoperatively) and 10% were worse (fortunately, no one in this group had useful preoperative voluntary motor activity).

4. Relief of pain

Pain which accompanies spasticity (70% of the cases in our series) can, most often, be favourably influenced by MDT, whatever its mechanism may be, i.e., somatogenic, neurogenic, or both. 60% of our patients became pain-free after surgery, and 40% found their pain reduced to a moderate or slight level. These percentages are close to those obtained through similar procedures for pure somatogenic or neurogenic pain.

Interestingly enough, vaso-motor disturbances – supposedly more or less related to pain – when present, were improved in parallel with pain relief.

Four patients experienced new post-operative pain considered to be neurogenic and related to surgery. For 3 of them, this was only a change in the quality of the pain experienced pre-operatively. For the last one, who had no pain before MDT, progression of his disease (MS) was probably the cause of this new pain.

5. Modifications of sensations

MDT constantly produces a decrease in sensation, as clearly observed in patients in whom cutaneous and deep sensations were normal or near normal preoperatively.

This decrease was slight in 40% of the patients, marked in 40% and severe in 20%. It affected both the extralemniscal and, to a lesser extent, the lemniscal modalities.

Whereas the effect on thermal and pin-prick sensations is expected, since it is directly related to the anatomical rationale of MDT, the impairment of nonthermoalgesic sensations – mainly tactile, but also vibratory and proprioceptive – appears somewhat surprising. This can be explained by the destruction of axons belonging to pathways other than the classical dorsal column presynaptic system, and carrying tactile information, more than by creation of a significant lesion of dorsal column afferents. This conclusion is supported not only by our postoperative clinical examinations, but also by electro-physiological investigations (Jeanmonod et al. 1989).

6. Effects on urinary function

MDT performed bilaterally in the conus medullaris, at the S2 and S3 (and sometimes in addition S4) segments, is able to reduce spasticity of the bladder. But clinical improvement, as well as clearcut modifications at urodynamic examinations, can only be noticed if there is no irreversible sclerosis of the urinary system.

In our series, neuro-urological improvement was noted in only 6.3% of patients. These weak effects of MDT on bladder hyperreflexia, sphincteric dyssynergia, and urinary urgency may be explained in several ways. First of all, the lower sacral roots often were not operated upon, because neuro-urological problems were never by themselves an indication for surgery. Secondly, and probably most importantly when a large number of lower sacral roots were, however, operated upon, the absence of effects was due to chronic fixed sclerotic lesions of the bladder and sphincters.

As the value of MDT in the field of neuro-urology cannot be evaluated in this series of patients, we have recently initiated a new series of appropriately selected cases affected with pure neurological bladder dysfunction without irreversible sclerosis. The initial, still unpublished, results of this work are very promising.

Since MDT could impair preserved uro-genito-anal functions in globally spastic paraparetic patients, there is the possibility of limiting the procedure to the lumbar spinal cord segments with the addition of a complementary selective neurectomy of the tibial nerve (Sindou and Mertens 1988), as was done with success for two of our patients in order to alleviate the spasticity of their feet.

7. Results on functional status

Efficacy of MDT, as judged by the patient's comfort and quality of life, is a combined result of the effects on spasticity, mobility, and pain.

After surgery for spasticity in the *hemiplegic upper limb*, all the patients improved, the gain amounting to one or two grades, except in one case . But the functional status reached post-operatively, was closely dependent on pre-operative function (Tables 4 and 5). In all the patients in the group without any useful motor function, passive mobilization became easy and painless; voluntary movements reappeared in half of them but were not practically useful. In the group with slight preoperative active mobility, motor function improved significantly, mainly in the shoulder and elbow.

The effects of MDT in the patients with spasticity in the *lower limbs* were dramatic, as evidenced by the global functional score (GFS) study (Table 6 and Fig. 12). As a matter of fact, the mean value of the scores (0 = normal, 20 = total dependance) went from 15.58 to 3.56. The serious pre-operative condition of our patients obviously limited the post-operative functional recovery. The gain remained, nevertheless, highly significant and contented most of these formerly severely disabled persons. We have found the GFS very useful in selecting patients for MDT. The threshold at which surgery is deemed to be indicated is 10/20. The GFS is simple, easily reproducible over

Table 4. Functional score for hemiplegic patients with spasticity in the upper limb

Grade	Description
I	Absence of useful active mobility, and uneasy and painful passive mobilization, making it difficult to dress and wash
II	Easy passive mobilization, but without any useful voluntary movements
III	Slight, but useful voluntary motor function
IV	Good active mobility with the possibility of prehension in the hand and fingers

Table 5. Comparison between pre and post-operative functional status in hemiplegic patients with spasticity in the upper limb (see Table 4 for explanation of the grading system)

Pré-op	Post-op I	II	III	IV	Total
IV					0
III				4	4
II		1			1
I		6	5		11
Total	0	7	5	4	16

Table 6. Global functional score for paraplegic patients with spasticity in the lower limb(s). This score developed by Millet et al. (1981) quantifies five components that are directly influenced by spasticity, abnormal postures, and articular limitations, and are parts of the patient's every day life. The score goes from 0 to 4 each component with a total of 20/20 denoting a bedridden and totally dependent patient. A score of 10/20 was seen to correspond reproducibly to the threshold between a decent and an unacceptable condition, and thus as the lowest position at which to consider surgery

Pain
  0 absent
  1 rare and mild
  2 frequent; minimal disability
  3 marked and frequent; marked disability
  4 permanent and severe

Spasms
  0 absent
  1 rare and mild spasms, only during mobilization; no disability
  2 frequent, spontaneous but moderate spasms; moderate disability
  3 frequent, spontaneous and marked spasms; marked disability, some problems for sitting or lying
  4 almost constant and severe spasms; severe disability, major problems for sitting or lying

Sitting position
  0 normal
  1 mild difficulty
  2 moderate to marked difficulty, causing reduction of sitting periods
  3 severe difficulty, patient has to be tied down in position
  4 impossible

Body transfers
  0 normal
  1 mild difficulty
  2 moderate difficulty
  3 marked difficulty, need for a person helping
  4 severe difficulty, need for two persons helping

Washing and dressing
  0 normal
  1 mild difficulty
  2 moderate difficulty
  3 marked difficulty, need for a person helping
  4 severe difficulty, need for two persons helping

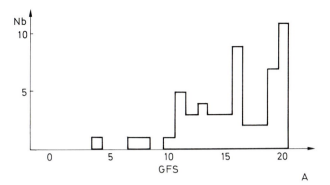

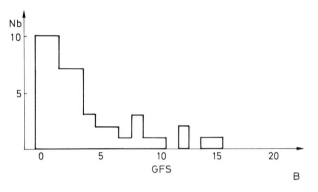

Fig. 12. Distribution of pre (**A**) and post-operative (**B**) *global functional scores* (GFS) in patients with spasticity in the lower limbs. *Nb* number of patients (see Table 6 for explanation of the scoring system)

time and by different examiners. It gives a reliable quantification of the over all abilities for the patient (Millet et al. 1981).

Complications

MDT has the inherent risks of any open surgical procedure. In the series of operations for spasticity in the *upper limb* (16 cases), there were no death and no general complication. One patient suffered hypotonia and a partial but permanent loss of mobility in the leg ipsilateral to the cervical procedure. This impaired standing and walking.

In the series of patients operated on for spasticity in the *lower limbs* (53 cases), the complication rate was high, due to their precarious condition. Delayed but spontaneous wound healing was seen in 18.9%. Two patients (3.8%) had a transient leakage of CSF. Cutaneous (28.3%), respiratory (22.6%), digestive (11.3%), urinary (3.8%), thromboembolic (3.8%) and septic (1.9%) complications were noted. Death occurred in 5 patients (9.4%) and was due to pulmonary emboli in 1 patient, respiratory problems in 3 and cutaneous problems in 1. Two MS patients presented with an acute but transient increase of their pre-existing neurological symptoms during the post-operative period, whereas 2 others suffered post-operative exacerbation of their disease as revealed by new clinical signs.

These complications were minor in 26.4%, moderate in 5.7% and severe in 13.2%. The majority of these complications were observed in patients with very advanced MS. They occurred at the beginning of the series, at a time when patient selection was not rigorous enough. Comparison of these complication rates with those obtained when the same procedure was used for pain, in less debilitated patients, indicates clearly that the high rate of risk is due to the very precarious clinical condition of the patients referred in this series.

Discussion

Consideration of the results shows that MDT can restore functional abilities and improve everyday activity without significant loss in its effectiveness over time, in most cases. This long-term efficacy might be related to the large number of spinal segments operated upon, and also to the specific modulatory action of MDT on tone regulation structures. The procedure is supposed to suppress the majority of excitatory inputs while maintaining most inhibitory ones. In other words it would *"retune" the tone regulation structures towards inhibition*, as could be the case for chronic pain. This "retuning" probably takes place due to section of the large myotatic fibers participating in the monosynaptic stretch reflex, and, may be more significantly, through an interruption of the so-called "flexor reflex afferents", the presence of which in animals has so authoritatively been described by Lundberg (1979) and Eccles et al. (1961).

Until now, indications were restricted to *patients suffering from severe, harmful spasticity* with extensive sensory-motor deficits. In most patients, surgery covered a large number of spinal cord segments. The reason was not only to deal with the peripheral overlap of cord segments but also to treat the abnormally widespread muscular responses to stimulation of each of the dorsal roots. These abnormal responses could well be due to the extensive destructions of the descending inhibitory pathways induced by the causal disease processes and/or to subsequent plastic adaptations.

Spasticity and its harmful consequences (abnormal postures, articular limitations...) were *significantly decreased in more than three-fourth of the patients*. In the upper limb, the results were better in the shoulder and elbow than on flexors of wrist and fingers. As far as lower limbs were concerned, our data show that the best outcome was in patients with pure spinal cord lesions, followed by MS, the poorest results being for patients with cerebral lesions. A severe cord lesion can be supposed to interrupt a large number of suprasegmental descending tracts to the more caudal cord

segments, thus leaving a large number of vacated, postsynaptic sites open to occupation by sprouting segmental afferent neurons (McCouch et al. 1958). Under these conditions, spasticity can be thought to be associated with an excessive influence of excitatory segmental inputs on tone regulation reflex arcs. These inputs are the specific targets of MDT, which will thus produce a swing of the balance towards inhibition, with a subsequent decrease or suppression of spasticity. On the other hand, to produce spasticity, a cerebral lesion must cause damage to descending inhibitory systems predominantly or exclusively. The remaining facilitative descending components would constitute the preponderant substrate for this sort of spasticity. These suprasegmental projections are not the target of MDT and will be spared, with a consequent less favourable outcome.

The long term *relief of both somatogenic and neurogenic pain* after MDT, and the infrequent production of painful post-operative deafferentation phenomena emphasizes a strong modulatory effect of MDT on the function of the dorsal horn.

When an excess of spasticity or pain causes a loss of mobility, a successful MDT *may improve the patient's voluntary movements*. Conversely, when the lack of mobility is a direct result of impairment of the central structures only and is not due to the disabling influence of spasticity or pain, the postoperative functional improvement may offer the patient comfort, but return of voluntary movement is doubtful.

For localized and severe spasticity in the upper limb, there is no really effective surgical alternative to MDT. In his report entitled "On the indications and results of the excision of posterior spinal nerve roots in men", published in 1913, Foerster (1913) mentioned 23 cases of spastic paralysis of the arm treated by resection of the posterior cervical roots from C4 to T2 except C6, or from three-fifths to four-fifths of the fascicles composing each root including C6. In contrast to paraplegia, he concluded that for spastic hemiplegia of the arm "in the majority the result was not good, as satisfactory improvement being obtained in only a few cases", and he did not recommend posterior rhizotomy as a valuable procedure for spasticity in the upper limb. Many years later, Kottke (1970) and Heimburger et al. (1973) reported successful decreases of spasticity in the upper limbs after posterior cervical rhizotomy of C1 to C3 and the upper rootlets of C4. Their series consisted of 6 and 15 patients, respectively, who were suffering from cerebral plasy. In both, lessening of spasticity was observed not only in the neck, but in the arms and in the spine and legs. This was attributed to the abolition of the tonic reflexes of the neck. Similarly favourable distant effects were noticed by Ouaknine (1980) and Gros et al. (1967) in their series of Little's disease treated with lumbosacral posterior rhizotomies. Improvement in spine, arms and even speech were considered by the authors as "related to a quantitative reduction in the stimulations transmitted by the intersegmentary connections through the spinal cord interneurons". As far as we know, no other attempt to use neuro-ablative procedures at the spinal level was made to alleviate spasticity in the upper limbs. Recently selective fascicular neurectomies of the motor nerves – associated or not with orthopaedic operations – have been performed by us and others (see chapter on Selective peripheral neurotomies).

In disabled spastic adults with severe paraplegia, the choice of MDT seems to us more justified than the other surgical procedures available. Selective peripheral neurotomies are effective for very localized forms of spasticity only. The other surgical procedures directed to the spinal cord (longitudinal myelotomies, Bischof 1951) or the spinal roots-especially the so-called selective dorsal rhizotomies whatever their technical modalities may be: percutaneous (Uematsu et al. 1974) or open [sectorial (Gros 1979, Privat et al. 1976), functional (Fasano et al. 1976) or partial (Fraioli and Guidetti 1977)] present more or less the same general risks as MDT. The mean useful results of these latter procedures are between 75 and 80%, close to the rates obtained in this MDT study and others in the literature. It must be mentioned that these dorsal rhizotomies have been applied mainly in children disabled by cerebral palsy, a clinical situation very different from ours. For this reason, it is difficult to compare data from these studies with our own, in some details. Neurostimulation techniques are useful mainly against moderate spasticity. Finally intrathecal infusion of antispastic drugs is promising, but the data are incomplete about its long term results.

The *originality of MDT* is that it is performed at the junction between the peripheral and central parts of the somatosensory system – a position which allows sectioning of specific components of this system, thanks to their spatial segregation; and this acts upon gating mechanisms by influencing their modulatory activity towards inhibition. Post-operative, post-mortem anatomical studies in three cases enable us to

confirm that the action of MDT is not mainly due to a massive destruction of the dorsal horn, as is the case with the more recently introduced Drez operations using radio-frequency (Nashold et al. 1976, Nashold and Ostdahl 1979) or laser lesions (Levy et al. 1983, Powers et al. 1984). On clinical and physiological grounds, it can be argued that the extremely low percentages of post-operative motor deficits and the preservation of the activity of the dorsal column-lemniscal system, as well as the relative preservation of the large caliber afferent fibers indicates that the goal of placing a restricted lesion is at least partially reached.

The sum of data collected here and in the domain of chronic pain (Sindou and Daher 1988) allows one to envisage in the *near future the application of MDT to spastic patients who have less widespread, massive symptoms and who retain significant motor function.*

References

Bischof W (1951) Die Longitudinale Myelotomie. Zentralbl Neurochir 2: 79–88

Denny-Brown D, Kirk EJ, Yanagisawa N (1973) The tract of Lissauer in relation to sensory transmission in the dorsal horn of spinal cord in the macaque monkey. J Comp Neurol 151: 175–200

Dimitrijevic MR, Nathan PW (1967a) Studies of spasticity in man: some features of spasticity. Brain 90: 1–30

Dimitrejevic MR, Nathan PW (1967b) Studies of spasticity in man: analysis of stretch reflex in spasticity. Brain 90: 333–358

Dimitrijevic MR, Nathan PW (1968) Studies of spasticity in man: analysis of reflex activity evoked by noxious cutaneous stimulation. Brain 91: 349–369

Eccles J, Eccles R, Magni F (1961) Central inhibitory action attributable to presynaptic depolarization produced by muscle afferent volleys. J Physiol 159: 147–166

Fasano VA, Barolat-Romana G, Ivaldi A, Sguazzi A (1976) La radicotomie posterieure fonctionnelle dans le traitement de la spasticité cérébrale. Neurochirurgie 22: 23–34

Foerster O (1913) On the indications and results of the excision of posterior spinal nerve roots in men. Surg Gynecol Obstet 16: 463–474

Fraioli B, Guidetti B (1977) Posterior partial rootlet section in the treatment of spasticity. J Neurosurg 46: 618–626

Gros C, Ouaknine G, Vlahovitch B, Frerebeau P (1967) La radicotomie sélective postérieure dans le traitement neurochirurgical de l'hypertonie pyramidale. Neurochirurgie 13: 505–518

Gros C (1979) Spasticity: clinical classification and surgical treatment. In: Krayenbühl (ed) Advances and technical standards in neurosurgery, vol 6. Springer, Wien New York, pp 55–97

Heimburger RF, Slominski A, Griswold P (1973) Cervical posterior rhizotomy for reducing spasticity in cerebral palsy. J Neurosurg 39: 30–34

Jeanmonod D, Sindou M, Mauguière F (1989) Intraoperative spinal cord evoked potentials during cervical and lumbo-sacral micro-surgical DREZ-tomy (MDT) for chronic pain and spasticity. Acta Neurochir [Suppl] 46: 58–61

Kottke J (1970) Modification of athetosis by denervation of the tonic neck reflexes. Dev Med Child Neurol 12: 236–237

Levy WJ, Nutkiewicz A, Ditmore M, Watts C (1983) Laser-induced dorsal root entry zone lesions for pain control: report of three cases. J Neurosurg 59: 884–886

Lundberg A (1979) Multisensory control of spinal reflex pathways. In: Granit R, Pompeiano O (eds) Reflex control of posture and movement. Elsevier, Amsterdam (Prog Brain Res 50: 11–28)

McCouch GP, Austin GM, Liu CY (1958) Sprouting as a cause of spasticity. J Neurophysiol 21: 205–216

Melzach R, Wall PD (1965) Pain mechanism. A new theory. Science 150: 971–979

Millet MF, Mortamais J, Sindou M, Eyssette M, Boisson D, Bourret J (1981) Neurochirurgie dans les paraplégies spastiques et douloureuses de la sclérose en plaques. Résultats à moyen terme de la radicellotomie postérieure sélective dans 12 cas. In: Simon L (ed) Actualités en Rééducation Fonctionnelle et Réadaptation serie 6. Masson, Paris, pp 76–85

Nashold BS, Urban B, Zorub DS (1976) Phantom relief by focal destruction of substantia gelatinosa of Rolando. In: Bonica JJ, Albe-Fessard D (eds) Advances in pain research and therapy, vol 1. Raven Press, New York, pp 959–963

Nashold BS, Ostdahl PH (1979) Dorsal root entry zone lesions for pain relief. J Neurosurg 51: 59–69

Ouaknine G (1980) Le traitement chirurgical de la spasticité. Union Med Can 109: 1–11

Powers SK, Adams JE, Edwards MSB, Boggan JE, Hosobuchi Y (1984) Pain relief from dorsal root entry zone lesions made with argon and carbon dioxide microsurgical lasers. J Neurosurg 61: 841–847

Privat JM, Benezech J, Frerebeau P, Gros C (1976) Sectorial posterior rhizotomy. A new technique of surgical treatment of spasticity. Acta Neurochir 35: 181–195

Sindou M (1972) Etude de la Jonction Radiculo-medullaire postérieure: la Radicellotomie Postérieure Sélective dans la Chirurgie de la Douleur. Thesis, Lyon

Sindou M, Lapras C (1982) Neurosurgical treatment of pain in the Pancoast-Tobias syndrome: selective posterior rhizotomy and open antero-lateral C2-cordotomy. Adv Pain Res Ther 4: 199–209

Sindou M, Goutelle A (1983) Surgical posterior rhizotomies for the treatment of pain. In: Krayenbühl H (ed) Advances and technical standards in neurosurgery, vol 10. Springer, Wien New York, pp 147–185

Sindou M, Daher A (1988) Spinal cord ablation procedures for pain. In: Dubner R, Gebhart GF, Bond MR (eds) Proceedings of the Fifth World Congress on Pain, Pain Research and Clinical Management, vol 3. Elsevier, Amsterdam, pp 477–495

Sindou M, Mertens P (1988) Selective neurotomy of the tibial nerve for treatment of the spastic foot. Neurosurgery 23: 738–744

Sindou M, Jeanmonod D (1989) Microsurgical DREZ-otomy for the treatment of spasticity and pain in the lower limbs. Neurosurgery 24: 655–670

Sindou M, Fischer G, Goutelle A, Mansuy L (1974a) La radicello-tomie postérieure sélective. Premiers résultats dans la chirurgie de la douleur. Neurochirurgie 20: 391–408

Sindou M, Fischer G, Goutelle A, Schott B, Mansuy L (1974b) La radicellotomie postérieure sélective dans le traitement des spasticités. Rev Neurol 130: 201–215

Sindou M, Quoex C, Baleydier C (1974c) Fiber organization at the posterior spinal cord-rootlet junction in man. J Comp Neurol 153: 15–26

Sindou M, Fischer G, Mansuy L (1976) Posterior spinal rhizotomy and selective posterior rhizidiotomy. Prog Neurol Surg 7: 201–250

Sindou M, Millet MF, Mortamais J, Eyssette M (1982) Results of selective posterior rhizotomy in the treatment of painful and spastic paraplegia secondary to multiple sclerosis. Appl Neurophysiol 45: 335–340

Sindou M, Mifsud JJ, Faivre G, Remec JF, Boisson D, Eyssette M, Goutelle A (1984) Neurochirurgie de la spasticité chez le malade hémiplégique. Lyon Med 251: 325–331

Sindou M, Pregelj R, Boisson D, Eyssette M, Goutelle A (1985) Surgical selective lesions of nerve fibers and myelotomies for the modification of muscle hypertonia. In: Sir Eccles J, Dimitrijevic MR (eds) Recent achievements in restorative neurology: upper motor neuron functions and dysfunctions. Karger, Basel, pp 10–26

Sindou M, Mifsud JJ, Boisson G, Goutelle A (1986) Selective posterior rhizotomy in the dorsal root entry zone for treatment of hyperspasticity and pain in the hemiplegic upper limb. Neurosurgery 18: 587–595

Uematsu S, Udvarhelyi GB, Benson DW, Siebens AA (1974) Percutaneous radiofrequency rhizotomy. Surg Neurol 2: 319–325

Correspondence: Prof. M. Sindou, M.D., D.Sc. Biol., Department of Neurosurgery, Hopital Neurologique Pierre Wertheimer, 59 Boulevard Pinel, F-69003 Lyon, France

Longitudinal myelotomy for spasticity

L.V. Laitinen

Sophiahemmet Hospital, Stockholm, Sweden

In 1951, the Austrian neurosurgeon Wilhelm Bischof described the new method of longitudinal myelotomy for the treatment of severe spasticity of the legs (Bischof 1951). His aim was to interrupt the spinal reflex arc between the anterior and posterior horns within the spinal cord. Bischof carried out the operation through a T-10 to T-12 laminectomy. The dura was opened and a bilateral longitudinal lateral incision was made, at the level of the L-1 to S-2 roots. In his second patient the lateral incision was made so deep that the knife cut the reflex arcs on both sides of the cord. Bilateral relief of spasticity was reported.

One year later Bischof performed a unilateral lateral cervical myelotomy in a patient with a left spastic hemiparesis after cerebral haemorrhage (Bischof 1952). He extended the spinal cut from C-6 to T-1. Not only did a total flaccidity of the left upper extremity result, but also the spasticity of the left leg disappeared.

In order to avoid complete interruption of the corticospinal fibers, Pourpre (1960) modified the Bischof myelotomy. Through a laminectomy of T-9 to L-1, he opened the dorsal fissure of the spinal cord. From the dorsal opening he extended a stylet knife in a lateral direction and cut the connections between the dorsal and ventral horns. Bischof (1967), and many others after him, used the dorsal longitudinal myelotomy for the treatment of intractable spasticity of the legs (Benedetti and Colombo 1981, Ivan et al. 1967, Laitinen and Singounas 1971, Moyes 1969, Yamada et al. 1976).

In 1973, I described a stereotactic instrument, the myelotome, to make the intramedullary sections more accurate and less traumatic for the patient (Laitinen 1973). In this paper the method and its results will be reported.

Operative technique

Preoperatively, the individual position of the conus medullaris is verified by lumbar myelography. Then a laminectomy of T-10 to T-12 or L-1 is carried out under general anesthesia. The dura is opened and the myelotome is fixed between the spinous processes, usually at the level of T-9 and L-1 (Fig. 1). The spinal cord is punctured in the midline, about 8.5 cm cranial to the conus medullaris, and the myelotome needle is inserted to a desired depth, which is preset according to the dimensions of the cord. Through the needle a stylet knife is extruded in a lateral direction, again to a preset depth equal to 3/4 of the hemi-cord (Fig. 2). In this position the needle is rotated 60 degrees so that the connections between the posterior and the anterior horns are severed. With the needle inside the cord the knife is withdrawn, and the needle is rotated by 180 degrees to the other side of the cord. The knife is again introduced, and a 60-degree rotation performed. The knife is withdrawn and the needle pulled out of the cord. The cord is then punctured about 8 mm more caudal and the same procedure is repeated. With 7–8 punctures the spinal reflex arc is cut for a cord length of 6 cm, so that 2.5 cm of the conus remains intact.

This technique saves as much as possible of the commissural region transmitting the nociceptive and thermal crossing fibres. By limiting the lateral cut to 3/4 of the cord, sectioning of corticospinal tract offshoots to the motor neurones is minimized. In

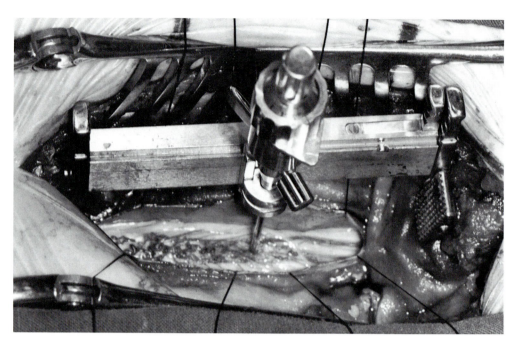

Fig. 1. The myelotome fixed between the spinous processes T-9 and L-1. The cord has been punctured in the midline

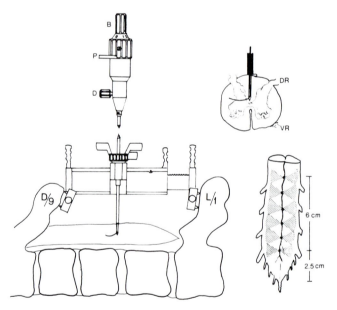

Fig. 2. A schematic illustration of stereotactic longitudinal myelotomy

patients with a total sensory and motor loss, the lateral rotations can be larger, almost to 180 degrees.

Results of myelotomy

This type of surgery has been carried out in 25 patients (Table 1). Twelve patients suffered from multiple sclerosis, six from spinal cord injury, five from cerebral palsy, one from spastic hemiplegia and one from spinal tumour. Fourteen were male and 11 were female. Their ages ranged from 11 to 62 years.

In this series, there were *no surgical complications*. Sometimes minor haemorrhage emerged from the puncture holes, but it always stopped spontaneously.

Table 2 shows the *effects of myelotomy on spasticity*. Sixty per cent of the patients had complete relief of spasticity. In 36 per cent some residual spasticity was seen in one or both legs. Within a year some muscular tone returned in most patients, but it was seldom spastic and was not associated with reappearance of tendon reflexes.

Table 3 shows that longitudinal myelotomy often had a positive *effect on the motility of the legs*, when

Table 1. The clinical material

Cause of Spasticity	Longitudinal myelotomy		
	No. of cases	Sex	Age (yrs)
Spinal injury	6	5 M	25–54
		1 F	
Cerebral palsy	5	3 M	11–23
		2 F	17–22
Multiple sclerosis	12	7 F	28–47
		5 M	32–45
Cerebral ischaemia	1	1 M	62
Spinal tumour	1	1 F	50
Total	25	14 M/11 F	11–62

Table 2. Effect of stereotactic longitudinal myelotomy on spasticity of the lower limbs

Diagnostic Group	Longitudinal myelotomy (effect on spasticity)			
	No. of Cases	Good	Result Fair	Poor
Spinal injury	6	4	1	1
Cerebral palsy	5	–	5	–
Multiple scelerosis	12	9	3	–
Cerebral ischaemia	1	1	–	–
Spinal tumour	1	1	–	–
Total	25	15	9	1

Table 3. Effect of stereotactic longitudinal myelotomy on motility of the lower limbs

Preoperative motility	Longitudinal myelotomy (effect on motility)	
	No. of cases	Postoperative motility
Paraplegia	15	some walking 5 / paraplegia 10
Paraparesis	7	much improved 2 / slightly improved 5
Involuntary	3	some voluntary 2 / involuntary 1

Table 4. Effect of stereotactic longitudinal myelotomy on cutaneous sensibility

Preoperative sensibility	Longitudinal myelotomy (effect on sensibility)	
	No. of cases	Postoperative sensibility
NIL	6	NIL
Hypaesthesia/hypalgesia	11	unchanged 3 / impaired 8
Normal	8	normal 5 / slightly impaired 2 / much impaired 1

Table 5. Effect of stereotactic longitudinal myelotomy on the urinary bladder

Preoperative bladder	Longitudinal myelotomy (effect on bladder)	
	No. of cases	Postoperative bladder
Normal	3	normal 3
Good automatic function	7	good automatic function 4 / Poor automatic function 2 / incontinence 1
Poor automatic function	5	poor automatic function 4 / incontinence 1
Incontinence	10	poor automatic function 3 / incontinence 7

the spasticity disappeared. This effect was common in patients with multiple sclerosis, where severe spasticity seemed often to hide voluntary movements. The improvement was most obvious in the seven patients with some voluntary residual motility before myelotomy; slight to moderate improvement was recorded.

Table 4 shows that longitudinal myelotomy very often impaired the residual *cutaneous sensations*. In the 11 patients with preoperative hypaesthesia/hypalgesia, the sensibility deteriorated in eight, and in the eight patients with "normal" preoperative sensibility three showed postoperative deterioration.

Table 5 shows that longitudinal myelotomy had a harmful transitory *effect on bladder function* in four patients (27%), who preoperatively had a good or fair automatic function. In three patients out of ten with preoperative incontinence some automatic function was observed postoperatively. This improvement may have resulted from active bladder training.

Discussion

This study confirms the previous findings that longitudinal myelotomy is a good form of treatment for severe spasticity of the legs (Benedetti and Colombo 1981, Bischof 1951, 1967, Ivan et al. 1967, Laitinen and Singounas 1971, Moyes 1969, Pourpre 1960, Tönnis and Bischof 1962, Yamada et al. 1976). In 1971 Laitinen and Singounas reported on nine patients operated on (Laitinen and Singounas 1971). They concluded that open dorsal longitudinal myelotomy was the method of choice in the treatment of severe spasticity of the legs. Nevertheless, they found the method "crude". The free-hand technique often led to asymmetrical and poorly placed sections inside the cord, with recurrence of spasticity being fairly common. Haemorrhages inside the cord were not infrequent. In order to refine the technique Laitinen (1973) developed the stereotactic myelotome to be used at open laminectomy.

The present study indicates that the results of "stereotactic" myelotomy are better than those obtained earlier by the open free-hand technique. Particularly the improvement of voluntary motility has become more frequent than before. The cutaneous sensory deficits have also diminished.

Yamada et al. (1976) used a special knife to place the intraspinal cuts more precisely. They also reported an improved postoperative motility of the legs, when the spasticity had disappeared.

Few studies have been published where the results of different spinal interventions, such as the posterior rhizotomy of Foerster (1908) the selective posterior rhizotomies of Fasano et al. (1976) and Gros et al. (1967) and the micro-DREZotomy of Sindou et al. (1974) were compared. According to my personal experience, the results of selective posterior rhizotomies and longitudinal myelotomy are similar. However, the stereotactic longitudinal myelotomy only takes 90 minutes, whereas selective rhizotomy of Fasano et al. (1976) in my hands usually takes four hours when all posterior fascicles of the rootlets L-1 to S-1 have been stimulated bilaterally and about two thirds of them cut. Benedetti and Colombo (1981) found that longitudinal myelotomy gave better results for the spasticity in flexion than for spasticity in extension. They reported that selective posterior rhizotomy of Gros et al. (1967) gave better results than open free-hand myelotomy. I am not aware of studies where the results of Sindou's procedure (Sindou et al. 1974) were compared with those obtained by other spinal methods. However, it seems likely that the three methods, longitudinal myelotomy, selective posterior rhizotomy and selective posterior rhizotomy in the DREZ, all may achieve more or less similar results.

References

Benedetti A, Colombo F (1981) Spinal surgery for spasticity (46 cases). Neurochirurgia 24:195–198

Bischof W (1951) Die longitudinale Myelotomie. Zbl Neurochir 11:79–88

Bischof W (1952) Die longitudinale Myelotomie, erstmalig zervikal durchgeführt. Zbl Neurochir 12:205–210

Bischof W (1967) Zur dorsalen longitudinalen Myelotomie. Zbl Neurochir 28:123–126

Fasano VA, Barolat-Romana G, Ivaldi A, et al (1976) La radicotomie postérieure fonctionnelle dans le traitment de la spasticité cérébrale. Premières observations sur la stimulation électrique per-opératoire des racines postérieures et leur utilisation dans le choix des racines à sectionner. Neurochirurgie 22:23–34

Foerster O (1908) Ueber eine neue operative Methode der Behandlung spastischer Lähmungen mittels Resektion hinterer Rückenmarkswurzeln. Ztschr Orthop Chir 22:203–223

Gros C, Ouaknine G, Vlahovitch B, et al (1967) La radicotomie sélective postérieure dans le traitement neuro-chirurgical de l'hypertonie pyramidale. Neurochirurgie 13:505–518

Ivan LP, Paine KWE, Hunt TE (1967) Experience with Bischof's myelotomy. Can J Surg 10:191–195

Laitinen LV (1973) A myelotome for the treatment of spasticity. Acta Neurochir (Wien) 29:267

Laitinen L, Singounas E (1971) Longitudinal myelotomy in the treatment of spasticity of the legs. J Neurosurg 35:536–540

McCouch GP, Austin GM, Liu CN, et al (1958) Sprouting as a cause of spasticity. J Neurophysiol 21:205–216

Moyes PD (1969) Longitudinal myelotomy for spasticity. J Neurosurg 31:615–619

Pourpre MH (1960) Traitement neuro-chirurgical des contractures chez les paraplégiques posttraumatiques. Neurochirurgie 6:229–236

Sindou M, Fischer G, Goutelle A, et al (1974) La radicellotomie postérieure sélective dans le traitement des spasticités. Rev Neurol 130:201–216

Tönnis W, Bischof W (1962) Ergebnisse der lumbalen Myelotomie nach Bischof. Zbl Neurochir 23:29–36

Yamada S, Perot PL Jr, Ducker TB, Lockard I (1976) Myelotomy for control of mass spasms in paraplegia. J Neurosurg 45:683–691

Correspondence: Prof. L.V. Laitinen, M.D., Ph.D., Sophiahemmet Hospital, Box 6505, S-11486 Stockholm, Sweden

Destructive stereotatic procedures for spasticity directed to the brain and the cerebellum

J. Siegfried

AMI Klinik Im Park, Zürich, Switzerland

The introduction of new techniques in the neurosurgical treatment of spasticity has resulted in the abandonment of destructive therapeutic lesions in the cerebrum and in the cerebellum. Nevertheless a review of these methods will be given briefly as they were popular 25 years ago and the reasons for their abandonment will be emphasized.

Stereotactic cerebral lesions

1. Ventrolateral thalamotomies

Stereotactic lesions in the ventrolateral part of the thalamus reduce rigidity but not spasticity. However, it has been emphasized by Narabayashi (1982) that the so-called spastic cases in cerebral palsy usually have a mixture of spasticity with great rigidity, when the brain damage is localized and the children are of almost normal intelligence. In these cases, the thalamotomies improve the hypertonicity. On the contrary, spastic cases with idiocy have more signs of spasticity with less rigidity, suggesting a more diffuse brain damage. Stereotactic thalamotomies in these conditions are disappointing. Since the largest series of Narabayashi and others deal with cerebral palsy cases having complex neurological symptoms, results on spasticity alone are not given. The results of operation were analysed more in terms of general improvement, and these were mostly relative.

Method

Only stereotactic techniques allow circumscribed deep cerebral structures to be destroyed without damaging the function of important nearby regions. Many stereotactic frames can be used for making a therapeutic lesion. The thalamic target is calculated radiologically after ventriculography. High-frequency coagulation probably produces the safest lesion, the amount of tissue coagulation is controlled and complications, mostly haemorrhages, minimized by using a pure sinusoidal high-frequency current and a thermoregulated electrode (Riechert and Spuler 1982).

Discussion

In earlier operations for the treatment of motor disorders, parts of the motor cortex or of the pyramidal tracts (pyramidotomy) were removed or interrupted. The alleviation of symptoms was offset by the development of paralysis. As the palsy improved, the primary symptoms, in particular the tremor, reappeared. The transfer of operative site from the precentral cortex to the ventrolateral thalamic nuclei was made in order to interrupt uncontrolled afferent motor impulses passing across the pallidum and the thalamus into the cortex. By this means, injury to the efferent tracts emerging from the motor cortex was avoided. The ventrolateral thalamic nuclei (V.o.i., V.o.a. and V.o.p.), which possess no descending fibers of their own, have connections to the motor cortical fields. These are principally 4 Gamma, 5 a Alpha, 4 s and 6 a Beta. These tracts have, according to Hassler, a two-way course and must be considered as belonging to the extrapyramidal system. Hassler was the first to suggest carrying out an elimination of certain nuclear areas of the ventrolateral thalamus for the treatment of extrapyramidal motor disturbances (Hassler 1959). Experience showed that an interruption of the afferents to the motor cortex was sufficient to abolish disturbed motor movements (Hassler and Riechert 1954), without necessarily resulting in signs of a pyramidal tract lesion. Ventro-lateral thalamotomy, by interrupting the neuronal chain coming from the cerebellum has proven since then its very high value in the treatment of tremor (extrapyramidal and cerebellar). Other extrapyramidal symptoms like rigidity will also be markedly improved. Pyramidal spasticity will, however, not be influenced. In cerebral palsy, the extrapyramidal signs commonly observed are, according to Narabayashi (1982): rigidity in rigid-type cases, rigidity in the spastic-type cases and rigidity in severe dystonic-type cases. These symptoms can be somewhat improved by ventrolateral thalamotomy, but pure spasticity cannot. There is no rationale for a thalamotomy in the treatment of spasticity.

2. Pulvinarotomy

In 1971, evidence was presented by Cooper et al. (1971) that the pulvinar contributes to motor function. In his first extensive clinical study, Cooper reported the results of 10 operations for spasticity resulting either from a cerebro-vascular or traumatic lesion. Four of these patients had previously undergone ventrolateral nucleus surgery, two had cerebellar decortication and dentate nucleus ablation, and two had surgery in the nucleus lateralis posterior (LP) prior to or in addition to the pulvinectomy. Seven of these 10 patients showed marked relief of spasticity. None of them were rendered hypotonic. Three failed to improve (Cooper et al. 1974). This series, however, seems difficult to interpret, since most of the patients underwent other stereotactic operations as well. Fraioli, with a limited experience with spastic cases, did not report very encouraging results (Fraioli and Guidetti 1976). Other reports of stereotactic pulvinarotomy alone for spasticity with long-term follow up are rare, suggesting that this procedure has limited usefulness. In addition, for a series of 22 patients operated on by us between 1969 and 1972 using stereotactic pulvinarotomy in the treatment of intractable pain, we never observed a diminution of muscular tone postoperatively (Siegfried 1977).

Method

Pulvinarotomy has always been done stereotactically using the same technique as for ventrolateral thalamotomy. However, while the nucleus ventro-intermedius or the nucleus ventro-oralis posterior have clear coordinates, the pulvinar is a rather large

mass, so that a lesioning can be done in several different places. It seems that the midpoint of the outlined pulvinar was usually chosen.

Discussion

More than 20 years ago, Walker called the pulvinar the "terra incognita" of the thalamus (Walker 1961); today we still have minimal knowledge concerning the function of this structure. Stereotactic lesions in the human pulvinar were first reported by Kudo et al. (1966) for the reduction of chronic pain. An integrative role of this complex in transferring afferent impulses from one system to another and disseminating them to extensive neocortical areas, as required probably in the elaboration of the painful experience, was then suggested (Cooper et al. 1973). The pulvinar has been shown to be a polysensory complex with neuronal pools responding to multiple sensory stimuli (Kreindler et al. 1968); its role in motor integration has not been clearly reported. Thus, to date, we have no significant physiological or anatomical evidence to support the clinical observation of the role of the pulvinar in control of spasticity. Therefore, pulvinarotomy in the treatment of spasticity has been completely abandoned.

Stereotactic cerebellar lesions

1. Lesion of nucleus fastigii

Based upon the animal experiments of Moruzzi and Pompeiano (1956) and Batini and Pompeiano (1957), where ipsilateral release from the rigidity of decerebration was obtained by destruction of one nucleus fastigii, Hassler and Reichert performed in 1960 an electrocoagulation of the ipsilateral nucleus in a cerebral palsied patient (Hassler and Reichert 1961). The hypertonicity disappeared postoperatively and active and passive movements were again performed. Some days later, the hypertonia reappeared although it was less marked than before and much less painful. One year later, this improvement was still present, and was estimated to be about 50%. We do not know if this target in the treatment of spasticity has been pursued.

2. Dentatotomy

The first trial of selective destruction of the dentate nucleus was made by Delmas-Marsalet and Van

Bogaert (1935). The indication was not spasticity, but a parkinsonian symptomatology. The dentate nucleus was destroyed by means of a hook introduced through a small burr hole. Unfortunate complications of myoclonus, nystagmus, severe swallowing difficulties, right-sided hemiplegia and anaesthesia, aggravation of tremor, and finally the death of the patient on the ninth postoperative day discouraged further new approaches to this nucleus for several years. Toth, after opening the posterior fossa, later performed the same operation in three patients with Parkinson's disease (Toth 1961). In all three patients, homolateral rigidity was decreased, and, in two, tremor was ameliorated while it was aggravated in the third.

The first stereotactic dentatotomy in a patient with cerebral palsy was performed by Heimburger in 1963 and reported in 1965 (Heimburger and Whitlock 1965). This resulted in a renewal of interest in the stereotactic approach to this nucleus in the treatment of certain functional disorders, particularly spasticity resulting from cerebral palsy. Between 1965 and 1969, there were many publications on this topic, but dentatotomy never became as popular as thalamotomy in cases of tremor. Later, interest in dentatotomy declined markedly, mainly after evaluation of long term results. Analysing 109 stereotactic electrocoagulations of the dentate nucleus in 50 patients, most with cerebral palsy, over a period of more than 10 years (most patients underwent a bilateral dentatotomy), we reported in 1988 a more realistic appreciation of the results. In only 30% of the cases was a clear improvement in the spasticity obtained, while in 50% of cases nursing and rehabilitation were facilitated. While the operation could be performed without complications and an unexpected neurological deficit did not occur, stereotactic dentatomy never completely suppressed the spasticity and spectacular results were never observed (Siegfried and Verdié 1977). Its place in the actual state and in the future of functional neurosurgery is questionable, but its limited use today cannot be ignored.

Method

The stereotactic approach to the dentate nucleus is performed with the stereotactic frame mounted upside down. A visualization of the fourth ventricle is obtained by fractional pneumo-encephalography, allowing the drawing of a base-line passing through the fastigium which is perpendicular to the line tangent to the floor of the fourth ventricle. The target point is 10 mm behind the floor of the fourth ventricle, 5 mm below the base-line and 14 mm lateral to the midline (Siegfried 1982, Siegfried et al. 1970). The orientation of the dentate nucleus is anteromedial to posterolateral. The electrode is introduced at such an angle that the axis of the electrode corresponds with main axis of the dentate nucleus in the frontal and sagital planes.

Discussion

In the depth of the white matter of the cerebellum, dorsal and dorsolateral to the fourth ventricle, are four nuclei on each side. From medial to lateral they are nucleus fastigii, nucleus globosus, nucleus emboliformis and nucleus dentatus. The anatomy of the largest nucleus, the nucleus dentatus is known: the dorsomedial, microgyric, magnocellular region and the ventrolateral, macrogyric, parvicellular region (Demole 1927). According to Hassler (1950), the cerebello-rubral fibers to the small-celled part of the red nucleus come from the ventral part (small-celled or parvicellular) of the dentate nucleus. Jansen showed that all nuclear divisions send fibers rostrally beyond the mesencephalon, but that approximately two-third of these fibers are derived from the dentate nucleus, while the last third seems to be composed of almost an equal number of fibers from the nuclei emboliformis, globosus and fastigii. While approximately one half of the fibers from the dentate nucleus to the brachium conjunctivum passes beyond the red nucleus, little more than 10% of the fibers from the nucleus interpositus (N. globosus and emboliformis) do so (Jansen and Jansen 1965). This observation gives an indication of the functional difference between the two nuclei in question. Angaut and Bowsher (1965) did not find degenerative lesions in the red nucleus after stereotactic lesions of the dentate nucleus of the cat, but only after destruction of the nucleus interpositus. The connections of the dentate nucleus with the thalamus are very rich. According to different authors, it is the parvicellular region of the nucleus dentatus which projects into the thalamus, and particularly into the ventrolateral part of the thalamus (Bowsher et al. 1965, Hassler 1950). The efferent projection from dentate and interpositus nuclei in primates into the nucleus ventrolateralis thalami were also found by Mehler et al. (1958). We can then suggest, that the ventrolateral part of the dentate nucleus belongs in part to the same neuronal system as the ventrolateral part of the thalamus and this hypothesis is supported by the partial success of the dentatotomies in cases of extra-pyramidal disease like Parkinson's disease or involuntary movements disorders. In these cases the clinical effect is sometimes comparable to ventrolateral thalamotomies, but to a lesser degree. But, since the spasticity can be improved by the ventrolateral dentatotomy but not after a ventrolateral thalamotomy, we must also be acting on another neuronal system not yet demonstrated.

Conclusion

The main reasons for the abandonment of destructive lesions to the brain and the cerebellum in the treatment of spasticity are the relatively poor results obtained and the lack of rationale. Only dentatotomy could be demonstrated to have some favourable clinical effects. However, in comparison with other neurosurgical methods, its indication is today questionable.

References

Angaut P, Bowsher D (1965) Cerebello-rubral connections in the cat. Nature (Lond) 208: 1002–1003

Batini O, Pompeiano O (1957) Chronic fastigial lesions and their compensations in the cat. Arch Ital Biol 95: 147–152

Bowsher D, Angaut P, Condé H (1965) Projection des noyaux cérébelleux sur le noyau ventrolatéral du thalamus: confrontations des résultats acquis par la technique anatomique et par la technique électro-physiologique. J Physiol (Paris) 57: 570–585

Cooper IS, Waltz JM, Amin I, Fujito S (1971) Pulvinectomy: a preliminary report. J Am Geriatr Soc 19: 553–554

Cooper IS, Amin I, Chandra R, Waltz JM (1973) A surgical investigation of the clinical physiology of the LP-pulvinar complex in man. J Neurol Sci 18: 89–110

Cooper IS, Amin I, Chandra R, Waltz JM (1974) Clinical physiology of motor contributions of the pulvinar in man: a study of cryopulvinectomy. In: Cooper IS (ed) The Pulvinar-LP complex. Thomas, Springfield, pp 220–232

Delmas-Marsalet P, van Bogaert L (1935) Sur un cas de myoclonies rythmiques continues déterminées par une intervention chirurgicale sur le tronc cérébral. Rev Neurol (Paris) 64: 728–740

Demole V (1927) Structures et connections de noyaux dentelés du cervelet. Schweiz Arch Neurol Psychiatr 20: 271–294

Fraioli B, Guidetti B (1976) Problèmes cliniques et possibilités neurochirurgicales actuelles dans le syndromes d'hypertonie et de dyskinésie. Neurochirurgie 22: 557–567

Hassler R (1950) Ueber Kleinhirnprojektionen zum Mittelhirn und Thalamus beim Menschen. Dtsch Z Nervenheilk 163: 629–671

Hassler R (1959) Gezielte Operationen gegen extrapyramidale Bewegungsstörungen. In: Schaltenbrand G, Bailey P (Hrsg) Einführung in die stereotaktischen Operationen mit einem Atlas des menschlichen Gehirns, Bd 1. Thieme, Stuttgart, S472–488

Hassler R, Riechert T (1954) Indikationen und Lokalisationsmethode der gezielten Hirnoperationen. Nervenarzt 25: 441–447

Hassler R, Riechert T (1961) Wirkungen der Reizungen und Koagulationen in den Stammganglien bei stereotaktischen Hirnoperationen. 32: 97–109

Heimburger RF, Whitlock CC (1965) Stereotaxic destruction of the human dentate nucleus. Confin Neurol 26: 346–358

Jansen J, Jansen J (1955) On the efferent fibers of the cerebellar nuclei in the cat. J Comp Neurol 102: 607–632

Kreindler A, Crighel E, Marinchesus C (1968) Integrative activity of the thalamic pulvinar lateralis posterior complex and inter-relations with the neocortex. Exp Neurol 22: 423–435

Kudo T, Yoshii N, Shimizu S, Aikawa S, Nakehama H (1966) Effects of stereotaxic thalamotomy to intractable pain and numbness. Keio J Med 15: 191–194

Mehler WR, Vernier VG, Nauta WJH (1958) Efferent projections from dentate and interpositas nuclei in primates. Anat Rec 130: 430–431

Moruzzi G, Pompeiano O (1956) Crossed fastigial influence on decerebrate rigidity. J Comp Neurol 106: 371–384

Narabayashi H (1982) Choreoathetosis and spasticity. In: Schaltenbrand G, Walker EA (eds) Stereotaxy of the human brain. Thieme, Stuttgart New York, pp 532–543

Riechert T, Spuler H (1982) Instrumentation of stereotaxy. In: Schaltenbrand G, Walke EA (eds) Stereotaxy of the human brain. Thieme, Stuttgart New York, pp 350–363

Siegfried J (1977) Stereotactic pulvinarotomy in the treatment of intractable pain. Prog Neurol Surg 8: 104–113

Siegfried J (1982) Stereotaxic cerebellar surgery for spasticity. In: Schaltenbrand G, Walker EA (eds) Stereotaxy of the human brain. Thieme, Stuttgart New York, pp 562–564

Siegfried J, Verdié JC (1977) Long-term assessment of stereotactic dentatotomy for spasticity and another disorders. Acta Neurochir [Suppl] 24: 41–48

Siegfried J, Esslen E, Gretener U, Ketz E, Perret E (1970) Functional anatomy of the dentate nucleus in the light of stereotaxic operations. Confin Neurol 32: 1–10

Toth S (1961) The effect of removal of the nucleus dentatus on the parkinsonian syndrome. J Neurol Neurosurg Psychiatry 24: 143–154

Walker AE (1961) Internal structure and afferent-efferent relations of the thalamus. In: Purpura DP, Yahr M (eds) The thalamus. Columbia University Press, New York, pp 1–12

Correspondence: Prof. Dr. J. Siegfried, AMI Klinik Im Park, Seestrasse 220, CH-8002 Zürich, Switzerland

Other treatments

The spastic bladder and its treatment

C. Beneton[1,2], **P. Mertens**[2] with the collaboration of **A. Leriche**[3], and **M. Sindou**[2]

[1]Centre Médical Germaine Revel, Saint Maurice sur Dargoire, [2]Hôpital Neurologique, Lyon, and [3]Hôpital Henry Gabrielle, Saint Genis Laval, France

Introduction

Spastic bladder and its complications on the upper urinary tract, is a frequent occurrence after spinal cord lesions.

In normal subjects the bladder, when stimulated by filling, sends messages to the micturition center located in the sacral spinal cord at the S2 to S4 levels (principally S3) and hence to the brain. At the appropriate time, the brain sends its release message down to the bladder through the micturition center (Blaivas 1982) (Fig. 1).

When the pathways between the micturition center and the brain are impaired, the bladder is no longer under voluntary control. Voiding becomes, thus, reflexive, with the message to empty coming only from the micturition center. There is no more voluntary inhibition from the brain.

In addition, the threshold for the release of the detrusor reflex is lowered, resulting in detrusor hyperreflexia. If spasticity is chronic, the bladder wall thickens, becomes hypertonic and its capacity is permanently reduced. This bladder dysfunction leads to vesico-ureteral reflux and renal damage.

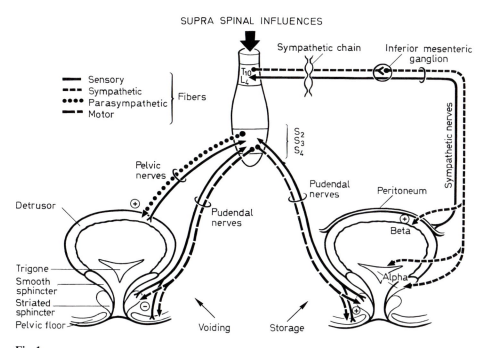

Fig. 1

Table 1. Terminology

–*Normal bladder capacity*: 350 ml to 500 ml (first normal desire to void: 200 to 300 ml).

–*Residual urine*: volume of fluid remaining in the bladder immediately after completion of micturition. It is commonly estimated by palpation, catheterisation, radiography, ultrasonics (Bates et al. 1979).

–*Cystometry capacity*: volume at which the patient has a strong urge to void or develop urinary incontinence (Bates et al. 1979, Blaivas et al. 1982).

–*Uninhibited detrusor contractions*: sudden involuntary increase in detrusor pressure, usually described as having more than 15 cm water, but often of lesser magnitude (Blaivas et al. 1980, 1982).

–*Hyperactivity with detrusor hyperreflexia*: uninhibited contractions elicited at a low volume of urine and at a low pressure (Buzelin 1984).

–*Hyperactivity with detrusor hypertonicity*: uninhibited contractions elicited at a low volume of urine and high bladder pressure (Buzelin 1984).

–*Detrusor sphincter dyssynergia*: characterized by an involuntary contraction of the striated urethral sphincter during an involuntary detrusor contraction leading to a "conflicting" bladder (Bates et al. 1979, Blaivas et al. 1982).

–*Bladder neck obstruction*: characterized by a delay and/or a failure in bladder neck opening, synchronous with detrusor contraction, due to dyssynergia of adrenergic smooth muscle, or organic obstruction (fibrous narrowing of the bladder neck).

Clinical signs

The spastic bladder, because of involuntary contractions, fails to store urine adequately. Therefore, the symptoms most commonly experienced by the patient are:

–urinary frequency, that is, an increase in the number of voidings during the day and the night;
–urinary urgency, the feeling of having to empty the bladder immediately, combined with an inability to hold urine once the urge to void is felt;
–urge incontinence, the involuntary loss of urine associated with an uncontrollable urge to void during the day and night (Bates et al. 1979).

Urodynamic evaluation
(Bates et al. 1979, Blaivas et al. 1982)

This procedure consists of simultaneous recordings of intra-vesical and intra-urethral pressure, associated with the measurement of the intra-abdominal pressure using a rectal catheter, and an electromyography of the striated urethral sphincter.

Radiographic contrast medium can be used as the infusant for cystometry, so that the entire process can be monitored under fluoroscopy.

Cystometry: is the graphic representation of intra-vesical pressure as a function of volume. The bladder is infused with fluid or gas through a catheter. During the bladder filling, the patient is instructed to report his sensations to the examiner.

The parameters studied at cystometry are:

–the volume at which the patient has the first desire to void and the maximum cystometric capacity which is the volume at which the patient has a strong desire to void.
–the detrusor pressure which corresponds to the intra-vesical pressure due to active and passive forces in

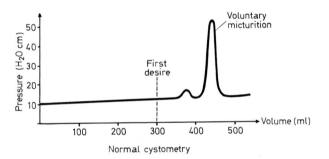

Normal cystometry

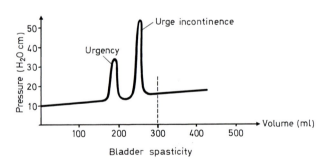

Bladder spasticity

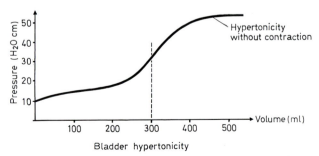

Bladder hypertonicity

Fig. 2

the bladder wall. It is determined by substracting intra-abdominal pressure from intravesical pressure.

–the compliance, which indicates the change in volume in relation with the change in bladder pressure. A low compliance bladder is one that has a steep filling curve indicating hypertonicity of the detrusor. A high compliance bladder accepts a large volume of urine without significant rise of pressure.

In the spastic bladder, cystometry demonstrates:

–a hyperactivity with uninhibited detrusor contractions during the filling phase (Fig. 2),
–a decrease of the cystometry capacity,
–reflex detrusor contractions triggered by suprapubic tapping.

Further testing consisting of injections of IV or IM anticholinergic agents or sacral anaesthetic blocks using lidocaine, allows one to differentiate hyperactivity with detrusor hyperreflexia, from hyperactivity with detrusor hypertonicity. Anticholinergic agents or anaesthetic blocks, in suppressing hyperactivity, increase bladder capacity and compliance in the former situation, while not in the latter. A decreased compliance persisting after these tests indicates an alteration of the bladder wall (fibrosis).

Radiographic visualization of the bladder during storage and voiding shows:

–a bladder of small size (Fig. 3),
–bladder trabeculations and diverticuli, a vesico-ureteral reflux provoked by bladder contractions in cases of long-term dysfunction.

Management of the spastic bladder

I. Prevention: It is of paramount importance to recall that nociceptive factors such as urinary tract infections, bladder stones, pressure sores, constipation etc..., increase bladder spasticity and must be prevented, or, if present, treated first (Archimbaud et al. 1976).

II. Pharmacological treatments (Fig. 4): 1) Anticholinergic agents which inhibit the parasympathetic system, i.e. decrease transmission of impulses from the micturition center to the detrusor, suppress the uninhibited contractions and thus increase bladder capacity. Anticholinergic drugs, routinely used are Propantheline (Blaivas et al. 1980), Oxybutinin, Hexocyclium, Imipramine. 2) Beta-adrenergic agents which are supposed to relax the detrusor are not used, because of lack of practical effectiveness. 3) Myorelaxants (like Benzodiazepam...) or lidocaine injections of the striated sphincter, may be useful for treating sphincter dyssynergia known to exacerbate bladder spasticity.

III. Urological procedures (Leriche and Leriche 1983): Bladder neck obstruction or striated sphincter hypertonicity, increasing bladder spasticity, must be treated before it leads to progressive upper urinary tract deterioration. In males, bladder neck obstruction requires incision or transurethral resection, while striated sphincter hypertonicity is treated with external sphincterotomy, if medical treatment and lidocaine injections fail. Should this result in a loss of urine, the patient can be equipped with an external collecting device. In females, because of the lack of an effective external drainage device, intermittent catheterization is generally preferred.

IV. Neurological procedures. Neurosurgical procedures for spastic bladder aim at increasing bladder

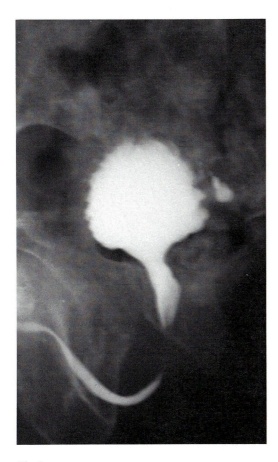

Fig. 3

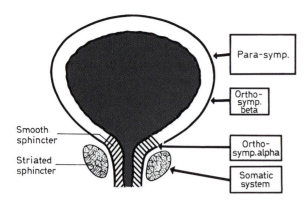

Smooth sphincter

Striated sphincter

Para-symp.

Ortho-symp. beta

Ortho-symp.alpha

Somatic system

Fig. 4

capacity and suppressing uninhibited contractions to prevent leakage of urine, while preserving what sphincteric and sexual functions are present.

In patients with complete neurological deficits, this can be achieved by using destructive procedures. Decrease in bladder tone generally creates bladder retention which necessitates permanent or intermittent catheterization. In patients who retain neurological functions, surgery has to be conservative. If ablative procedures are chosen they must be as selective as possible.

Before deciding on a neurosurgical procedure, testing with local anaesthetic blocks is mandatory to evaluate the functional state of the bladder and to determine the targets to be operated upon (Hawkes et al. 1983).

1. Diagnostic blocks

These consist of injections of short (lidocaïne) or long-lasting (bupivacaïne) local anaesthetics, under fluoroscopic control, using cystometry and urethral, ano-rectal, pressure monitoring.

–*Sacral nerve blocks* of S2, S3, S4 roots are performed at the level of the anterior foramen, through a posterior foramen approach. They interrupt both the parasympathetic pathways and the somatic innervation of the pelvis. They aim at determining which one of these roots gives a predominant innervation for the detrusor (Torrens 1974).

–*Pelvic nerve blocks* are performed directly in the trigonal and retrotrigonal region, through a trans-vaginal approach in females and a latero-prostatic approach in males. They aim at interrupting the autonomic innervation to obtain detrusor release.

–*Pudendal nerve blocks* are performed above and below the ischial spine or in the pudendal canal, on one or both sides. They are effective when there is a decrease in the urethral pressure profile. Bilateral pudendal blocks, although releasing the striated sphincter, do not create incontinence if the bladder neck is normal.

2. Destructive procedures

Long-lasting or permanent effects on spasticity can be obtained by achieving destruction of nerve fibers with the injection of neurolytic agents (70% alcohol or 0.6% phenol solutions), percutaneous thermocoagulation or other ablative open procedures. The targets can be the pelvic nerves, the sacral roots or the dorsal root entry zone.

A) Pelvic neurotomies

Techniques for chemical neurolysis are the same as for diagnostic blocks.

Surgical neurectomies can be performed either through 1) a parasacral approach, which allows one to cut all the pelvic parasympathetic nerves in the sacro-rectal space, or 2) a sub-pubic approach with section of the nerves in the intervesicorectal (or vesicovaginal) space. The latter is more selective, due to the preservation of the automatic rectal innervation.

The methods directed at the pelvic nerves are technically difficult, especially because of a frequent local fibrosis. In addition they are often followed by incomplete and/or transient effects. Therefore sacral rhizotomies are more commonly used.

B) Sacral rhizotomies

The approach for *chemical neurolysis* or *radiofrequency thermo-coagulation* of the sacral roots, is the same as for diagnostic blocks. Of the 10 cases of detrusor hyperreflexia treated with thermo-coagulation of several of the sacral roots, Young and Mulcahy reported (1980), seven as having good results, i.e., an increased bladder capacity, (follow up: 1 year on average).

Open selective sacral rhizotomies can be used for bladder spasticity, either by obtaining a peripheral paralysis using ventral root sections or by creating an areflexic bladder with dorsal rhizotomies. These selective procedures are based on the use of microsurgical techniques, and intraoperative electro-stimulation for differentiation of the motor and sensory rootlets.

For *ventral rhizotomies*, the approach is to the conus medullaris through a L1 to L2 laminectomy or at the level of the sacral canal itself. There are more difficulties in differentiating the motor rootlets from the sensory ones in the latter. The fascicles giving detrusor contraction at low threshold stimulation are cut; they generally belong to S2 and S3 roots (and also S4 to a variable degree) on one or both sides. The fascicles giving a motor response in the lower limbs or anorectal contractions are spared. Of the 11 patients with uninhibited bladder and incontinence in whom Torrens and Griffiths (1976) performed selective sacral ventral rhizotomies, 7 were improved (follow up: 3 months). Toczek et al. (1978) reported 5 such cases with similar results and noted that better results were obtained in patients with a complete neurological lesion and with a more complete interruption of bladder innervation. Of the 6 patients with multiple sclerosis tested by Rockswold et al. (1978), 3 had a successful result.

For *dorsal rhizotomies*, the approach is performed at the level of the conus medullaris or the cauda equina. A variable amount of the dorsal roots from S2 to S5 are cut, according to the data obtained from the intraoperative stimulation testing. To keep reflex erection, S2 has to be preserved, at least on one side. This technique produces anaesthesia in the corresponding cutaneo-mucous territories. In a recent review of 45 cases who underwent dorsal sacral rhizotomies for spastic bladder, Saurwein and Dersh (1989) reported a good result (complete continence) in 40, a partial one in 4, and a failure in one (follow up: 5 years). 82% good results were reported by Barat and Egon (1989) (follow up: 2 years).

C) Sacral Microsurgical Drez-Tomy (MDT)

MDT, a method first developed for the treatment of pain and/or spasticity in the limbs (Sindou 1972) (see chapter 23) can also be applied to spastic bladder.

The target of the procedure is the ventro-lateral region of the Dorsal Root Entry Zone (DREZ) at the S2, S3 and S4 spinal segments. MDT selectively interrupts the nociceptive and myotatic afferent fibers while sparing the tactile and proprioceptive ones. MDT has the advantage of preserving, at least partially the sensory functions as compared to the classical dorsal rhizotomies. In addition, with this method, dorsal roots are easy to differentiate from motor ones. But identification of the landmarks between the S1 and the S2 roots, and between the other sacral roots, is difficult and needs intraoperative electrical stimulation. Our results in 15 patients with disabling spastic bladders are very encouraging since all these patients experienced disappearance of their urge incontinence after surgery (follow up: 1 to 3 years).

3. Neurostimulation procedures

A) Spinal cord stimulation (SCS)

Developed in the seventies for the treatment of certain types of pain, SCS has shown some effectiveness in spastic syndromes, such as those encountered in multiple sclerosis or spinal cord degenerative diseases (see chapter 11). Only a few authors have reported detailed studies about the effects of SCS on bladder spasticity. Whereas Dooley et al. (cited in Khoury et al. 1987) and Meglio et al. (1980) mentioned good results, others like Hawkes et al. (1983) are less enthusiastic as only 3 of their 18 cases became continent after SCS.

Our personal experience is that SCS is able to decrease hypertonia in the bladder as well as in the lower limbs of paraplegic patients, but only when the spasticity is mild and if the dorsal columns have kept enough functional fibers.

B) Sacral ventral root stimulation for bladder continence

If peripheral motor fibers are intact, stimulation of the ventral sacral roots, with intradural or extradural electrodes, can be used in a continuous mode to enhance the striated sphincter contraction and thus to obtain bladder continence (Toczek et al. 1978). The rationale for such a method is that provoked contractions of the striated sphincter inhibit detrusor activity. As the sphincter has a lower threshold of excitabity than the detrusor, it is thus possible to make a selective stimulation of the sphincter without detrusor contraction. Of the 11 paraplegic patients, in whom Brindley et al. (1982) performed a permanent stimulation of the anterior sacral roots, 7 had a decrease in urinary leakage (follow up: 2 years).

C) Neurostimulation for micturition

In the sixties, several methods using neuro-stimulation were attempted to produce active micturition in patients. Stimulation was at the level of the pelvic nerves, the detrusor, the striated sphincter and also the conus medullaris. The latter introduced by Nashold in 1972 (Nashold et al. 1977) consists of implanting a bipolar electrode inside the conus medullaris at the level of the micturition center. All these methods have been replaced by the technique of ventral root stimulation developed by Brindley et al. (1982) and Tanagho (Schmidt and Tanagho 1985).

This technique consists of an intermittent stimulation of the ventral roots to create an active micturition. When stimulation stops, the striated sphincter has a quick release in base tone for approximatively 2 seconds, while detrusor has a slower decrease in tone, keeping a contraction for 20 seconds. Evacuation of the bladder is thus possible during the interval after stimulation stops. Several successive stimulations can totally empty the bladder.

To achieve better continence by decreasing detrusor spasticity and to avoid catheterization, dorsal rhizotomies or a micro-surgical DREZ-tomy can be combined with electrode placement for ventral root stimulation at the same surgical session.

In a recent Symposium on "sacral ventral root stimulation by Brindley's technique", held in Le Mans in 1989, a 116 case series with a 80% success rate, was reported, i.e. micturition with less than 70 cc of urinary residue after micturition.

4. Intrathecal baclofen infusion

Intrathecal administration of Baclofen with implantable pumps, developed to treat spasticity in the lower limbs (Penn and Kroin 1987) (see chapter 13), has also been reported to improve bladder spasticity. This conservative method is promising, although Baclofen may induce urinary retention. It still needs longer follow-ups and more patients at least in the field of bladder spasticity.

Conclusion

It is of importance to keep in mind that all these procedures directed at the nervous system are effective only as long as the bladder has little or no irreversible fibrotic degeneration. These procedures are able to reduce detrusor hyperactivity and hyperreflexia, but have only limited effects when the bladder has become hypertonic. They have almost no effect when the bladder is fibrotic. It is thus easy to understand that urodynamic evaluation is necessary to determine, prior to surgery the exact functional status of the urinary tract, and to predict the effects of this type of surgery.

In conclusion, it must be emphasized that early treatment of the spasticity of the bladder, not only to save renal functions, but also to relieve urinary frequency, urinary urgency and urge incontinence. The latter are psychologically so distressing and socially disturbing to be of paramount importance. If not treated early enough, spasticity of the bladder can evolve towards detrusor hypertonicity and fibrosis, and be responsible for intractable incontinence and irreversible renal damage.

Acknowledgement

We are grateful to Mrs. Béatrice Leriche who helped us in the redaction of this article.

References

Archimbaud JP, Leriche A, Ejazy M (1976) Les dysfonctionnements vésico-sphinctériens neurologiques. E.M.C.- Paris, Tome III 18237 A 10

Barat M, Egon G (1989) Communication on results synthesis. In: Congress on Sacral Ventral Root Stimulation. Brindley's technique. Le Mans, November 24–25

Bates P, Bradley WE, Glen E, Griffiths D, Melchior H, Rowan D, Sternling A, Zinner N, Hald T (1979) The standardization of terminology of lower urinary tract function. J Urol 121: 551

Blaivas JG (1979) A critical appraisal of specific diagnostic techniques in clinical neuro-urology. Krane R, Sirdey M (eds) Little, Brown and Co Boston-chap 5

Blaivas JG (1982) The neurophysiology of micturition: a clinical study of 550 patients. J Urol 127: 958

Blaivas JG, Labib KB, Michalik SJ, Zayed AA (1980) Cystometric response to propantheline in detrusor hyperreflexia: therapeutic implications. J Urol 124: 259

Blaivas JG, Awad SA, Bissada N, Khanna OP, Kranz RJ, Wein AJ, Yalla S (1982) Urodynamic procedures: recommandations of the urodynamic society. I. Procedures that should be available for routine practice. Neuro-urol Urodyn 1: 51

Brindley G, Polkey CE, Rushton DN (1982) Sacral anterior root stimulators for bladder control in paraplegia. Paraplegia 20: 365–381

Brindley GS, Polkey CE, Rushton DN (1984) Sacral anterior root stimulators for bladder control in paraplegia: the first 40 cases. In: Proceedings of the 14th Meeting of International Continence Society, Innsbruck, 1984, pp 53–54

Buzelin JM (1984) Urodynamique, Bas appareil urinaire. Masson, Paris

Hawkes CH, Beard R, Fawcett D, Paul EA, Thomas DCT (1983)

Dorsal column stimulations in multiple sclerosis: effects on bladder and long term findings. Br Med J 287: 793–795

Khoury S, Buzelin JM, Richard F, Sussey J (1987) Physiologie et pathologie de la dynamique des voies urinaires. Fondation Internationale pour l'Information Scientifique

Leriche A, Leriche B (1983) La chirurgie neuro-urologique dans la sclérose en plaques à propos de 60 patients. 6e congrès SIFUD, Montpellier, pp 104–118

Meglo M, Cioni B, D'Amico E, Ronzoni G, Rossi F (1980) Epidural spinal stimulation for the treatment of neurogenic bladder. Acta Neurochir 54: 191–199

Nashold BS, Grimes J, Friedman H, Semans J, Avery R (1977) Operative stimulation of the neurogenic bladder. Neurosurgery 1: 218, 220

Penn R, Kroin J (1987) Long term baclofen infusion for treatment of spasticity. J Neurosurg 66: 181–185

Rockswold G, Chou S, Bradley W (1978) Reevaluation of differential sacral rhizotomy for neurological bladder disease. J Neurosurg 48: 773–778

Sauerwein D, Dersh U (1989) Communication in the congress on: sacral anterior root electrostimulation. G.S. Brindley's technique. Le Mans, November 24–25, 1989

Schmidt RA, Tanagho EA (1985) Restoration of continence in low thoracic spinal injury via sacral nerve stimulator. J Urol 133(4): 180 A (Abstract)

Schmidt R (1986) Advances in genito-urinary neurostimulation. Neurosurgery 19: 1041–1044

Sindou M, Jeanmonod D (1989) Microsurgical DREZ-otomy in the treatment of spasticity and pain in the lower limbs. Neurosurgery 24: 665–670

Toczek S, Mc Cullough D, Boggs J (1978) Sacral rootlet rhizotomy at the conus medullaris for hypertonic neurogenic bladder. J Neurosurg 48: 193–196

Torrens M (1974) The effect of selective sacral nerve blocks on vesical and urethral function. J Urol 112: 204–205

Torrens M, Griffith H (1976) Management of the uninhibited bladder by selective sacral neurectomy. J Neurosurg 44: 176–185

Torring J, Petersen T, Klemar B, Sogaard I (1988) Selective sacral rootlet neurectomy in the treatment of detrusor hyperreflexia. J Neurosurg 68: 241–245

Young B, Mulcahy J (1980) Percutaneous sacral rhizotomy for neurogenic detrusor hyperreflexia. J Neurosurg 53: 85–87

Correspondence: Dr. C. Beneton, Centre Médical Germaine Revel, Saint Maurice sur Dargoire, F-69440 Mornant, France

Orthopedic surgical corrections of spastic disorders

A. Bardot with the collaboration of **A. Delarque**, **G. Curvale**, and **J.C. Peragut**

Service de Réadaptation, CHU Timone, University of Marseille-Aix en Provence, Marseille, France

In the last 20 years, early treatment of neurologically disabled patients with drugs and modern neuromuscular rehabilitation methods has considerably reduced the need for surgery. It is now indicated under more clearly defined conditions (Katz 1988). Surgery, whatever its may be, must take into account the notion of useful spasticity. Disharmony in the intensity of muscular hypertonia creates articular imbalance requiring selective treatment. This selectivity can only be achieved by neurological and/or orthopedic surgery, usually after muscular blocking tests. The orthopedic procedures can act in two ways: 1. in reducing spasticity by means of muscle relaxation resulting from tendon lengthening; 2. in restoring the biomechanical conditions required for suitable articular function in cases of irreducible deformity.

Basic surgical techniques

Surgical techniques include soft tissue procedures, osteotomies, and articular surgery (arthrodesis).

1. Musculotendinous surgery can refer to lengthening of the "muscle-tendon assembly" or to tendon transfers. Current techniques for correcting excessive shortness, are muscular disinsertion (Fig. 1), myotomy, tenotomy and lengthening tenotomy (Fig. 2). The result of these various techniques is an unequivocal achievement of a more functional position. Such techniques do not increase the motion of the muscle in question and they sometimes reduce it, especially if they are repeated on the same muscle. In one circumstance: the patellar tendon surgery may be undertaken to shorten the muscle-tendon assembly. In the patient with cerebral palsy it is the only example of a tendon which lengthens when its muscle shortens. Its surgical shortening can augment lengthening of the hamstring tendons (Fig. 3).

Tendon transfer has a different goal: normalizing the articular orientation when it has been deviated by muscular imbalance. Tendon displacement or bifurcation, with care taken not to invert its mechanical effect in the sagittal plane, may be an efficient procedure for reorientating an articular movement. However – contrary to what one can observe in cases of flaccid paralysis-, it is difficult to predict the results of transfer in central disorders. Pre-operative electromyography can give an approximation, but does not exclude the possibility of failure. It is generally risky to transfer a tendon to its antagonist in the sagittal plane, in order to palliate the inefficiency of a muscle or to reinforce its action; therefore we carefully avoid transferring a flexor to an extensor or vice versa.

2. Osteotomies may be indicated to correct bone deformities due to a morphogenetic pathology of growth (for example: femoral derotation osteotomy to correct excessive anteversion in patients with cerebral palsy) or to treat stiffened articulations with irreducible abnormal postures (Fig. 4).

3. Articular surgery is especially indicated in patients with severe spasticity in the foot or the wrist. Arthrodesis is chosen in two circumstances: when there are osteoarticular structural deformities that osteotomy cannot correct – this is a resection arthrodesis-, or when articular imbalance cannot be correct in a stable and lasting manner by tendon surgery alone (Fig. 5). Arthrodesis must not be performed until the end of growth.

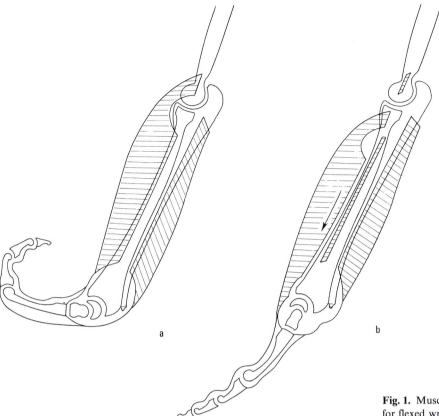

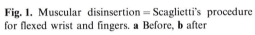

Fig. 1. Muscular disinsertion = Scaglietti's procedure for flexed wrist and fingers. **a** Before, **b** after

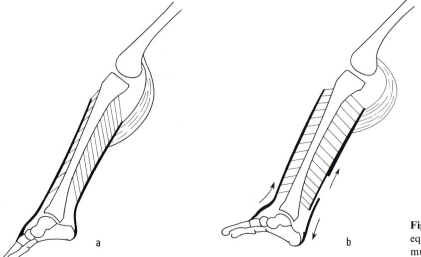

Fig. 2. Tendon lengthening of the heel cord for equinus. **a** Before, **b** after. *N.B.* As in Fig. 1, muscle fibers of the two antagonist muscular groups are shortened after operation.

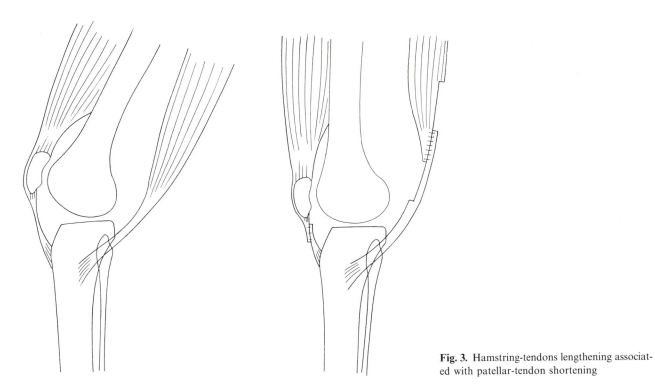

Fig. 3. Hamstring-tendons lengthening associated with patellar-tendon shortening

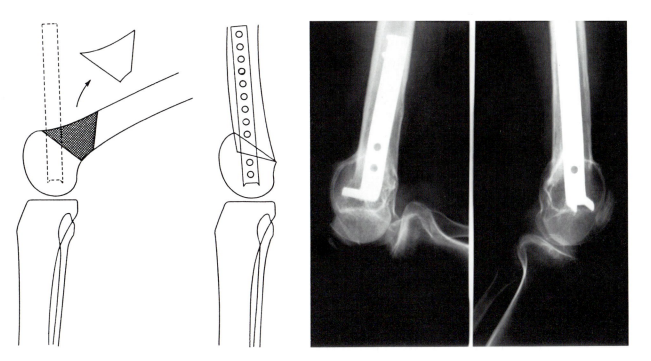

Fig. 4. Supracondylar femoral osteotomy for irreducible flexed knee

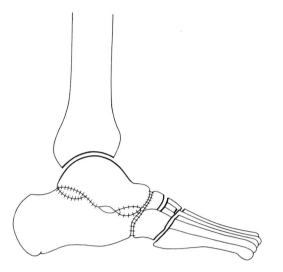

Fig. 5. Hind-foot arthrodesis (the same technique is named "triple arthrodesis" in English and "double arthrodesis" in French). With this technique, the ankle remains free

Spasticity in children

In children, morphogenesis of the osteoarticular system is rigorously conditioned by the mechanical forces that control it. Of those forces, muscular tension plays a leading and permanent role. This tension is sustained by two mechanisms: hypertonia and 'contracture' (Bleck 1979). This second phenomenon is a result of growth asynchronism in length between the striated muscle fibers and the long bones resulting in a relative shortness of muscles compared to the skeleton (Tabary et al. 1971, Tardieu et al. 1971). In spastic children, these two mechanisms are aggravated by an imbalance between two antagonist muscular groups for one given articulation. In the lower limb, there is a prevalence of adductors for the hip, flexors for the knee, plantar flexion muscles for the foot; inverse imbalance is much rarer. In the upper limb, the wrist is in flexion-adduction and pronation, and the elbow is flexed. Permanence of this imbalance, in addition to the discomfort they cause, determine the osteoarticular structural deformities which must be prevented. Medical treatment has no effect on imbalance. The effects of alcohol nerve blocks are transitory. Neurotomies are effective but must be used with caution in children. Orthopedic surgery – provided it be appropriate – may be the treatment of choice (Bleck 1979, Cahuzac 1977).

1. For the lower limbs, *orthopedic surgery* is indicated in the following order of frequency: the hip, foot, and knee.

For the *hip,* the usual problems that develop in spastic children and teenagers are the following isolated, or associated, deformities: adduction, flexion, and internal rotation. Their ultimate complication is spastic hip dislocation. Early diagnosis, and appropriate careful rehabilitation, can appreciably reduce their incidence. Early verticalization, at 8 to 10 months, is one of the best preventive measures. When these measures fail, orthopedic surgery is indicated, almost always on soft tissues: muscular disinsertions, myotomies, tenotomies. Muscle section of the long adductor, short adductor, gracilis – which frees abduction – can be usefully complemented by neurotomy of the anterior branch of the obturator nerve. Sectioning of these muscles, also, in part, frees extension. When the deformity is in flexion, upper sectioning of the tensor fascia lata, sartorius, and rectus femoris is generally sufficient. Tenotomy of the psoas, recommended by Bleck (1979), has been rejected by many authors (Cahuzac 1977). The treatment of spastic dislocation of the hip requires complementary bone surgery: subtrochanteric derotation-varization femoral osteotomy, acetabuloplasty, or Salter or Harris pelvic osteotomy. In cases of advanced dislocation, the therapeutic decision can range from no surgery at all to cervicocephalic femoral resection. When the hip's internal rotation deformity causes intoed gait, a derotation diaphysis femoral osteotomy may be considered if there is a serious handicap, representing a serious obstacle to comfortable walking.

As for the *knee,* the most common deformity is the flexion. When it is irreducible in a child who can walk, surgery can be considered (Cahuzac 1977). But when making a choice among the numerous techniques, care should be taken to avoid over correction resulting in hyperextension.

One of these techniques, the Eggers's procedure (Eggers 1952), consists of transferring all the hamstring tendons, from their distal tibial and fibular insertions, proximally to the femoral condyles. The hyperextended knee – genu recurvatum – is a common postoperative disadvantage of this technique, often as a result of overlooked quadriceps' spasticity which was hidden by the hamstring's contracture before surgery. The complete Eggers operation has been abandoned by all. However, a part of this procedure can still be used; it consists of transferring the semi-tendinosus onto the femur, while lengthening of other hamstrings: semi-membranosus, biceps. The gracilis is usually tenotomized. For severe knee-flexion deformity, it is also necessary to use a Z-plasty cutaneous incision, and to resect the popliteal aponeurosis: thus, inversion of the Z-flaps – impossible if aponeurosis is not resected – allows a relaxed cutaneous suture. This posterior liberating surgery must sometimes be completed by a shortening of the ligamentum patellae when the patella is in very high position.

Foot deformities in children with cerebral palsy are frequent indications for surgery. The most common problem is the equinus deformity. Not unfrequently its conservation may be necessary for the standing position. When very severe, it must be treated either by acting on the gastrocnemius if it is the sole cause or by tendo-achilles (heel-cord) lengthening. It is wiser to conserve a 5° equinus. Varus or valgus should only be approached with great care in children with cerebral palsy. Tendon transfers are uncertain in the long term and can cause regrettable hypercorrections. Calcaneus osteotomy may be indicated, during the growth period, for severe varus deformity. Arthrodesis (almost always triple: subtalar and midtarsal) should not be performed until bone maturation has been completed. This articular surgery is preferred for the varus deformity which is usually painful. Valgus deformity is awkward but usually painless and does not prevent the patient from walking.

2. *Orthopedic surgery* for spasticity **in the upper limb** of patients with cerebral palsy should only be considered with great caution (Sharrard and Baker 1977). Tendon lengthening or displacement, arthrodesis of the first intermetacarpal space, wrist or phalanges, can give the patient better use of the hand.

3. *The* **proper age for surgery** is a question of common sense (Bleck 1979, Cahuzac 1977, Lambard 1981). Before the age of walking, orthopedic surgery is only urgently indicated for prevention of hip dislocation or for major equinus deformity of the foot. Later on, time of surgery is conditioned by the severity and speed of deterioration, and with the concern of preventing scoliosis in the lower oblique pelvis.

Orthopedic surgery must not by-pass surgical destructive procedures on the nerves. As a matter of fact, if nerve resections are done inadequately, neurotomies can be followed by a recurrence of spastic deformity; and if done excessively, walking children can functionally deteriorate. If only one – third or one – fourth of the motor units remain after tibial neurotomy, there is a risk of delayed decompensation in the form of triceps paralysis, as observed in "delayed

post-poliomyelitis syndrome". This may lead to destabilization of the standing position.

Spasticity in adults

Orthopedic surgery for spasticity in adults should be considered according to the etiology of the spasticity (Bardot et al. 1989).

Cerebral palsy in adulthood

Surgery can be justified for certain delayed consequences indirectly due to spasticity, especially at the hips where early coxarthrosis may be the consequence of insufficient treatment during childhood, or in the feet when equino-varus deformities with painful and deformed toes are present.

Para and tetraplegias

1. *In the lower limbs*, orthopedic surgery may be indicated for complete and definitive lesions, either for the patient's comfort or for treatment of deformities which are the cause of pressure sores (Guillaumat and Le Mouel 1989). For comfort, it is undertaken for fixed deformities which neurosurgery cannot correct, i.e. section of adductors for flexion-adduction of the hip, of hamstrings for a residual flexed knee, of the Achilles tendon for a major equinus deformity. When a pressure sore persists because of by a bony prominence, operation of the causal deformity becomes necessary. One must always choose simple techniques which do not require plaster casts. For an incomplete lesion in a patient able to walk, surgery can be undertaken, but only when it is certain that ambulation will not be adversely effected.

2. *In the upper limbs* of tetraplegics, functional tendon surgery, under very precise conditions, can appreciably increase autonomy (Maury et al. 1981). Möberg (1975) was the first to undertake this surgery, the aim of which is restoration of some elementary functions of the upper limb, such as pollici-digital pinch or "key-grip", or elbow-extension. These techniques consist of tendon-transfers, and tenodesis with or without arthrodesis. Conceived of as palliative treatments for lesions of the peripheral nervous system they can also be applied to patients with central nervous lesions, provided the muscles to be transferred be not spastic. As a matter of fact, even mild spasticity in a muscle selected to be transferred, is a contra-

indication to this surgery. If necessary, suppression of spasticity in such muscles can be achieved by a neuro-surgical procedure (peripheral neurotomy or surgery in the corresponding dorsal roots or dorsal root entry zone) prior to tendon transfers.

Head trauma patients

Major deformities in head trauma patients are not only the consequence of spasticity, but also of long periods of complex motor disorders, during which it is often difficult to prevent abnormal posture. Once neurological stability has been obtained, a program of orthopedic surgery can be established to improve the patient's function, if a sufficient level of voluntary mobility is recovered (Barouk et al. 1989, Chantraine and Taillard 1989). Even if walking is impossible, surgery may be justified, to increase comfort in the sitting or lying position, especially in patients who have recovered good cognitive functions.

Hemiplegias

1. When *upper limb* functions are useless, due to permanent motor deficits, severe sensory disturbances, and/or harmful co-contractions of muscles (syncineses). Orthopedic surgery can only offer the benefit for comfort and aesthetics. The procedures are limited to simple lengthening tenotomies on the wrist and finger flexors. It is necessary to inform the patient that muscular relaxation will be strictly anatomical and non-functional.

When the hand is functional but hindered by hypertonia, our preference is to first carry out an alcohol block of the hypertonic muscles, generally the wrist and finger flexors. If the effects of the block are temporary, which is most frequently the case, a more permanent effect can be obtained using the classical lengthening and tendon transfer techniques. Lengthen-

ing involves the flexor carpi radialis, flexor carpi ulnaris, and flexor pollicis longus. For long finger flexors, the proximal end of each flexor digitorum profundus tendon is transferred on the distal end of the corresponding flexor digitorum superficialis tendon (Fig. 6). Each lengthening should be made with such precision that, under anaesthesia, residual muscular tension maintains each finger in a slightly flexed position.

2. Surgery is rarely indicated in the *lower limb* of hemiplegic patients; spasticity is usually in the hip and knee in extension, and consequently helpful for walking.

When the foot has an excessive spasticity, surgery can be strongly recommended (Asencio et al. 1989, Bardot et al. 1989, Martin et al. 1989). Neurosurgery is preferable if there is no fixed muscular contracture or articular deformity. Orthopedic surgery is indicated when the equinus deformity is irreducible, the varus makes stance unstable, or the foot is irreducibly deformed.

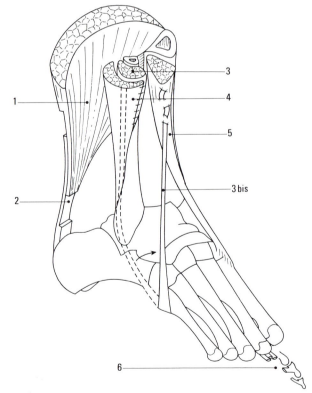

Fig. 7. Our procedure for tendon surgery in spastic equino-varus hemiplegic foot. *1* triceps surae; *2* heel cord lengthening; *3* peroneus brevis; *3bis* its tendon, freed from the muscle, is attached to tibialis anterior; *4* peroneus longus, untouched; *5* tibialis anterior; *6* toe flexors tenotomy

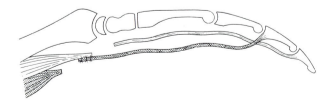

Fig. 6. Flexors digitorum lengthening in the hemiplegic hand: the proximal end of flexor profundus is sutured to the distal end of superficialis

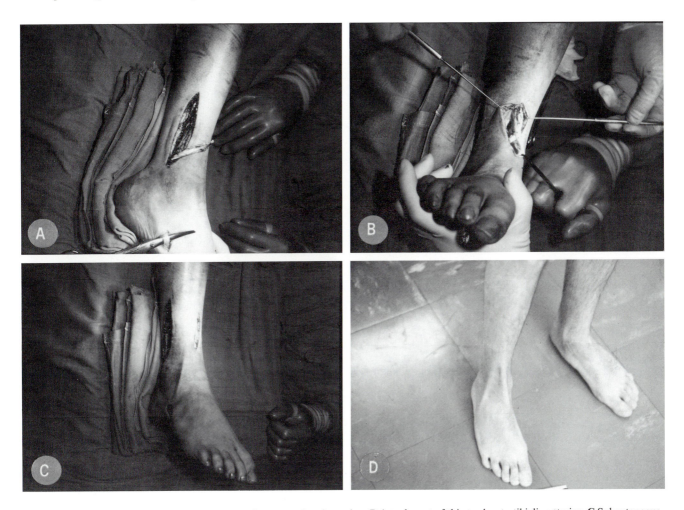

Fig. 8. Surgical views and results. **A** Dissection of peroneus brevis-tendon. **B** Attachment of this tendon to tibialis anterior. **C** Subcutaneous transferred tendon. **D** Result

The choice of the technique is based upon a kinesiological analysis of the bare foot when standing, walking and lying down. In the standing and walking positions, muscle behaviour in each phase is studied in the foot and in the toes. Examination of the foot in the lying position evaluates the force of the tibialis anterior and the irreducibility of the deformities.

For irreducible equinus deformity, Achilles tendon lengthening using any current technique is indicated. This may be sufficient if the equinus is pure in stable stance.

The generally associated varus deformity which causes problems with stance can be corrected by tendon transfer or by triple arthrodesis (subtalar and mid-tarsal). There are several techniques available for tendon transfer: complete lateral transfer of the bifurcation of the tibialis anterior, or fixation of the distal tendon of the peroneus brevis onto the tibialis anterior (Figs. 7 and 8). These procedures, each with

comparable results, are only effective if the preoperative kinesiological examination shows definite activity and sufficient force of the tibialis anterior in stance and swing phase. Triple arthrodesis is preferable to tibialis anterior transfer in the following cases: inactivity of this muscle in the standing position, insufficient muscle force, or a young and active patient. It must be avoided in patients for whom 10 weeks of immobilization in a cast presents risks (elderly or vascular patients).

Contracture of toes is usual after tendo-achilles lengthening in hemiplegic patients, so much so that prophylactic treatment is routine for us (at every achilles-tendon lengthening). Flexed toes are an indication for flexor tenotomy, either in the leg through the skin incision performed for the surgical approach of the achilles tendon, or percutaneously on the plantar side of each toe.

This type of surgery of the hemiplegic foot has become popular over the last 10 years. Its results have been reported elsewhere (Asencio et al. 1989, Barouk et al. 1989, Chantraine and Taillard 1989, Katz 1988). Its indications remain relatively rare, given the considerable number of hemiplegic patients, thanks to results obtained by modern rehabilitation methods.

Conclusion

Orthopedic surgery is one of the methods for the treatment of the consequences of spasticity. It has its own indications, limits and risks. It should only be undertaken after evaluation by a team of specialists with an expert surgeon and followed up by an experienced rehabilitation team.

References

Asencio G, Pelissier J, Privat J-M, Galouye P, Bertin R, Megy B, Leonardi C (1989) Chirurgie neuro-orthopédique du membre inférieur dans l'hémiplégie vasculaire. In: Bardot A, Pelissier J (eds) Neuro-Orthopédie des Membres Inférieurs chez l'Adulte. Masson, Paris, pp 91–98

Bardot A, Delarque A, Curvale G (1989) Spasticité et chirurgie orthopédique. In: Bardot A, Pelissier J (eds) Neuro-Orthopédie des Membres Inférieurs chez l'Adulte. Masson, Paris, pp 15–20

Bardot A, Delarque A, Costes O, Curvale G, Groulier P (1989) La chirurgie palliative du pied de l'hémiplégique adulte. In: Bardot A, Pelissier J (eds) Neuro-Orthopédie des Membres Inférieurs chez l'Adulte. Masson, Paris, pp 86–90

Barouk LS, Richer R, Deliac M, Laurent F (1989) La chirurgie du membre inférieur de l'hémiplégie séquelle de traumatisme crânien. In: Bardot A, Pelissier J (eds) Neuro-Orthopédie des Membres Inférieurs chez l'Adulte. Masson, Paris, pp 104–110

Bleck EE (1979) Orthopaedic management of cerebral palsy. Saunders, Philadelphia, pp 87–207

Cahuzac M (1977) L'enfant infirme moteur d'origine cérébrale. Masson, Paris, pp 141–305

Chantraine A, Taillard W (1989) Allongement du tendon d'Achille chez le traumatisé crânien spastique. In: Bardot A, Pelissier J (eds) Neuro-Orthopédie des Membres Inférieurs chez l'Adulte. Masson, Paris, pp 98–103

Eggers GW (1952) Transplantation of hamstring tendons to femoral condyles in order to improve hip-extension and to decrease knee-flexion in cerebral palsy. J Bone Joint Surg [Am] 34/A: 827–830

Guillaumat M, Le Mouel MA (1989) La chirurgie orthopédique des membres inférieurs chez le paraplégique adulte. In: Bardot A, Pelissier J (eds) Neuro-Orthopédie des membres inférieurs chez l'adulte. Masson, Paris, pp 129–135

Katz RD (1988) Management of spasticity. Am J Phys Med 167: 108–116

Lombard M (1981) Infirmité motrice cérébrale. In: Médecine de Rééducation. Flammarion Médecine, Paris, pp 350–363

Martin JC, Vogt JC, Lecocq J, Vautravers Ph (1989) Traitement chirurgical du pied varus équin spastique de l'adulte et de l'adolescent. In: Bardot A, Pelissier J (eds) Neuro-Orthopédie des membres inférieurs chez l'Adulte. Masson, Paris, pp 106–116

Maury M, Le Coeur P, Guillaumat M (1981) La main du tétraplégique et sa chirurgie. In: La paraplégie. Flammarion Médecine Sciences, Paris, pp 530–540

Möberg E (1975) Surgical treatment for absent single hand-grip and elbow-extension in quadriplegia. J Bone Joint Surg [Am] 57 A/2: 196–206

Sharrard WJW, Baker RH (1977) La main spastique. Evaluation pour traitement par intervention sanglante. Cah CDI 73: 17–34

Tabary JC, Goldspink G, Tardieu C, Lombard M, Tardieu G, Chigot P (1971) Nature de la rétraction musculaire des I.M.C Mesure de l'allongement des sarcomères du muscle étiré. Rev Chir Orthop 57: 463–470

Tardieu G, Tabary JC, Tardieu C, Lombard M (1971) Rétraction, hyperextensibilité et "faiblesse" de l'I.M.C., expressions apparemment opposées d'un même trouble musculaire. Consequences thérapeutiques. Rev Chir Orthop 57: 505–516

Correspondence: Prof. A. Bardot, Orthopedic surgeon, Centre d'Eludes et de Recherches en Réadaptation, 92 rue Auguste-Blanqui, F-13005 Marseille, France

Indications

Indications for surgery to treat adults with harmful spasticity

M. Sindou and **P. Mertens**

Department of Neurosurgery, Hopital Neurologique, Lyon, France

I

Spasticity in adults may result from a variety of CNS diseases and is frequently associated with, or masked by symptoms such as dystonia, dyskinesia, motor weakness or sensory disturbances. To evaluate the exact role which spasticity is playing in a disability, there must be a quantitative description of not only the spasticity present, but also of the other motor and sensory disorders involved in the disability. There must also be a differentiation of spasticity which is hampering limb function versus spasticity which is being used to augment function (e.g. extensor spasticity in a paretic leg which allows weight bearing).

Spasticity is a velocity dependent resistance to muscle stretching which can be differentiated from muscle or joint capsule contracture by repetitively stretching a muscle rapidly and comparing any range limitation demonstrated with the range limitation seen when slowly stretching the muscle. If there is any remaining doubt after this testing as to the cause of the limitation in limb movement, the individual may be tested under a brief anesthesia using curare or a similar muscle relaxant. The degree of limitation in mobility during anesthesia is indicative of muscle and joint contracture and this examination could then be compared to the examination in the awake patient.

Surgery should only be considered after the individual has been closely examined for signs of conditions which would aggravate his or her spasticity; e.g. urinary tract infections, decubitus ulcerations, long bone fractures, etc. There must also be a review of the individual's current therapy and medications to ensure that there has been an adequate trial with these agents.

Before undergoing surgery, the patient must be carefully examined not only with the spasticity being quantified using classical clinical scales, but also the individuals' functional abilities being scored. It is also helpful to obtain electrophysiologic evaluations including H-reflex measurements and EMG's.

Once it has been elected to treat a person's abnormal postures surgically, there must be a determination of whether the abnormal posture is due to spasticity (which would be treated by a neurosurgical procedure) or whether the abnormal posture is due to osteo-articular and/or musculo-tendinous limitations (which would be dealt with by an orthopedic procedure).

II

Whatever surgical procedure is selected, its goal should be to diminish the excessive hypertonia without suppressing useful muscle tone or limb function. What follows is a description of techniques which may be employed:

Spinal Cord Stimulation (SCS) is useful in treating spasticity of spinal cord origin such as multiple sclerosis or other degenerative diseases such as Strumpell–Lorrain syndrome. SCS is effective only when the spasticity is mild and if the dorsal columns have retained enough functional fibers. This can be tested for with a clinical sensory examination and Spinal Evoked Potential (SEP) recordings. Other targets for stimulation have been tried (e.g. deep brain and cerebellar) and have not been found to yield reliable functional improvement.

Intrathecal Baclofen administration is indicated for para- or tetraplegic patients with severe and diffuse spasticity. Because of its reversibility, this method can be performed prior to considering an ablative procedure. The technique does have the disadvantages of being costly and requiring frequent (q 1–2 month) clinic visits for refilling and reprograming of the pump. This leads to the further disadvantage of a geographical and pyschological dependence. As with any implanted device, it can malfunction or become infected, necessitating its removal. Therefore intrathecal baclofen is not a panacea.

Neuro-Ablative techniques are indicated for severe spasticity which is localized to the limbs of paraplegic, tetraplegic or hemiplegic patients.

Motor point and nerve blocks, as well as percutaneous thermo-rhizotomies or intrathecal chemical rhizotomies offer reduction in spastic tone on a temporary basis. When the spasticity returns, they can be repeated.

The open, destructive procedures which seek to produce a permanent alleviation of the spasticity must be selective and target abnormal circuits while preserving those necessary for the more normal sensory and motor functions.

When spasticity is localized to muscles or muscle groups innervated by a small number of or single peripheral nerve(s), peripheral neurotomy may be used. The main indication for this technique is to treat the spastic hip or foot in the lower limb, or the spastic elbow or hand in the upper limb. A preliminary field block of the targeted nerve(s) using a long acting anaesthetic agent such as Bupivacaine can be used prior to the neurotomy to evaluate its potential effects on limb function as the anaesthetics effect on the nerve(s) will result in a reversible decrease in muscle

Table 1. Indications for neurosurgery in paraplegias

Types of spasticity	Operative procedures
Non-ambulatory patients (with flexions, spasms and/or hip dislocation)	
In poor conditions:	
• General anesthesia and/or open surgery not allowed	⟶ Intrathecal chemical rhizotomy
• General anesthesia, open surgery allowed	
• Bladder catheter dependant, no sexual function	⟶ Myelotomy
• Automatic bladder and/or sexual function present	⟶ Combined neurotomies of: obturator n., knee flexor sciatic br., tibial n.
In good conditions:	Thermo-rhizotomy
• Pump implantation not possible	Microsurgical drez-tomy or dorsal rhizotomies (≠ types)
• Pump implantation possible (intrathecal test)	⊖ ⟶
	⊕ ⟶ Intrathecal baclofen administration
Ambulatory patients	
With person helping:	
• Diffuse regional spasticity (i.e., entire lower limbs)	⟶ Consideration of dorsal rhizotomies or limited MDT
• Focalized spasticity	
• Hip (add. and/or flex.)	⟶ Obturator neurotomy
• Knee (flex.)	⟶ Knee flexor sciatic branches neurot.
• Foot (equinus and/or varus)	⟶ Tibial neurotomy
• Combined localizations	⟶ Combined neurotomies
Autonomous:	
• Focalized spasticity	
• Mild regional spasticity	
(Dorsal columns) Functional	⊕ ⟶ Spinal cord stimulation
Non-functional	⊖ ⟶ No neurosurgical treatment
Special situations	
Sp. resistant to dorsal rhiz. or MDT (if totally paralyzed)	
• if bladder catheter	⟶ Chemical rhizotomy
• if automatic bladder	⟶ Ventral rhizotomy
Patients with irreducible extension	⟶ MDT or dorsal rhizotomy (≠ types)
Spastic bladder	⟶ MDT or rhizotomies

tone in the nerve's myotome. In addition to helping the medical team assess the effect to be expected with the neurotomy, the use of the reversible nerve block will give the patient a better appreciation of what will be gained with the procedure.

For paraplegic patients with severe spasticity affecting the entire limb bilaterally there are several procedures to choose from: dorsal rhizotomies (including the selective, partial, sectorial, and functional), longitudinal myelotomy, and microsurgical Drezotomy (MDT). Our preference is for the MDT operation which is done at the spinal segments corresponding to the myotomal levels disabled by the harmful hypertonia. We favor this procedure because it not only selectively interrupts the afferent myotactic and flexor reflex fibers but it also acts on the gating mechanisms within the spinal cord by shifting the modulatory activity towards inhibition. MDT is also our choice when treating spasticity which affects the entire upper limb. This is because the technique preserves to a large degree the afferent fibers of the lemniscal system allowing much more retention of tactile and proprioceptive sensation than other ablative procedures.

It is our present tendency to combine several types of neuro-ablative procedures in one patient. A frequent combination is the peripheral section of the flexor nerves of the wrist and fingers with a cervical MDT,

in case of spasticity in flexion of the upper limb. Another example is a tibial neurotomy associated with a lumbar MDT, to avoid operating on the sacral segments in patients with good genito-sphincterian functions.

Orthopedic procedures (tendon lengthenings, joint reconstructions) can reduce spasticity secondarily by relaxing the muscle and/or diminishing pain. Orthopedic procedures should not however be considered primary treatments for spasticity. Rather, physical and pharmacological therapies are applied first to treat spasticity and then neurosurgical procedures are considered if the noninvasive techniques fail to control the spasticity. It is not unusual for muscle retractions/contractures and/or ankyloses, considered irreversible, to improve or completely resolve after the spasticity has been successfully treated and follow up kinestherapy applied. In this setting, the orthopedic procedures are used to treat fixed deformities after maximal treatment for the spasticity has been applied and an adequate period for post-treatment kinestherapy has been allowed.

In the developing field of functional surgery for the treatment of spasticity a rigid protocol for its use cannot be given. Each patient must be comprehensively evaluated and treatment recommendations made based on the individuals unique needs. Every surgeon will choose his own way according to his experience and bearing in mind the goal(s) to be reached for the patient: increased comfort, the prevention of limb deformities, and the improvement of function. We have summarized our preferences for the treatment of spastic paraplegics, tetraplegics and hemiplegics in Tables 1–3.

Table 2. Indications for neurosurgery in hemiplegias

Types of spasticity	Operative procedures
Lower limb	

Spastic foot
• Equinus, clonus
• Varus
• Flexion of toes
	→ Neurotomy of tibial nerve
	   Soleus (gastrocnemius) branches
	   Posterior tibialis branch
	   Flexor fascicles
	   ⊕ Orthop. surg., if needed

Tonic ambulatory foot	→ Discussion: neurotomy of tibial nerve or no surgery at all.
Upper limb	
Entire limb (or shoulder and elbow alone)	→ C_5–T_1 microsurgical drez-tomy (or C_5–C_7 MDT)

Entire limb
with severe hypertonia
of wrist and finger flexors
	→ C_5–T_1 MDT with neurotomy
	   of flexor fascicles of the median
	   (and ulnar) nerve(s)

Isolated spastic hyperflexion of wrist and fingers	→ Neurotomy of median (and ulnar) flexor branches
Isolated hand in pronation	→ Neurotomy of median branches
Isolated flexion of elbow	→ Neurotomy of musculo-cutaneous n. ⊕ Combined orthop. surg., if needed.

Table 3. Indications for neurosurgery in tetraplegias

Types of spasticity	Operative procedures
	Try:
Spinal cord, brain stem, bihemispheric lesions	→ Spinal cord stimulation, if dorsal column: functional and test ⊕
	→ Intrathecal baclofen administration with programmable implanted pump, if test ⊕
	Before deciding:
	→ Neuroablative procedures in lower and/or upper limbs
	→ Complementary orthopedic surgery, if needed

Correspondence: Prof. M. Sindou, M.D., D.Sc. Biol., Department of Neurosurgery, Hopital Neurologique, 59 boulevard Pinel, F-69003 Lyon, France

Indications for surgery to treat children with spasticity due to cerebral palsy

R. Abbott

Division of Pediatric Neurosurgery, New York University Medical Center, New York, U.S.A.

The indications for treating spasticity in children affected with cerebral palsy will be discussed for each of the functional groups as outlined in Table 1 and defined in the chapter on childhood spasticity. It should be noted that catagorization of all patients into one of several specific functional groups with associated treatment recommendations is not always possible. Some patients may possess a set of characteristics which bridge several of these groups. Each case must be individually evaluated with deviations from the "norm" considered. An appropriate treatment plan is then designed based upon each child's clinical status.

Table 1. NYUMC patient groups

–Group I	Independent ambulators
–Group II	Ambulators dependent on assistive devices (canes, crutches, walkers)
–Group III	Quadraped crawlers either reciprocal or nonreciprocal (i.e., bunny hoppers)
–Group IV	Commando or belly crawlers
–Group V	Totally dependent, no locomotive abilities

Group I: independent ambulators

Children in this group are ambulatory and exhibit good strength and control in their leg muscles. They can be a very rewarding group to treat, the goal being to improve the efficiency and cosmesis of their walking. If the intervention is to be considered for this group, it is best delivered as soon after the child has demonstrated the ability to work with a therapist and before contractures develop within the hypertonic muscles. This is usually in the age range from three to seven years. Neurological surgery aimed at disrupting spastic reflex circuits, may be beneficial for older individuals in this group; but frequently it needs to be performed in conjunction with tenotomies because of shortened muscles.

Depending upon the degree of underlying strength and control in the leg musculature, one can aggressively seek to eliminate as many abnormally responsive afferent limbs of reflex circuits as can be identified. For this reason selective functional rhizotomy, where all abnormally responsive circuits are cut, is particularly effective in normalizing muscle tone. Once this is accomplished the child is ready for the reeducation in muscle use through a physiotherapy program.

Concern can be raised regarding the use of a destructive lesion to treat children functioning at such a high level. Two nondestructive alternatives can be discussed: intrathecal baclofen and functional electrical stimulation (FES). As there are side-effects with the use of baclofen intrathecally (e.g., depressed cognition, muscle fatigue), the general consensus is that until the baclofen therapy has been evaluated in more severely involved children, it should not be used to treat children functioning at high levels. With regards to FES,—given the small response rate [2 out of the 18 ambulatory, spastic diplegics treated between the ages of 5 and 7 by Dimitrijevic (personal communication)]– its use to treat spastic diplegia cannot be supported.

Group II: ambulators dependent on assistive devices

Group II can be a difficult group to improve functionally with neurosurgical treatment. While the majority of children in this group require assistive devices to supplant missing strength in the legs, some will require the devices to replace missing protective reactions, poor trunk control or a combination of the three. Occasionally, a young child will present for evaluation who is early on in the development of the functional skill of ambulation. Because these children have not perfected these skills they only require the temporary use of an assistive device.

The goal in group II is to lessen children' dependence upon assistive devices. The child with poor trunk control or lack of protective reaction but good underlying strength in the antigravity muscles can safely undergo a functional rhizotomy. Children who are to some degree dependent on the hypertonicity present in their quadriceps to weight bear should not undergo a functional rhizotomy. A sectorial posterior rhizotomy as performed by Frerebeau and Privat of the Montpellier group seems to be successful in preserving functionally useful spasticity in these children and is preferable to the functional dorsal rhizotomy. The "diffusion" of muscle activity in response to stimulation of abnormal afferent rootlets as described by Fasano must be considered in all cases. This diffusion implies that muscle hypertonicity can be due to an abnormally modulated root or rootlet at a distant spinal segment. The cutting of these abnormal afferents at segments other that those within the myotomes of the antigravity muscles could conceivably affect the tone of these muscles in an adverse way.

Group III: quadraped crawlers

This is a group which demands surgical treatment, typically during mid-childhood to early adolescence. The goal for this group of quadriped crawlers is assisted ambulation. A functional dorsal rhizotomy will decrease hypertonicity present in the leg musculature and allow for better alignment in the standing position for the child with adequate muscle strength. With this will come the possibility of meaningful training in ambulatory skills. The child who exhibits quadriceps weakness can be considered for a sectorial posterior rhizotomy or a combination of the functional and sectorial rhizotomies.

Children in this group can frequently present at young ages (<3 years) with x-rays demonstrating progressive hip dislocation. The goal of intervention for these children then changes to one which will halt the progressive orthopaedic deformity. There are four options when faced with this clinical situation. An aggressive stretching program with or without use of a hip abduction night splint should be initially tried in the hopes that time can be bought allowing the child to mature. If this fails then the choices of

percutaneous nerve block of the obturator nerve, adductor tenotomy or a functional dorsal rhizotomy can be considered. Rhizotomy is the preferred invasive therapy since it preserved muscle strength while dealing with the disfiguring hypertonicity.

Group IV: commando crawlers

This group is comprised of the spastic quadriplegics with minimal locomotive ability. These children are very compromised, and lack the basic brainstem reflex circuits for protective reactions or postural control. Because of these deficiencies little can be expected in the way of functionally important ambulation regardless of the type of treatment delivered. The treatment goal is to ease their care taking and to improve functioning in the sitting position by improving their stability. In striving for these goals one must take care not to compromise the current abilities of the child (e.g., the ability to assist in transferring from a bed to a chair) by eliminating functionally useful spasticity. The standard neurosurgical treatment for this group is a posterior rhizotomy. Of interest could be intrathecal baclofen; as suggested by Zierski (personal communication). But further study of the efficacy of intrathecal baclofen for this group of patients is needed.

Group V: totally dependent children

These are the maximally involved children who are unable to locomote and often severely impaired cognitively. Treatment goals are simply seeking to improve their comfort and to allow easier handling by their caretakers. Again, posterior rhizotomy is the standard neurosurgical treatment; but there is a need, as with group IV, for exploring the efficacy of intrathecal baclofen for treatment of this group of patients.

Asymmetrical spasticity

Asymmetrical spasticity presents a special problem for effective treatment. While posterior rhizotomies seem to be effective in treating spastic hemiplegia secondary to head or spinal cord injury, there is hesitancy in using posterior rhizotomies to treat spastic hemiplegic cerebral palsy. Sindou's microsurgical DREZotomy might be considered in this situation.

In these asymmetrical spasticities, a special mention has to be made, concerning the interest of selective peripheral neurotomies, especially of the obturator and tibial nerves, for the spastic hip and the spastic foot, respectively.

Conclusion

We are still young with our experience in treating this varied group of children with spasticity due to static encephalopathy. Our knowledge base is incomplete at this time. It is with a great deal of care that the above recommendations have been made. These recommendations must be accompanied with a warning that each child undergo a detailed evaluation for the development of a individual tailored treatment plan. A clinician who attempts to treat these children according to ridgid patient classifications and standardized treatment formulas will be risking a serious functional lost in their patients.

Correspondence: Prof. R. Abbott, Division of Pediatric Neurosurgery, New York University Medical Center, 550 First Avenue, NY 10016, U.S.A.

Conclusion

Advancement in medical technology has allowed both a reexamination of the classical ablative techniques and the introduction of such reversible therapies as chronic neurostimulation and intrathecal drug administration to treat disabling spasticity. While pharmacologic and physio-therapies should be the initial therapies, surgical treatments have a place in the management of disabling spasticity. Their use should not be viewed as a failure. Further, neurosurgical procedures have an important place in the surgical management. Significant advancements have been made in functional neurosurgery since the work of Foerster in the early part of this century. Ablative procedures have become much more selective with the introduction of microsurgical techniques and intraoperative physiologic monitoring. These advances have allowed a more precise identification of lesioning targets. With this increasing array of therapies which can be used in treating an individual's spasticity, it becomes increasingly important to appreciate what is being targeted by the treatment and why.

The classical orthopedic surgeries are to be used to correct irreducible deformities. While a muscle can be relaxed with many of these procedures, the neuronal circuits participating in driving the spasticity remain in place and can cause further problems. It is for this reason that we advocate considering functional neurosurgery as the front line treatment in treating spasticity and that orthopedic surgery be employed to treat limb deformity and muscle retractions (contractures) which have resulted from long standing spasticity.

Associated – when needed – with neurosurgery, orthopedic surgery can contribute to considerably improving the functional status of a large number of patients.

We would again stress that surgically treating spasticity is not without danger. So when a given therapy is considered, questions to be asked are not only how well it will treat the spasticity present, but how this will translate into a functional improvement and at what risk to the limb's functional power and sensation. This type of evaluation is best carried out by a multidisciplinary team skilled not only in the surgical treatments being considered but also in physiotherapy and neurorestorative biology.

Neurosurgical procedures target spasticity and pain in these patients and in doing so attempt to correct abnormal postures, increase the patient's comfort and prevent bone and joint deformities. In individuals who have useful function, these procedures in conjunction with postoperative kinestherapy attempt to improve the control and mobility of the limb.

The authors of this book have presented the basic anatomic, chemical and physiologic knowledge as well as the technique of assessing spasticity. We feel these need to be appreciated in order to minimize the risks and maximize the benefits in treating spasticity surgically. Although we readily admitted that this is not an exhaustive discussion of these topics, we hope that the reader comes away with an appreciation that spasticity requires a multidisciplinary approach in its treatment.

M. Sindou
R. Abbott
Y. Keravel

April 1990

Frank Rattay

Electrical Nerve Stimulation

Theory, Experiments and Applications

1990. 136 figures. IV, 264 pages.
Soft cover DM 98,–, öS 686,–
ISBN 3-211-82247-X

Prices are subject to change without notice

Functional electrical stimulation is the most important application in the field of clinical treatment with currents or magnetism. This technique generates artificially neural activity in order to overcome lost functions of the paralized, incontinent or sensory handicapped patient. Electricity and magnetism also is used in a lot of other cases, e.g., to stimulate bone growth or wound healing. But in contrast to these applications, the basic mechanism of the artificial excitation of nerve and muscle fibers have become known in the last few years.

Although many textbooks are concerned with the natural excitation process there is a lack in information on the influence of an applied electric or magnetic field. This book, written for students and biomedical engineers, should close the gap and furthermore, it should stimulate to design new instrumentation using optimal strategies.

Contents: Preface. – Abbreviations and Symbols. – Table of Important Constants and Typical Parameters. – Functional Electrical Nerve Stimulation – A Way to Restore Lost Functions. – Functional Design of the Nervous System. – The Excitability of Cells. – The Space Clamp Experiment of Hodgkin and Huxley – Non-Propagating Action Potentials. – Modeling the Membrane. – Propagation of the Spike. – Extracellular Stimulation of Fibers. – Current-Distance Relations for Monopolar Electrodes and for Ring Electrodes. – Repetitive Firing and Fiber Reactions to Periodic Stimuli. – Control of the Neuromuscular System. – Case Studies: Nerve Cuff Electrodes, Stimulation by Magnetic Fields. – Electrostimulation of the Auditory Nerve. – References. – Author Index. – Subject Index.

Springer-Verlag Wien New York

J. D. Pickard, F. Cohadon,
J. Lobo Antunes (eds.)

Neuroendocrinological Aspects of Neurosurgery

Proceedings of the Third Advanced Seminar in Neurosurgical Research, Venice, April 30–May 1, 1987

Acta Neurochirurgica / Supplementum 47

1990. 60 figures. VII, 128 pages.
Cloth DM 158,–, öS 1106,–
Reduced price for subscribers
to "Acta Neurochirurgica":
Cloth DM 142,–, öS 995,–
ISBN 3-211-82160-0

Contents: B. J. Everitt and T. Hökfelt: Neuroendocrine Anatomy of the Hypothalamus. – J. D. Vincent and G. Simonnet: Neurohormonal Communication in the Brain. – I. Assenmacher: Central Control of Circadian and Ultradian Neuroendocrine Rhythms. – J. Lobo Antunes and K. Muraszko: The Vascular Supply of the Hypothalamus-Pituitary Axis. – M. D. Page et al.: A Clinical Update on Hypothalamic-Pituitary Control. – R. Fahlbusch et al.: Clinical Syndromes of the Hypothalamus. – G. Teasdale: Pituitary Tumours: Problems and Questions. – P. Lees: Intrasellar Pressure. – I. Lancranjan: The Medial Treatment of Prolactin and Growth Hormone-Secreting Pituitary Tumours. – R. M. Buijs: Vasopressin and Oxytocin Localization and Putative Functions in the Brain. – St. Lightman: Central Nervous System Control of Fluid Balance: Physiology and Pathology. – V. Walker: Fluid Balance Disturbances in Neurosurgical Patients: Physiological Basis and Definitions. – G. Neil-Dwyer et al.: The Stress Response in Subarachnoid Haemorrhage and Head Injury. – E. F. M. Wijdicks et al.: Hyponatremia and Volume Status in Aneurysmal Subarachnoid Haemorrhage. – R. J. Nelson: Blood Volume Measurement Following Subarachnoid Haemorrhage. – T. Dóczi et al.: Central Neuroendocrine Control of the Brain Water, Electrolyte, and Volume Homeostasis. – M. Brock: The Hypothalamus: New Ideas on an Old Structure.

G. Broggi, J. Burzaco, E. R. Hitchcock,
B. A. Meyerson, S. Tóth (eds.)

Advances in Stereotactic and Functional Neurosurgery 8

Proceedings of the 8th Meeting of the European Society for Stereotactic and Functional Neurosurgery, Budapest 1988

Acta Neurochirurgica / Supplementum 46

1989. 58 figures. VIII, 114 pages.
Cloth DM 140,–, öS 980,–
Reduced price for subscribers
to "Acta Neurochirurgica":
Cloth DM 126,–, öS 882,–
ISBN 3-211-82120-1

The present work comprises selected papers from a much larger group of interesting and important communications to the European Society for Stereotactic and Functional Neurosurgery. They represent modern views on a wide variety of stereotactic surgical topics from internationally acclaimed experts in this field. The neurosurgeon who has little or no acquaintance with this fruitful sub-speciality will be surprised to find very broad applications of the technique which is gradually replacing many conventional neurosurgical procedures.

Contents:

Preface – Epilepsy – Spasticity and Movement Disorder – Pain – Tumours – Vascular Diseases – Technical

Prices are subject to change without notice.

Springer-Verlag Wien New York
Moelkerbastei 5, P.O. Box 367, A-1011 Wien · Heidelberger Platz 3, D-1000 Berlin 33
175 Fifth Avenue, New York, NY 10010, USA · 37-3, Hongo 3-chome, Bunkyo-ku, Tokyo 113, Japan